A Reader in Promoting Public Health

Challenge and Controversy

Jenny Douglas
Sarah Earle
Stephen Handsley
Cathy E. Lloyd
and
Sue Spurr

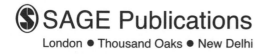**SAGE** Publications
London ● Thousand Oaks ● New Delhi

The Open
University

The Open University
Walton Hall
Milton Keynes
MK7 6AA
United Kingdom
www.open.ac.uk

SAGE Publications Ltd
1 Oliver's Yard
55 City Road
London EC1Y 1SP

SAGE Publications Inc.
2455 Teller Road
Thousand Oaks, California 91320

SAGE Publications India Pvt Ltd
B-42, Panchsheel Enclave
Post Box 4109
New Delhi 110 017

British Library Cataloguing in Publication data

A catalogue record for this book is available
from the British Library

ISBN 1-4129-3074-X   ISBN 978-1-4129-3074-1
ISBN 1-4129-3075-8 (pbk)   ISBN 978-1-4129-3075-8 (pbk)

Library of Congress Control Number: 2006925449

Typeset by C&M Digitals (P) Ltd., Chennai, India
Printed on paper from sustainable resources
Printed and bound in Great Britain by The Cromwell Press Ltd, Trowbridge, Wiltshire

Contents

Acknowledgements

Every effort has been made to trace all the copyright holders, but if any have been inadvertently overlooked the publishers will be pleased to make the necessary arrangement at the first opportunity.

Chapter 4
Original text appeared as Chapter 3 in Blaxter, M. (ed.) (2004) *Health*. Cambridge: Polity Press Ltd. Reproduced with permission from Polity Press Ltd.

Chapter 5
Original text appeared as Chapter 3 in Sidell, M. et al. (eds) (2003) *Debates and Dilemmas in Promoting Health* (2nd edn). Basingstoke: Palgrave Macmillan. Reproduced with permission of Palgrave Macmillan.

Chapter 6
Geddie Watt, R. (2002). Emerging theories into the social determinants of health: implications for oral health promotion, *Community Dentistry and Oral Epidemiology*, 30 (1): 241–7. Reproduced with permission from Blackwell Publishing Ltd.

Chapter 7
Bambra, C., Fox, D. and Scott-Samuel, A. (2005) Towards a politics of health, *Health Promotion International*, 20 (2): 187–93. By permission of Oxford University Press.

Chapter 8
Reprinted from Bellis, M.A. et al. (2002) Healthy nightclubs and recreational substance use: from a harm minimisation to a healthy settings approach, *Addictive Behaviors*, 27 (6): 1025–35. © 2002 Elsevier Science Ltd. Reproduced with permission from Elsevier.

Chapter 16
This is a revised version of Urla, J. and Swedland, A.C. (1998) The anthropometry of Barbie, in J. Terry and J. Urla (eds), *Deviant Bodies*. Bloomington, IN: Indiana University Press. Reproduced with permisson from the authors.

Chapter 23
Box 23.1 is reprinted with permission from the American Public Health Association.

Chapter 24
Box 24.1 is taken from Global Health Watch (2005) *Global Health Watch 2005–2006: An Alternative World Health Report*. London: Zed Books.

Table 24.1 is taken from Drèze, J. and Sen, A. (2002) *India: Development and Participation, second edition*. By permission of Oxford University Press.

Chapter 25
Grove, N. and Zwi, A. (2006) Othering of refugees: social exlusion and public health, *Social Science and Medicine*, 62 (2006): 1931–42.

Chapter 26
Bandesha, G. and Litva, A. (2005) Perceptions of community participation and health gain in a community project for the South Asian population: a qualitative study, *Journal of Public Health*, 27 (3): 241–5. By permission of Oxford University Press, on behalf of Faculty of Public Health.

Chapter 29
Bridgen, P. (2004) Evaluating the empowering potential of community-based health schemes: the case of community health policies in the UK since 1997, *Community Development Journal*, 39 (3): 289–302. By permission of Oxford University Press.

Chapter 30
Mittlemark, M.B. (2001) Promoting social responsibility for health: health impact assessment and healthy public policy at the community level, *Health Promotion International*, 16 (3): 269–74. By permission of Oxford University Press.

Introduction: Challenge and Controversy in Promoting Public Health

Cathy E. Lloyd

At many levels and in a wide range of settings, multidisciplinary public health has become the focus for much national, international, regional and local policy and practice. As the term 'multidisciplinary' implies, a broad range of disciplines are represented in this area of health action, from sociology and psychology, through to epidemiology, health policy, and economics. Multidisciplinary public health is practised by a wide range of individuals, including public health specialists, nurses, health visitors and community workers, as well as by lay people. Indeed, a vast array of policy and practice can be said to fall under this broad umbrella term. Furthermore, as this Reader will demonstrate, the involvement of people in promoting public health includes not just professionals from a range of settings, but also the lay public, with all the challenges and controversy that this may imply. This Reader encapsulates this range of settings, disciplines and practice in a series of chapters which focus on the theory, the practice and the place of promoting public health.

Part I of the Reader introduces some of the key challenges and debates within multidisciplinary public health in the 21st century, and considers some of the controversies within the field today. A range of theoretical perspectives, concepts and approaches are debated, not only in contemporary terms, but also by looking back at the history and political roots of public health. Drawing on the theme of continuity and change, many of the chapters in this part of the book highlight the importance of understanding the past in order to make sense of the future. It goes on to open up the debate around what is health, exploring definitions of both 'health' and 'public health' from differing perspectives and concluding with a discussion of the inherently political nature of health.

The chapters in Part II have been written to challenge the concept of public health and its current meaning in practice. The issue of diversity, in terms of setting as well as individual difference, is approached in a range of ways to explore the deconstruction and reconstruction of public health. The implications of current efforts to promote public health are considered in terms of contemporary approaches to multidisciplinary practice. The tensions which surround the ethical practice of public health and underpinning values are explored. At one extreme, this part of the Reader explores issues of life and death and their significance to public health. At another, this part of the Reader also considers the role of individual choice and autobiographical reflection in public health action.

Part III of the Reader focuses on research, and seeks to make explicit the links between research and knowledge about health. The chapters included here help demonstrate the ways in which health issues are defined, how research informs policy, and how multidisciplinary public health initiatives are planned, carried out and evaluated. These chapters highlight the different methods and underpinning methodologies that can be used, and challenge assumptions about the utility of quantitative and qualitative data and the nature of evidence when promoting public health.

Part IV of this volume moves into the realm of public policy and explores the potential for promoting public health, taking a global perspective. International strategies and the impact of actions at the global level on national and local public health are highlighted, as are the links between social and economic inequalities and health. These chapters make explicit the need for public health practitioners to recognise the political nature of policy-making and the distribution of wealth and power if they are to impact upon the underpinning causes of social and economic inequalities in health.

Current UK policy focuses on working alongside local communities to promote health, and this is echoed at the international level too. Part V of this Reader considers the implementation of policy in local communities and investigates multidisciplinary public health practice at a local level. The chapters in Part V make important contributions to current debates around the effectiveness of local initiatives to promote public health, as well as challenging how community-based health interventions are assessed and evaluated. However, the primary focus of this section is on the potential of participatory and community-action approaches to promoting public health.

The collection of chapters in this Reader has been put together with the aim of providing a wide-ranging, thought-provoking volume, which covers theory and practice, the local and the global, and the personal and political. It is hoped that, together, these chapters will challenge current thinking and confront some of the controversies that arise when promoting public health.

Part I
Back to the Future: Reflections on Multidisciplinary Public Health

Introduction

Sarah Earle

It is increasingly recognised that public health policy and practice can be enhanced by drawing on contemporary theoretical approaches and perspectives, and by being aware of its historical and political roots. Public health is often criticised for ignoring the lessons that can be learned from history: looking back to the past and forward to the future. It is often described as atheoretical and apolitical. Multidisciplinary public health action can, and does, occur with little recourse to the concepts, models, theories or politics that can help to explain what happens on the ground. In Part I of this Reader on promoting public health, some of these concepts, theories and approaches are presented.

In Chapter 1, Iqbal Sram and John Ashton reflect on public health in the new millennium. They look back to the past as they write a memo to Sir Edwin Chadwick following the anniversary of the 1848 Public Health Act. They describe the Act as a 'monumental legacy' which laid the foundations for public health action. However, they note that while great strides have been taken to promote public health, there exist considerable disparities in health across the globe and considerable differences in morbidity and mortality between social and ethnic groups across the United Kingdom. They highlight the challenges posed by globalisation and increasing environmental degradation, and argue that the state must play a key role in promoting and protecting the public's health.

In Chapter 2, Jenny Douglas continues to explore continuity and change in promoting public health. She begins by documenting the political influences which led to the 1848 Public Health Act, and the subsequent development of an infrastructure which became dominated by a biomedical approach to public health. The chapter outlines the development of the New Public Health and reflects on the emergence of health promotion. Taking a more global perspective, it then considers different definitions of health promotion. Finally, Jenny Douglas charts the renaissance of public health in the UK and the tension and conflict between health promotion and public health. By exploring changing roles and functions, this chapter considers the development of modern multidisciplinary public health.

Chapter 3 considers the place of social marketing in the future of public health. In this chapter, Jeff French argues that it is the dawn of a new age of individualism: a phase in civic development which places the citizen at the centre of promoting public health. He notes the clash of ideological positions between the democratic free market approach of most governments and the paternalistic, collectivist stance supported by many public health professionals. Unlike Iqbal Sram and John Ashton, Jeff French does not call for greater state responsibility for health. Instead, he argues that the state will adopt a less paternalistic approach to public health, and will become increasingly characterised by a more liberal, free-market economic approach. He concludes by arguing that social marketing will emerge to rival the collective paternalist approach that has, so far, dominated the history of public health policy.

It is important to explore the nature and history of public health policy and action, but very little can be achieved without some discussion and critical reflection on the question 'what is health?' There are many ways to explore experiences of health, and in Chapter 4 Mildred Blaxter draws on classic surveys to explore lay concepts of health. She begins the discussion by arguing that health is not an observable or easily measurable phenomenon. She maps changes in approach to lay concepts of health, all of which have impacted on approaches to the role of the lay person in promoting public health. She notes that health cannot be defined solely in relation to the absence of disease, but that it is a subjective experience grounded in the everyday.

Although public health and, to some extent, health promotion, have been dominated by biomedical and epidemiological approaches to health, in Chapter 5 Moyra Sidell examines Antonovsky's salutogenic approach. By exploring the health of older people, Moyra Sidell argues that the 'sense of coherence' theory can be used to understand the cumulative effects of social inequalities on older people's health. She argues that rather than focusing on what stops older people from getting sick, the question should be 'what helps them to be healthy in spite of disease?' She explores how meaningfulness, comprehensibility and manageability in the daily lives of older people can assist in maintaining their health.

Over recent years many attempts have been made to develop theoretical approaches and models of health promotion. Drawing on some of these, in Chapter 6 Richard Geddie Watt focuses on oral health promotion and evaluates whether these theoretical approaches and models can be applied to this emerging field. As in the previous chapter, Richard Geddie Watt explores the role of salutogenesis, concluding that a focus on salutogenic factors and settings can usefully focus attention away from disease and risk behaviours. He draws on a life-course perspective to show how useful it is to reflect on the relationship between individuals and environments over time, and argues that a life-course perspective can pinpoint windows of opportunity for promoting oral health. Finally, Richard Geddie Watt evaluates theories of social capital, concluding that community development can enhance social networks and increase the capacity of individuals and groups to achieve good health.

The last chapter in Part I carefully develops the case for a politics of health to sit outside the traditional approach that equates health with health care. Clare Bambra, Debbie Fox and Alex Scott-Samuel argue that health is both implicitly and explicitly political, but that the politics of health have been marginalised and ignored by policy-makers and practitioners. They suggest that health is political because whether it is seen to be a commodity or a resource, some people enjoy more of it than others. They also argue that it is political because its social determinants are shaped by political action and inaction. Finally, they suggest that health is a human right and a condition of citizenship and, thus, very much a political issue. To conclude, they argue that an explicit acknowledgement of the politics of health will lead to more effective health promotion practice and policy, and a more realistic evidence-driven, public health.

Chapter 1

Millennium Report to Sir Edwin Chadwick

Iqbal Sram and John R. Ashton CBE

To mark the 150th anniversary of the 1848 Public Health Act, Iqbal Sram and John Ashton write a memo to Edwin Chadwick, the architect of the 1848 Act, on the state of the public health at the end of the millennium.

Dear Sir Edwin,

We live in a world which you would have envied. You played a dominant role in laying the foundations of this world. A clean and secure water supply for the population at large, coupled with the separate disposal of their sewage and waste, were the central planks of your crusade to protect public health in your day. However, Sir Edwin, we enter a caution here. The harmonious world referred to is, in essence, the 'first world'. The insanitary conditions which you were determined to eradicate still persist over large parts of the globe.

It will not have escaped your notice that it is 150 years since the enactment of the 1848 Public Health Act (An Act for promoting the Public Health), for you were its chief architect.[1] You subscribed to the contemporary laissez-faire doctrines in the management of economic affairs, having worked closely with the economist Nassau Senior in the reform of the poor laws, which dated back to Elizabethan times.[2] In the social policy arena you battled hard and successfully against those who wished to extend and entrench that approach to a wide range of public policy areas. Your energy and determination secured support for state intervention for public health protection from the major perceived health hazards of the day,[3] in particular the acute infectious diseases. You attributed these to insanitary conditions due to poor and sometimes non-existent drainage and disposal of urban waste and sewage. It is said that in this context you were mainly concerned with the plight of the able-bodied urban poor. Because you were convinced that many deaths among the urban inhabitants were avoidable,[3] you started by identifying the problem and its size and its cause.[4] The next stage was to find a workable solution. Here you were

The first part of this chapter, the original letter, is from: Sram, I. and Ashton, J. (1998) 'Millennium report to Sir Edwin Chadwick; *British Medical Journal*, 317: 592–6 (29 August). The 'update' is newly commissioned material.

greatly assisted by the civil engineers of the day.[3] You then proceeded to build support for your evidence-based proposals. Although the provisions of the 1848 Act fell short of your expectations, its historic significance was clear. The idea that the state can act in an enabling capacity could now be tested.[5, 6]

Summary points

- The state has a key role in promoting and protecting public health
- Public health today faces a number of challenges posed by globalisation and must develop appropriate responses
- Public health should focus on promoting sustainable economic and social development of individuals and communities
- Urgent action should be taken in the short term to narrow the health inequalities; priority should be given to measures to raise low incomes
- An independent public health commission should be established to monitor the effects of public policies on health and to offer proactive and independent advice on public health to government and other public bodies

---

Monumental legacy

Sir Edwin, your legacy is monumental. Your claim that the major threats to human health originate from the environment now enjoys widespread professional and popular support. Although the world and the public health challenges have changed since 1848, the foundations that you laid continue to guide today's practitioners. It is disappointing to report that in spite of your leadership, we still have disproportionate levels of ill health in our cities.[7] Like the towns in your day, our cities are hazardous places in which to live. Inequalities in health experience and outcomes persist and are associated with avoidable deaths.[8] In the 1990s nearly 90,000 people die each year before they reach their 65th birthday. Of these, more than 25, 000 die of heart disease, stroke, and related illnesses and 32,000 die of cancer.[9] Differences in health associated with social class exist not only for mortality but also for morbidity.[10] In your day, Sir Edwin, the excess deaths occurred mainly among the labouring classes in the towns. Today these chiefly occur among social classes IV and V–the partly skilled and unskilled occupations–of the registrar general's classification system. (You are of course familiar with this system as you had many interesting debates with its designer, William Farr.[11])

Update

Dear Sir Edwin,
Although only eight years have passed since our last communication with you, you will note that we are now in a new millennium. The historian in you will have noted that the

turn of the centuries tend to somehow result in a rapid turn of events. Thus at the beginning of the 18th century we had the continent of Europe convulsed by the Napoleonic Wars, and the corresponding period of the 19th century was marked by the Boer and the First World wars. In keeping with form, the beginning of this century was marked by [the terrorist acts of] 11th September 2001 and the Iraq War in 2003.

Major wars tend to have a profound impact on a nation and its society. The impact manifests itself in the changes in foreign and domestic policy and in the parameters and criteria used to conduct economic policy. In addition, the rapid and global expansion and integration of the world economy have posed fresh challenges to public health at the international, national, regional and local levels. The challenges arise due to increasingly intensive exploitation of scarce natural resources (thereby raising the question of sustainability), increased and accelerating movement of capital, goods and services. The rationalist in you would have deduced that risks to public health due to the potential to carry and transmit microbes are high and, unless checked by a 'fit for purpose' system, could materialise at periodic intervals and result in damage to public health.

You lived in an era of non-mechanised public transport, although you did witness the beginnings of the emergence of the modern railway system, which relied on power from fossil sources. Sir Edwin, you will be surprised to learn that today we tend to rely on the same sources of energy as in your day. The consensus is that unless we manage these energy sources intelligently and look for other more sustainable sources there is a real danger that we will exhaust the traditional sources. There is also a danger that inter-nation competition to secure supplies of fossil fuels from ever-diminishing reserves could lead to inter-nation rivalry resulting in full-scale military conflict in some cases.

Added to this is the ever-present danger that continued emission of carbon dioxide at current levels will lead to changes in climates across the globe due to rises in average temperatures. There is a strong view that a trend of rising temperatures is already evident. You will be pleased to note that many countries across the world appreciate the dangers associated with climate change but unfortunately at the present time there is no consensus on the best approach to address the issue on a long-term basis.

We are sure that you will agree that the desired consensus is harder to achieve when economic and political power is unevenly distributed among the countries of the world. Governments in the nation states also have to respond to competing interests. We are confident that your passion for public health would lead you to make a passionate and persuasive case for effective action on this issue.

Sir Edwin, we also draw your attention to the resource which you viewed as an important weapon in your campaign against communicable diseases of your time. You rightly placed great importance on water. Even though in your time the precise mechanisms for the transmission of infectious diseases were not known, you worked out that water could both be carrier of infectious agents but also that, given different circumstances, it could also be used as a device to aid the control and eradication of communicable diseases.

The rapid growth in population in many parts of the globe has dramatically increased the demand for water and this is resulting in a reduction in underground water reserves. In addition, due to changed patterns of rainfall, many of the great rivers are drying up. Many eminent commentators fear that there is a real danger that water shortages could become an everyday occurrence in many parts of the world. Some even foresee the shortages leading to full-scale wars between nations.

You rightly maintained that continued and sustained improvements in public health need the active involvement of the state. Sir Edwin, in the United Kingdom in the last eight years there has been a large increase in public investment to address under-achievement in primary and secondary education, decaying infrastructure in large cities and providing additional support to families with low incomes. These initiatives have short-term and long-term beneficial effects of improving public health.

Since our last communication there have been important developments in the United Kingdom in relation to public health. While the present constitutional arrangements for governing the constituent parts of the United Kingdom differ, it is interesting that the main thrust for policies and structures to deliver the public health agenda are broadly similar.

The major policy theme is to attack inequalities in the health experienced by members of different social classes and ethnic origins. The policy is underpinned by targets to reduce the gap in the health experience of the various population sub-groups. Target setting is frequently used to monitor and manage individuals and organisations in modern settings. While there is some debate on the effectiveness of the use of targets in improving performance, there is a body of evidence to suggest that the intelligent use of targets does improve performance and innovation, leading to greater efficiency. The areas with the worst health have been designated by local authority boundaries and named Spearhead areas. The aim is to focus resources on these areas with the view to improving health. There have been short-term gains in health but clearly on the long-term gains the judgement needs to be reserved.

At present, the health care and public health system is now underpinned by evidence-based standards and/or guidance mainly issued by the National Institute for Health and Clinical Excellence. Furthermore, the Department of Health also expects all NHS bodies to deliver services and care to minimum standards as set out in the Standards for Better Health. This system of checks and balances has an additional arm, that of assessing organisational performance and, when necessary, investigating episodes of serious organisational failure.

Sir Edwin, we live in an era of electronic communications and a mass consumer society. The influences of the national and international media are profound. The role of the expert and the professional is subject to constant challenge and change. Thes national governments are not often in control of issues which can either enhance or damage health. Lifestyle choices that individuals make often have a harmful effect on health. This clearly muddies the policy path to reducing health inequalities.

The present government's public health aims are encapsulated in the document *Choosing Health: Making Health Choices Easier* [Department of Health, 2004]. In the foreword to this document the Prime Minister says that 'We are clear that the Government cannot and should not pretend that it can "make" the population healthy. But it can and should support people in making better choices for their health and the health of their families. It is for the people to make the healthy choice if they wish to. *Choosing Health* sets out what this Government will do to help them'. You will no doubt agree that the role of public health practitioners in this era is to influence people to make the right choices.

The government also believes that it now needs to move from a centrally driven command and controlled approach to one which is more driven by professionals at a local level. Thus the government is introducing more reforms with a view to devolving more power to local organisations. The reforms are contained in the *Creating a Patient-led NHS* (Department of Health, 2005). There are many misgivings about both the content and the pace of changes to the structures needed to deliver the public health challenges of today. Your successors are now actively engaged in leading the debate to ensure that public health delivery systems emerge that are 'fit for purpose'.

Sir Edwin, human beings, through their collective social endeavours, ensure that their world is in a state of economic, social and cultural flux. The stage of development of these three elements has a profound influence on the health and well-being of individuals and societies. A 19th-century British prime minister once said that Britain has no permanent enemies or friends but permanent interests. Your enduring legacy is that public health professionals cannot afford to be wedded to a particular organisational form, structure or ideology. Effective public health practice requires a capability and capacity to respond to change. You can be assured that your legacy is in good hands.

Notes

1. Finer, S.E. (1952) *The Life and Times of Sir Edwin Chadwick*. London: Methuen.
2. Royle, E. (1997) *Modern Britain: a Social History 1750–1997* (2nd edn). London: Arnold.
3. Jones, K. (1994) *The Making of Social Policy in Britain, 1830–1990* (2nd edn). London: Athlone.
4. Midwinter, E. (1995) *The Development of Social Welfare in Britain*. Milton Keynes: Open University Press.
5. Evans, E.J. (1996) *The Forging of the Modern State: Early Industrial Britain 1783–1870* (2nd edn). London: Longman.
6. Hamlin, C. and Sheard, S. (1998) Revolutions in public health: 1848 and 1998? *British Medical Journal*, 317: 587–91.
7. *Proceedings of the First United Kingdom Healthy Cities Conference*. In: J. Ashton and L. Knight (eds) (1988), Liverpool: University of Liverpool, Department of Public Health.
8. Benzeval, M., Judge, K. and Whitehead, M. (1995) *Tackling Inequalities in Health: an Agenda for Action*. London: King's Fund.
9. Stationery Office (1998) *Our Healthier Nation: a Contract for Health*. London: The Stationery Office.
10. Denver, F. and Whitehead, M. (1997) *Health Inequalities*. London: Office for National Statistics.
11. Hamlin, C. (1995) Could you starve to death in England in 1839? The Chadwick–Farr controversy and the loss of the 'social' in public health. *American Journal of Public Health* 85: 856–65.

References

Department of Health (2004) *Choosing Health: Making Health Choices Easier*. London: The Stationery Office.
Department of Health (2005) *Creating a Patient–led NHS*. London Department of Health.

Chapter 2

Promoting the Public Health: Continuity and Change over Two Centuries

Jenny Douglas

Introduction

This chapter explores the origins of public health in the UK, documenting the political influences which led to the passing of the first public health Act in England and Wales in 1848. Although heralded as a turning point in the recognition of the role of poverty and environment in determining health status, the initial permissive public health act had to be strengthened by compulsory legislation and the development of a public health infrastructure which then became dominated by biomedical perspectives. The chapter will outline the more recent development of the 'new public health' and track the emergence of health promotion from the Ottawa Charter (WHO, 1986) to the Bangkok Charter (WHO, 2005). In exploring definitions of health promotion from the USA, Canada, and the UK, it will demonstrate the contested nature of health promotion, the divergence in understandings of health promotion and the relationship of health promotion to the 'new public health'.

Charting the renaissance of public health in the UK from 1988 to the present, the chapter looks at the development of modern multidisciplinary public health. The publication of UK public health strategies heralded a resurgence in public health, changes in the Faculty of Public Health Medicine to become the Faculty of Public Health and the development of competencies for public health. The influence of reports such as the Wanless Reports is explored and the relationship of health promotion to public health as part of multidisciplinary public health is examined. The conflicts and tensions that have emerged as a result of differences between policy and practice are interrogated as is the role that politics has played in developing public health in primary care organisations, local authorities and voluntary organisations.

The origins of public health in the UK

Politics and public health are inextricably linked. The origins of the first Public Health Act – An Act for Promoting the Public Health, 1848 – lay outside the health considerations and instead with the report of Edwin Chadwick on the state of poor people in England. Critics argue that Chadwick, as the architect and enforcer of the 1834 Poor Law, was not so much concerned with inequalities in health but with reducing costs caused by the death of male breadwinners from infectious diseases, which left families dependent on relief, and that it was in fact the Poor Laws themselves which caused ill health (Hamlin and Sheard, 1998). Whatever the historical reasons, the Public Health Act was passed in England and Wales in 1848 and was stimulated by a concern to improve sanitary conditions in thriving urban areas. A Central Board of Health was established which oversaw the implementation of the Act, although it had few powers and few resources. The Act did enable local people to get involved in health action, however, by allowing local health boards to be established if more than 10 per cent of the population petitioned for one. The Act therefore witnessed one of the first social movements of lay people in public health. Failing to produce the desired results, the 1848 Act was superseded by the 1866 Sanitary Act, which compelled local authorities to remove 'nuisance', and the Public Health Act of 1872, which created organised public heath services across England and Wales, dividing the two countries into urban and rural sanitary districts each with a public health board and its own Medical Officer of Health. Thus even in the 19th century there was a tension between reducing inequalities in health and establishing public health services. From the mid-19th century, however, public health became dominated by doctors and biomedical perspectives of health underpinned by the study of epidemiology.

The 'New Public Health' and health promotion

With the establishment of the World Health Organisation in 1948, notions of health started to change and move away from purely biological explanations. Recognising the limitations of a purely medical approach, Winslow, in a World Health Organisation monograph, defined public health as the 'Science and art of preventing disease, prolonging life and promoting physical health and efficiency through organised community efforts ... and the development of social machinery which will ensure to every individual in the community a standard of living adequate for the maintanence of health' (Winslow, 1951), thus moving away from a definition of public health which was located purely in public health services. The evolution of the 'New Public Health' and the birth of health promotion were inextricably intertwined and public health and health promotion have continued to influence each other over the ensuing decades. Both emerged in the 1970s with the publication of the Canadian health minister's report (Lalonde, 1974). While still placing emphasis on behavioural change, the Lalonde report pointed to the importance of the environment as well as biology and health services in maintaining and promoting health.

Health promotion – from Ottawa to Bangkok

From the mid-1980s, the role of health promotion as a movement for social and political change was elaborated in a series of health promotion conferences and charters, starting with the Ottawa Charter, which defined health promotion as 'the process of enabling people to increase control over the determinants of health and thereby improve health' (WHO, 1986). This definition became widely accepted across the world. However, in the USA, health promotion was defined as 'the science and art of helping people change their lifestyle to move toward a state of optimal health' (O'Donnell, 1986). The US definition of health promotion focused much more on lifestyles rather than on addressing the underlying determinants of health, and was further developed in 1989 to recognise that environments which support good health practice would probably have greatest impact in producing lasting changes (O'Donnell, 1989). While health promotion activities in Canada, Australia and the UK have attempted to focus on structural and organisational change, health promotion activities in the USA have been focused much more on lifestyle and behavioural change, utilizing health education approaches rather than an emphasis in healthy public policy. Here in the UK, however, critics have argued that although the terminology of 'health promotion' was used, until the development of the healthy cities movement, health promotion practice in the 1980s was very much dominated by health education approaches. By the 21st century the scope and role of health promotion in developing healthy public policy were widely acknowledged. At the 6th Global Conference in Bangkok, the Bangkok Charter for health promotion in a globalised world was adopted. The Charter, recognising the impact of globalisation in the 20 years succeeding the Ottawa Charter, called for strong political action from governments, international bodies and corporate and private organisations (WHO, 2005).

It is worth noting that at the same time as the 'New Public Health' was emerging at an international level, spearheaded by developments in Canada and the World Health Organisation, in the UK, the health and local government reorganisation of the 1970s dismantled the local authority 'public health empire' under the Medical Officer of Health and replaced it with NHS consultant-based community medicine (Berridge, 2001). So while the ideology of the new public health embraced the need to look beyond biomedical understandings of health and to focus on the social, economic and environmental determinants of health, public health services in the UK moved back into the narrow confines of the NHS.

Modern multidisciplinary public health in the 21st century

The WHO's definition of public health was re-stated and further developed in 1988 by the Committee of Inquiry into the Future Development of the Public Health Function: 'science and art of preventing disease, prolonging life and promoting health through organised efforts of society' (Acheson Committee Report, 1988). Initiated by a concern about the continual reorganisation of the NHS and the marginalisation of public health and health protection, the review of the public health function in England led to the change of terminology from 'community medicine' back to 'public health' and the re-stating of the broader role of public health to take action on the wider determinants of health. The Acheson Report also called for the appointment of a Director of Public Health in each district and regional health authority and the production of an annual report on the state of the public health of the population, although public health services remained in the NHS.

The first formal public health policy in England was *The Health of the Nation* (Department of Health, 1991). Although this policy set clear targets for reducing ill health, the report was heavily criticised for its focus on disease to the exclusion of an examination of inequalities in health. The election of a new Labour government in 1997 placed public health policy and practice high up on the agenda of health and social care agencies. It placed an emphasis on reducing inequalities in health and social inclusion and each of the countries in the UK published a public health policy which reflected this. While the scope and purpose of public health appeared to be huge and expanding, the concept of what constitutes 'public health' was still open to debate and challenge.

In England, The Chief Medical Officer's Project to strengthen the public health function (Department of Health, 2001), concluded that 'the aim is a strong, effective, sustainable and multidisciplinary public health function which is in good shape to underpin the delivery of the NHS Plan and to improve health and reduce inequalities' (Department of Health, 2001: 43). Recognising that people from a range of backgrounds contribute to the public health workforce, the report identified three different levels of involvement in public health: public health specialists from a variety of professional backgrounds, such as directors of public health and environmental health officers; public health practitioners, including nurses and health promotion specialists; and professionals whose work includes elements of public health, such as social workers, teachers and police officers.

Thus by the 21st century it was widely acknowledged that modern public health was multidisciplinary in nature and that an effective multidisciplinary public health workforce required that all public health workers were adequately trained. This gave rise to the question of competency to practise public health given that the public health workforce would be coming from diverse professional backgrounds. To this end, a competency-based framework for public health was developed in 2001 by Healthwork UK on behalf of a tripartite Steering Group comprising the Faculty of Public Health Medicine, the Multidisciplinary Public Health Forum, and the Royal Institute of Public Health and Hygiene, supported by the health departments of the four UK countries (Faculty of Public Health, 2005). National Standards for Specialist Practice in Public Health were produced and a voluntary register for public health specialists was established. The voluntary register for generalist specialists opened in 2003 and by 2006, 80 generalist public health specialists were registered. This was extended in 2004 with the development of a set of competencies for public health practitioners, although no register was established for this group.

Critics of the competency-based framework argue that the voluntary register reinforced an artificial divide between specialists and practitioners and served to reinforce 'old' hierarchies – namely between medically trained public health specialists and other groups. Furthermore, it is argued that individual public health specialists or public health practitioners could not be expected to meet the competencies in all ten key areas, and that if a truly multidisciplinary approach were to be adopted, the competencies should be measured across a multidisciplinary public health team. Nevertheless, standards for defined specialists (e.g. health promotion, information specialists) have been devised and the voluntary register for defined specialists opened in 2006. In nursing, public health competencies are outlined in the third pathway for NMC registration (Nursing and Midwifery Council, 2003).

There has been keen debate about the boundaries between public health and health promotion. MacDonald (1998: 28) has stated that: 'the principles and content of modern health promotion are identical to those of the new public health'. However, as public health has risen up the political agenda, critics have argued that health promotion and health promotion specialists seem to be disappearing (Scott-Samuel, 2003). Health promotion specialists are a group of health professionals who have received limited attention in the academic literature on developing the public health workforce, although they make up the bulk of the multidisciplinary public health workforce (Department of Health, 2005). Despite the 20-year history of health promotion, new terms such as 'health improvement' or 'health development' are increasingly being used. For some, health promotion is seen as an integral part of the public health function.

Despite the rhetoric espoused by successive UK governments' public health strategies about the importance of a multidisciplinary public health workforce, differentials persist between the professional status and financial remuneration of different professional groups. While health promotion specialists make up the bulk of the multidisciplinary public health workforce in England and Wales, many health promotion practitioners point out that they do not receive the same remuneration or professional recognition as medically qualified public health practitioners.

Despite the reviews of public health in the four UK countries and the development of public health White Papers, it was the Wanless Reports which placed public health high up on the government agenda. In 2002 Derek Wanless, a former banker, produced a report for the Treasury that assessed resources that would be needed to provide high-quality health services (Wanless, 2002). This report examined future funding in the context of three possible future directions – 'slow uptake', 'solid progress' and a 'fully engaged' scenario – and set out an economic case for effective public health. A second report, *Securing Good Health for the Whole Population* (2004), looked at the cost of a fully engaged scenario and assessed the actions that would need to be taken to achieve the relative reductions in future demand for healthcare services and the improvements in the health of the population implied by the fully engaged scenario. The report concluded that one of the underlying reasons for the lack of progress on public health was a lack of political will and political importance attached to public health by successive governments (Wanless, 2004).

Continually changing organisational structures and positioning of public health has led to instability in the public health workforce. With the development of Primary Care Trusts (PCTs) in England in April 2001, each PCT was required to appoint a Director of Public Health. Although there was no requirement to appoint medically qualified directors, the majority of PCTs have appointed medical directors. This development led to a recognition of the importance of public health and an expansion in the multidisciplinary public health workforce. The Faculty of Public Health (2005) reported that a much larger public health workforce was needed. However, it was judged that the newly configured PCTs were not economically viable and in 2006 PCTs and strategic health authorities were reconfigured. Many practitioners fear that this, accompanied with a refocusing of resources in the NHS, will lead once more to the marginalisation of public health and health promotion and the gains that were made in the early part of the 21st century. There is the scope, however, for joint appointments of Directors of Public Health, with local authorities, particularly where newly formed PCTs are coterminous with their local authority. Such a move could place Directors of Public Health in a position to influence local authority agendas and the health of the local population.

Since the reforms of 1974, when public health services in the main were taken out of local authorities, the influence of public health has been greatly reduced. Although environmental health departments continued to have some statutory responsibilities for aspects of public health, limited resources meant that these responsibilities were discharged with a fairly narrow focus, with only a few environmental health departments developing a wider role in promoting public health. In the 1980s some local authorities set up 'Health

Units'(e.g. Lambeth), which were part of the egalitarian thrust of welfare policy. These recognised that individuals' health experiences were shaped by wider structural factors and that local authorities were better placed to take action on the determinants of health. The 1980s saw the development of the Healthy Cities Movement and many towns, cities and boroughs set up Healthy City Units (e.g. Sheffield, Liverpool, Camden). More recently, while some local authorities have used the Health Scrutiny Committee to call for action on inequalities in health, the role of local authorities on advocating for public health has been greatly diminished in the last two decades.

Many voluntary and community organisations have maintained a lobbying and campaigning role supporting public and lay activism around health issues. The widening social movement in health has been effective in challenging the UK governments on a range of public health policies. Organisations such as the UK Public Health Association, National Heart Forum, Action for Smoking on Health, Diabetes UK, the Sickle Cell Society, to name but a few, have been influential in changing the public health agenda and ensuring the continued involvement of the public.

One of the fundamental contentions of public health and health promotion is individual versus structuralist approaches. Individual approaches focus on encouraging people to change their behaviour and adopt healthy lifestyles. Structuralist approaches focus on changes in legislation, taxation, public policy, ecological or environmental measures. It can also be said that some health protection approaches, such as immunisation and screening, lie between a lifestyle approach and a structuralist approach as they involve both changes in behaviour and changes in service provision. These are sometimes referred to as upstream and downstream approaches, where upstream approaches represent structuralist approaches.

One of the reasons that it is very difficult to define public health is because it represents a number of different understandings of 'health' and the causes of health and illness. Public health can be seen from two ends of a very broad spectrum. One end of the polarity sees health as determined by biology or medicine. In the medical model the causes of ill health are seen to be due to disease or other medical concerns and the explanations of ill health are much more biological in nature. At the other end of the polarity poor health may be seen to be caused by a range of social, economic or political factors and hence the explanations of health and illness are much more sociological. Although the social model of health and the biomedical model of health are sometimes presented as oppositional perspectives, or two extremes of a binary divide, an understanding of both perspectives is essential to developing an understanding of health and health inequalities.

Conclusion

So how far have we got with promoting the public health in the 21st century? What is modern multidisciplinary public health? It is important for those people involved in promoting public health to have a historical perspective to understand the present and to recognise that what might appear to be a shift in the present may be a move to the past. The contention about definitions of public health in relation to addressing inequalities in health continues, as do the struggles surrounding its organisational positioning. Having experienced a renaissance in public health in the latter part of the 20th century and early part of the 21st century, practitioners fear that organisational changes to primary care trusts and strategic health authorities introduced in England in 2006 may once more relegate public health to the margins. Many authors argue that although there are public health strategies in each country of the UK, the fact that public health services are still located in the NHS restricts the potential of public health to act in the interest of the health of people. Despite the limitations of the 1848 Public Health Act, some public health practitioners have called for a 21st-century Central Health Board and a shift of public health services from the NHS back to local authorities, where action on the determinants of health can be more effective. More than ever there is a need to bring the politics back into public health as without political will and commitment the continuing widening inequalities in health in the 21st century will not be stemmed and public health will not be equipped to deal with the challenges of modern society and increasing globalisation.

References

Acheson Committee Report (1988) *Public Health in England: The Report of the Committee of Inquiry into the Future Development of the Public Health Function*, Cm 289. London: HMSO.

Berridge, V. (2001) Constructing Women and Smoking as a Public Health Problem in Britain (1950–1990s), *Gender and History*, 13 (2): 328–48.

Department of Health (1991) *The Health of the Nation*. London: The Stationery Office.

Department of Health (2001) *The Report of the Chief Medical Officer's Project to Strengthen the Public Health Function*. London: Department of Health.

Department of Health (2005) *Shaping the Future of Public Health: Promoting Health in the NHS*. London: Department of Health.

Faculty of Public Health (2005) *The Ten Key Areas for Public Health Practice*, http://www.fphm.org.uk/about_faculty/what_public_health/10key_areas.asp.

Hamlin, C. and Sheard, S. (1998) Revolutions in public health: 1848 and 1998?, *British Medical Journal*, 317: 587–91.

Lalonde, M. (1974) *A New Perspective on the Health of Canadians*. Ottawa: Ministry of Supply and Services.

MacDonald, T.H. (1998) *Rethinking Health Promotion: A Global Approach*. London: Routledge.

Nursing and Midwifery Council (2003) *Third Part of the New Register. Proposed Competency Framework for Specialist Community Public Health Nurses*. Consultation document. London: NMC.

O'Donnell, P. (1986) Definition of health promotion, *American Journal of Health Promotion*, 1 (1): 4–5.

O'Donnell, P. (1989) Definition of health promotion. Part III: Expanding the definition, *American Journal of Health Promotion*, 3 (3): 5.

Scott-Samuel, A. (2003) Specialist health promotion – can we save it?, *Public Health News*, 5 December.

Wanless, D. (2002) *Securing our Future Health: Taking a Long-term View*. London: HM Treasury.

Wanless, D. (2004) *Securing Good Health for the Whole Population: Final Report*. London: HM Treasury.

WHO (World Health Organisation) (1986) *Ottawa Charter for Health Promotion*. Geneva: WHO.

WHO (2005) *The Bangkok Charter for Health Promotion in a Globalised World*. Bangkok: WHO, http://www.who.int/healthpromotion/conferences/6gchp/bangkok_charter/en/.

Winslow, C.E.A. (1951) 'The cost of sickness and the price of health', *WHO Monograph*, 7: 28. Geneva: WHO.

Chapter 3

The Market-dominated Future of Public Health?

Jeff French

Introduction

This chapter explores the market-dominated future of public health. The proposition is put forward that in a world that is, and will increasingly be, characterised by liberal democratic free market economies, public health and health promotion practice will move from the current dominant ideological position of 'paternalistic collectivism' to embrace a model characterised more by individual rights and market solutions. It will be argued that 'social marketing' will emerge to rival 'collective paternalistic' public health as the dominant approach to improving health. It is argued that social marketing will assume increasing significance because its theoretical and ideological base better reflects liberal democratic free market government policy and the increasing demand from citizens to be given more power in shaping all forms of state-provided services, including public health and health promotion efforts.

What are we trying to achieve?

In the developed world we live in a society that has a long life expectancy and a high level of wellness (Sanders and Carer, 1985; WHO, 1991, 2003). We are in many respects working for health gain at the margins relative to the improvements brought about through sanitation, better nutrition, improvements in employment conditions, social infrastructure, improved medical services and better education (Doyal and Pennell, 1979; McKeown, 1979). Within many developed countries, however, there are growing relative health inequalities between rich and the relatively poor. The developing world, by contrast, faces a set of challenges relating to the development of the basic prerequisites and infrastructures for health, infectious disease and a rapidly growing epidemic of chronic disease.

In most health policy over the last twenty years, the word 'health' denotes not merely the absence of disease but also well-being and social justice. Health has also been promoted as a fundamental 'human right', at least since the 1974 World Health Organisation (WHO) Alma Ata declaration. WHO has argued that this 'right to health' can only be realised through the combined and coordinated action of all social and economic sectors. This is a reasonable proposition supported by a wealth of insights and evidence from many academic and practice fields. Health has been described as an emergent capacity arising from the integrated effects of somatic, social, economic and cultural activity. It is not something that can be attained solely from health sector-directed expenditure, or attempts to get people to live healthy lives.

If we accept that health is determined by such factors, the development of better health will need whole systems solutions. The whole systems solution, however, depends on how the system is conceived and the role of state-sponsored public health within this. There are very different views about the answers to these questions among public health practitioners and between governments, the commercial sector and citizens.

The growth of global paternalistic healthism

WHO and many public health practitioners have, for over thirty years, argued that prevention and treatment of disease should be viewed by all governments as their primary duty. In so doing the avoidance of disease is positioned as the driving force and the ultimate goal of the world's economic and political systems. Smith et al. (2003) have advocated that health actually constitutes the most important form of 'global health good'. Conceived in this way public health represents a radical socialist position calling for no less than a global, political and economic reorientation.

For those public health practitioners who hold such views, the goal of society is not seen as the promotion of individual freedom, collective prosperity or the accumulation of wealth. In fact many public health practitioners view markets and capitalism as a key part of the problem rather than being part of the solution to improving health. Protecting and promoting health is seen as the first and most important social activity. For such public health professionals, health as measured by the absence of disease is seen as the key indicator of social progress.

Public health conceived in this way has been criticised by Armstrong (1983, 1993, 1995), Fitzpatrick (2001) and others as representing the ever-expanding medicalisation of life. Kurtz (1987) has also argued that health has become the 'new religion' and public health workers are the new puritanical priests offering punishment for the 'bad' life and rewards for the 'good' healthy life.

This 'collective paternalistic' stance is in stark contrast to how health promotion is perceived by most governments. Minkler (1989) believes that for most governments, health promotion and public health are viewed as being largely about protection from infectious diseases, encouraging voluntary behavioural change, and a process of providing information about how to live healthy lives.

All democratic governments use an intervention mix of law, education and services to improve health. Governments are also responsible for developing regulated markets to act as an engine for collective and individual prosperity and increased well-being. This clear clash of ideological positions between the democratic free market position of most governments and the paternalistic collectivist stance supported by many public health professionals sits at the heart of the current theoretical and practical antagonism between public health advocates and elected administrations.

The impact of ideology on health promotion theory

Kelly and Charlton (1995) agree with the proposition outlined above that health promotion and public health have become a left of centre political campaign in which health is viewed as a moral right. Seedhouse (1997), in a more thorough review, has argued that the theoretical development of health promotion and public health is muddled, poorly articulated and devoid of a clear political philosophy. In political terms, public health and health promotion can, if we accept this criticism, mean whatever you want them to mean.

Peterson and Lupton (1996) have further criticised public health as a source of moral regulation and consequent state-sponsored control of individual freedoms. Stevenson and Burke (1991) are also critical of health promotion, arguing that it weakens and depoliticises action for social equality by turning what is a political and economic struggle into a technical professionally led intervention.

New individualism

During the last hundred years or so the state's influence on the lives and health of populations has grown in significance. The introduction of polices and legislation, education, universal suffrage, the establishment of new health and social services and professional groups to provide them have had a large impact on the prevention of disease and the promotion of better health. It is probably true, however, that this 'big state' approach has now moved past its zenith. We may be at the beginning of a new phase in civic development, one that seeks to place the citizen as consumer at the centre of attempts to maintain and further improve health (Birchall and Simmons, 2004; Lent and Arend, 2004).

This new individualism, rather than assigning the responsibility for good health to individual choices and behaviour, locates responsibility with both individuals and the providers of public and private organisations serving the public. The responsibility of these bodies is to place the needs and wishes of individuals at the centre of their planning and provision. Rather than 'blaming the victim', new individualism is about blaming service or product providers for failing to deliver what consumers require so that they can live the healthy and self-actualising lives that they demand.

A key commitment set out in *Choosing Health* (Department of Health, 2004), the English public health strategy, was to develop a more coordinated, personalised and choice-based approach to the promotion of positive health. The final Wanless review, which informed *Choosing Health*, made it clear that the most critical success factor in achieving what it called the 'fully engaged scenario', in which the majority of the population would be actively seeking to live healthy lives, would be a high degree of engagement of the population in taking steps to improve their health. Progress, it argued, demanded that a wide range of public and private sector organisations work together with communities and individuals to tackle health inequalities and promote positive health (Wanless, 2004).

Wanless argued that achieving the maximum attainable shift in behaviour and attitude would require a significant shift in the way public health was practised in England. Such a shift would require more effort being directed to working in partnership with the public, the private sector and further significant shift in current approaches to the coordination of action across government.

The public endorses this approach themselves. Research carried out by the King's Fund and Health Development Agency in 2004 found that 89 per cent of people agree that individuals are responsible for their own health and 93 per cent agree that parents are more responsible than anyone else for their children's health. There is equally strong demand from the public for more choice and 'voice' in the provision of services and falling trust in government and its institutions (OLR, 2002).

There is a public demand for more engagement in promoting health and recognition by the population and policy makers that the development of better health will require a move away from an isolated professionally dominated top-down approach. Future public health strategies will need, then, to recognise that people are powerful agents of their own health and that other sectors, including the 'not for profit' and 'for profit' sectors, have a key role to play in developing and maintaining health and well-being.

The rise of social marketing

Social Marketing is the systematic application of marketing concepts and techniques to achieve specific behavioural goals relevant to a social good. (French and Blair-Stevens, 2005: 4)

Due to the close ideological match between social marketing and liberal democratic imperatives it is probable that it will increasingly be selected by governments as a preferred public health intervention and strategy development approach. Social marketing is a highly systematic approach to health improvement that sets out unambiguous success criteria in terms of behaviour change. In this respect, social marketing stands in stark contrast to many health promotion interventions which demonstrate weak planning systems and poor evaluation. Social marketing will also be attractive to governments because of its emphasis on developing deep customer insight, choice and population segmentation to develop interventions that can respond to a diversity of needs.

In 1971 Kotler and Zaltman published 'Social marketing: an approach to planned social change'. This paper marked the first time the phrase 'social marketing' was used in an academic journal but, in reality, social marketing approaches were being applied from the 1960s onwards in both developed countries and as part of international development programmes in much of the developing world. Large-scale health promotion programmes, such as the Stanford Heart Disease Prevention Program in America, began to apply social marketing principles alongside other forms of health promotion interventions. During the 1980s a growing number of academic institutions established social marketing centres. The literature on both the theoretical and practice base of the discipline grew rapidly. Social marketing has over the last twenty years had a profound influence on the delivery of both national and local health promotion efforts in Canada, America and Australia, but much less so in the UK.

Social marketing has a number of defining principles and concepts, and it is widely accepted to be a systematic planning and delivery methodology drawing on techniques developed in the commercial sector, such as audience segmentation, but also drawing on experience from the public and not-for-profit sectors. Social marketing is focused on enabling, encouraging and supporting voluntary behaviour change among target audiences and the re-engineering of services and systems to support and facilitate change.

A central concept of social marketing is that of 'exchange'. Exchange recognises that if people are going to change their behaviour or collectively work for social change, they need to believe that the reward for such action is worth the price paid. The price paid is the financial, emotional and time cost of taking part in any change programme. This implies that any offers developed by those intent on assisting people to live healthier lives need to be developed on the basis of a deep understanding of the views, motivations and barriers encountered by target audiences.

The lack of social marketing capacity in the UK

Public health practice in the UK is highly regulated and codified by powerful professional groups who determine what effective practice is, what competencies are important, and which are pre-eminent. The dominance of the medical profession in the UK within public health has led to a situation in which the contributions of fields of practice outside the traditional focus of medical public health (epidemiology, infection disease control) have been relegated to subordinate positions. This has led to approaches such as social marketing not receiving the prominence that the evidence suggests it should have in actually delivering the solutions to the largely behaviourally related health problems that we face.

Social marketing has also probably failed to develop significantly in the UK due to a general antipathy towards 'markets' and market philosophy by public health practitioners and advisers, as discussed earlier in this chapter. A further factor that has slowed social marketing's development in the UK is the dominance of what can be called the 'campaign paradigm' or social advertising approach to health promotion over the last twenty years. This paradigm is characterised by an over-reliance on awareness-focused social advertising 'campaigns', to the exclusion of other forms of health promotion intervention. There are a number of drivers for this paradigm, including the perceived need of politicians to be seen to be taking action on public health issues, and a lack of understanding and knowledge about what health communication programmes can and cannot deliver.

Conclusions

Some argue that public health came into being over the last two hundred years as a humanitarian response to incompetent or complicit governments in league with the private sector. Other accounts paint a different view, of world development driven by trade and technological innovation with improved social conditions arising from these advances and a struggle led by the people, often in the face of the establishment.

In recent years the dominant public health ideology has been one of anti-market, paternalistic collectivism. Most democratic governments have, in contrast, increasingly supported a greater emphasis on individual rights and responsibilities, and the role of markets in bringing about social improvement. A resulting state of conflict flowing from these opposed ideological positions has existed between most governments and professional public health practitioners over the last thirty years. This antagonism runs deep and governments and their policies are often seen as a key part of the problem by many public health practitioners. Politicians often view with increased frustration the constant criticism from public health professions and their inability to deliver any significant impact on major health challenges. One of the emergent probable solutions to this uneasy relationship is the development and application of social marketing as an alternative to paternalistic professional-dominated approaches to population health improvement. Social marketing emphasises a target-driven, citizen-centric approach to the provision of public health interventions, a view held by most governments. Social marketing also stresses the importance of building alliances between the state, the for-profit sector, and NGO sector. Building delivery coalitions between sectors and marshalling all available expertise and resources to support behaviour change and the environmental conditions that enable it, represents one of the key features of a social marketing approach and is one that sets it apart from more traditional state-dominated attempts to improve the health of the nation.

References

Armstrong, D. (1983) *The Political Anatomy of the Body*, Cambridge University Press, Cambridge.

Armstrong, D. (1993) Public health spaces and fabrication of identity, *Sociology*, 27(3), pp. 393–410.

Armstrong, D. (1995) The rise of surveillance medicine, *Sociology of Health & Illness*, 17(3), pp. 393–404.

Birchall, J. and Simmons, R. (2004) *User Power: The Participation of Users in Public Services*. London: National Consumer Council.

Department of Health (2004) *Choosing Health: Making Healthier Choices Easier*, The Stationery Office, London.

Doyal, L. and Pennell, I. (1979) *The Political Economy of Health*, Pluto Press, London.

Fitzpatrick, M. (2001) *The Tyranny of Health: Doctors and the Regulation of Lifestyle*, Routledge, London.

French, J. and Blair-Stevens, C. (2005) *Social Marketing Pocket Guide*, National Consumer Council, London.

Kelly, M. and Charlton, B. (1995) The sociology of health promotion, in R. Bunton, S. Nettleton and R. Burrows (eds), *The Sociology of Health Promotion: Critical Analysis of Consumption, Lifestyle and Risk*, Routledge, London.

King's Fund and Health Development Agency (2004) *Public Attitudes to Public Health Policy*, King's Fund and Health Development Agency, London.

Kotler, P. and Zaltman, G. (1971) Social marketing: an approach to planned social change, *Journal of Marketing*, 35, pp. 3–12.

Kurtz, I. (1987) Health educators – the new puritans, *Journal of Medical Ethics*, 13(1), pp. 40–41.

Lent, A. and Arend, N. (2004) *Making Choices: How Can Choice Improve Local Public Services?*, New Local Government Network, London.

McKeown, T. (1979) *The Role of Medicine*, Basil Blackwell, London.

Minkler, M. (1989) Health education, health promotion and the open society: an historical perspective, *Health Education Quarterly*, 16(1), pp. 17–30.

OLR (2002) *It's a Matter of Trust: What Society Thinks and Feels about Trust*, Opinion Leader Research, London.

Peterson, A. and Lupton, D. (1996) *The New Public Health*, Sage, London.

Sanders, D. and Carer R. (1985) *The Struggle for Health*, Macmillan, Basingstoke.

Seedhouse, D. (1997) *Health Promotion, Philosophy, Prejudice and Practice*, Wiley, Chichester.

Smith, R., Beaglehole, R., Woodward, D. and Drager, N. (eds) (2003) *Global Public Goods for Health*, Oxford University Press, Oxford.

Stevenson, H. and Burke, M. (1991) Bureaucratic logic in new social movement clothing: the limits of health promotion research, *Health Promotion International*, 6(3), pp. 281–9.

Wanless, D. (2004) *Securing Good Health for the Whole Population: Final Report*, HM Treasury, London.

WHO (1974) *ALMA ATA Declaration*, World Health Organisation, Geneva.

WHO (1991) *World Health Statistics Annual*, World Health Organisation, Geneva.

WHO (2003) *The Solid Facts: the Social Determinants of Health*, 2nd edn, World Health Organisation, Europe, Copenhagen.

Wilkinson, R. (1996) *Unhealthy Societies: the Aflictions of Inequality*, Routledge, London.

Chapter 4

How is Health Experienced?

Mildred Blaxter

Lay concepts of health

[...] The topic of lay concepts of health and illness has been the focus of very active research and discussion. Kleinman (1980) distinguished three broad sectors of knowledge about health and illness:

- professional (orthodox, scientific, Western)
- alternative (folk, traditional, complementary)
- lay (popular, informal).

These overlap and their boundaries are, increasingly, flexible. Professional knowledge now includes much of the 'alternative'. Lay knowledge rests on both tradition and medical science. Indeed, it has been argued that, just as it is not practical to oppose illness and disease, so the label 'lay' concepts, though common as a shorthand, is not useful. Early definitions of lay attitudes to health, as those beliefs and practices explicitly derived from other cultural frames of knowledge, are not obviously applicable in modern Western societies, where lay accounts are usually filtered through internalized professional accounts. Lay beliefs can be better defined as commonsense understandings and personal experience, imbued with professional rationalizations.

The mid-twentieth-century interest in lay concepts was largely based on a wish to understand why people behaved as they did in choosing health-related actions or interacting with the profession of medicine. What 'folk' beliefs – especially among different ethnic or socio-economic groups – might intervene in efficient and 'compliant' collaboration with their doctors? Why was there resistance to medical procedures, or why were symptoms ignored? What 'wrong' beliefs required attention in health education?

Edited from: Blaxter, M. (ed.) (2004) *Health*, Cambridge: Polity Press, Chapter 3, pp. 45–53. Reproduced with permission from Polity Press Ltd.

If, in more recent decades, the approach to what is still called lay concepts is very much more complex, this is not to deny that residues of older or 'folk' concepts are still present in people's minds.

> Treatment of a Cold or Chill is your own responsibility; it is your own problem, and is less likely to mobilise a caring community around you than a Fever. As in all Hot–Cold and humoural [*sic*] systems, treatment aims primarily to fight cold with warmth, and to move the patient from 'Cold' (or 'colder' than normal) back to 'normal', by adding heat in the form of hot drinks, hot-water bottles, rest in a warm bed, and so on; and in giving him the means to generate his own heat, especially by ample warm food ('Feed a Cold, Starve a Fever'), as well as tonics and vitamins, which are also perceived as a type of nutriment. In addition, he must if necessary be shifted from the 'Wet' to the 'Dry' state – not by expelling or washing out the Fluids, but by drying them up. These Fluids are considered part of the body, and should be conserved, with the aid of nasal drops, decongestant tablets, inhalations, and drugs to solidify the loose stools. (Helman, 1978: 117–18)

Moreover, their doctor may be complicit in trying to talk in folk terms: a patient who presents a list of symptoms is often given a diagnosis in the everyday idiom of the folk model: 'You've picked up a germ', 'It's just a tummy bug – there's one going around'.

Research on lay concepts now goes much farther than this interest in folk ideas, however. It covers a number of essentially different questions. It may be, simply, how people (especially in different sections of society) define health. This is a difficult question to ask (or answer) in a direct form, and other issues may be used as indicators: what they see as the causes of ill health, how they think disease can be avoided, how they recognize other people as 'healthy', the accounts they give of their experiences of illness at particular times or over a life-time.

The questions may be asked by the qualitative method of interviewing people, in relatively unstructured or more structured ways, or by applying the methods of psychology such as tested 'instruments'. For large populations statistics can be applied to simple agree/disagree answers to statements about health, or some open-ended single question asking for a definition of health or combined answers to a range of questions about different aspects of health can be analysed. Each study may begin with different interests and hypotheses, and thus the analytic categories produced may be different: concepts of health cannot be 'reliably' measured in the same way as physiological or psychological attributes. Some common theses arise, however.

Surveys of lay definitions

A classic series of early studies was that of Claudine Herzlich in France in the 1960s, influenced by the work of Foucault and Muscovici's concept of 'social representations'. This approach to social psychology – examining the way in which individuals perceive the world as part of the more extensive systems of knowledge that society shares – saw subjectively perceived social representations both as the models which individuals use and as discourses in the public domain.

Herzlich (1973) identified three different metaphors to describe the way in which people talked about health and illness:

- *Illness as destroyer*, involving loss, isolation and incapacity:

  If I were very seriously ill, if nothing more could be done, then it would be family life wouldn't exist any more … (p. 106)

- *Illness as liberator*, a lessening of burdens:

  For me, illness is breaking off from social life, from life outside and social obligation, it's being set free.
  … It allows [people] to be what they were before and what they can't be because of social circumstances. (p. 114)

- *Illness as occupation*, freedom from responsibility, except for the need to fight the disease:

  From the moment you know what's in front of you it seems to me the only thing to do is to gather your strength and fight. (p. 119)

Turning to more explicit representations of *health*, Herzlich found three, which could co-exist in one person's account:

- *health in a vacuum*, or the absence of illness, an impersonal condition, recognized only when one becomes ill
- *health as a reserve*, or physical strength and the capacity to resist illness, something inherited or the outcome of a good childhood, a characteristic of the individual which protects against becoming ill
- *health as equilibrium*, balance, harmony and well-being, contingent upon events in life, a state often under attack in modern society.

These three are sometimes discussed in terms of health as having, doing and being.

Other work, among different groups of people, has found similar categories. A study of middle-aged women in a Scottish city, and their daughters, both in poor socio-economic circumstances (Blaxter and Paterson, 1982), found that health (especially for the older generations) was defined principally in terms of 'not being ill': health was either the absence of symptoms of illness, the refusal to admit their existence, the ability to define illnesses as normal ('at my time of life') or the determination not to 'lie down' to them. Health as a positive concept of well-being or positive fitness was absent in the older generation, and though their daughters were more conscious of fitness few had time or energy to devote much thought to it. A constant theme of these women's talk was the concept of illness as a state of spiritual or moral, rather than physical, malaise, associated with personality and a lack of moral fibre. If, in the face of this view, the experience of illness was inescapable – and, for the older generation in particular, it was – then the obvious residual category was one of health as simply chance.

Another study in Scotland (Williams, 1990), of older people, found similar concepts to those of Herzlich, and similar emphasis on the moral and functional aspects of health. Health was defined as the absence of disease, and illness has to be coped with in five broad ways:

- as controlled by normal living, by keeping up normal activity
- as a continuous struggle
- as an alternative way of life
- as a loss to be endured
- as release from effort.

All the work considered so far has noted that the concepts of health derived must be considered in the light of the particular groups being studied. A different type of study has attempted to obtain definitions from large populations, with, usually, a particular interest in looking at the differences between groups. D'Houtard and Field (1986), for instance, reported on a very large survey in France which simply asked the question 'What is, according to you, the best definition of health?' The answers were analysed into forty-one different themes:

- for 'higher' and 'middle classes, prominent themes were 'life without constraints', 'personal unfolding' and 'good physical equilibrium'
- for 'employees', they were 'watching oneself', 'being in a good mood', 'sleeping well', 'living as long as possible'
- for urban workers, themes were as for employees, but also particularly 'engaging in sports', 'having a normal appetite'
- for rural workers, they were 'being able to work', 'avoiding excess'.

In other words, those who did manual work found physical fitness and the ability to work to be key criteria, while those with non-manual occupations could see health as a more positive concept.

Another study in France, reported by Pierret (1993), used content analysis of both quantitative and qualitative methods with three sub-samples: residents of an 'old quarter' of Paris, residents of a 'new city', and farmers. The topic was introduced simply by 'I would like you to tell me about health, what it means to you'. Four 'registers' were found:

- health-illness, talk organized around health as not being ill
- health-tool, an impersonal view of health as a capital that everyone has, the principal form of wealth, to be used as a tool
- health-product, health as a personal value, with controllable and uncontrollable factors held in balance
- health-institution, health seen from a collective and political viewpoint, to be managed by society.

Which of these was favoured appeared to be related to the individual's social and occupational position. For instance, public-sector wage-earners tended to express health as collective and governmental; manual workers saw it in terms of not-illness or as a tool; farmers' illness and risk beliefs fell into a homogeneous world-view based on a cycle of life over which they had some control. Pierret observed that, 'In France, persons' relations to the State, in particular whether they work in the private or public sector, seem to be as important as social class origins' (1993: 22).

A nation-wide UK study, *Health and Lifestyles* (Blaxter, 1990), posed a similar open-ended question: 'What is it like when you are healthy?', also asking people to describe 'a healthy person' whom they knew. Replies were analysed to form five categories:

1 Health as not-ill

Here health is defined by the absence of symptoms or lack of need for medical attention, for example:

> Health is when you don't hurt anywhere and you're not aware of any part of your body. (woman of forty-nine)
>   A healthy person is someone who hasn't seen a doctor for fifty years. (woman of seventy, speaking of her husband)

Health was clearly distinguished from disease. One might be diseased, and ill, and therefore unhealthy, but equally one could be healthy despite disease: 'I am very healthy apart from my arthritis.' This definition of health was found to be a little more frequently used by the better educated and those with higher incomes, and was markedly associated with the speaker's own state of health. Those who themselves were in poor health were much less likely than those in good health to use the non-ill definition.

2 Health as physical fitness, vitality

Among younger people, health as physical fitness was very prominent. Young men, in particular, stressed strength, athletic prowess and the ability to play sports; 'fit' was by far the most common word used in these descriptions of health by men under forty. Women and older men used the word 'energy': sometimes physical energy was meant, and sometimes a psychosocial vitality which had little to do with physique, but often the two were combined. This, and the idea of 'healthy though diseased', has some affinity with Herzlich's 'health as reserve'. This concept was often expressed in ideas of heredity, or resistance, or recovering quickly from illness, for example:

> Both his parents are alive at ninety so he comes of healthy stock. (woman of fifty-one)
>   Health is when I feel I can do anything … nothing can stop you in your tracks. (man of twenty-eight)
>   Health is having loads of whump. You feel good, you look good, nothing really bothers you, life is wonderful, you seem to feel like doing more. (woman of twenty-eight)

3 Health as social relationships

Social relationships were also frequently associated with this definition of health, though almost always by women rather than men. For younger women, health was defined in terms of good relationships with family and children; for the elderly, this was redefined as retaining an active place in the social world and caring for others, for example

> You feel as though everyone is your friend. I enjoy life more, and can work, and help other people. (woman of seventy-four)

4 Health as function

Both health as energy and health as social relationships overlap with the idea of health as function – health defined as being able to do things, with less emphasis on a description of feelings. Health as function was more likely to be expressed by older men and women; the ability to cope with the tasks of life might, of course, be taken for granted among younger people. For men particularly, health was bound up with pride in being able to do hard work. For the elderly, health could mean being mobile, or self-sufficient, able to care for themselves or to continue to work, despite the inevitable ills of old age:

> Health is being able to walk around better, and doing more work in the house when my knees let me. (woman of seventy-nine)

5 Health as psychosocial well-being

This category was reserved for expressions of health as a purely mental state, instead of, or as well as, a physical condition. It was, in fact, the most common definition of health among all age groups except young men, and a definition expressed by over half of middle-aged women. It tended to be used rather more by those with higher education or non-manual jobs. It was a very holistic concept: 'happy', 'confidence', 'enjoying life' were words used to describe it, and 'health is a state of mind' or 'happy to be alive' were common statements. Examples of this definition of health include:

> … physically, mentally and spiritually at one. (woman aged forty-five, living in a religious community)
> Emotionally you are stable, energetic, happier, more contented and things don't bother you so. (woman aged twenty, secretary)
> I've reached the stage now where I say isn't it lovely and good to be alive, seeing all the lovely leaves on the trees, it's wonderful to be alive and to be able to stand and stare. (farmer's widow, aged seventy-four)

The way in which health was defined over the life-course differed, in not unexpected ways. There were also clear gender differences. At all stages, women gave generally more expansive answers than men and appeared to find the questions more interesting. These definitions were not exclusive, and many people combined several of the categories.

References

Blaxter, M. (1990) *Health and Lifestyles*. London: Routledge.

Blaxter, M. and Paterson, E. (1982) *Mothers and Daughters: A Three-Generational Study of Health Attitudes and Behaviour*. London: Heinemann.

D'Houtard, A. and Field, M. (1986) New research on the image of health. In C. Currer and M. Stacey (eds), *Concepts of Health, Illness and Disease*. Leamington Spa: Berg.

Helman, C. (1978) Feed a cold, starve a fever. *Culture, Medicine & Psychiatry*, 2: 107–37.

Herzlich, C. (1973) *Health and Illness*. London: Academic Press.

Kleinman, A. (1980) *Patients and Healers in the Context of Culture: An Exploration of the Borderland between Anthropology, Medicine and Psychiatry*. Berkeley and London: University of California Press.

Pierret, J. (1993) Constructing discourses about health and their social determinants. In A. Radley (ed.), *Worlds of Illness: Biographical and Cultural Perspectives on Health and Disease*. London: Routledge, 9–26.

Williams, R. (1990) *A Protestant Legacy*. Oxford: Clarendon Press.

Chapter 5

Older People's Health: Applying Antonovsky's Salutogenic Paradigm

Moyra Sidell

Introduction

If we take morbidity data as the yardstick, older people's health on the whole is not very good. Evidence from the General Household Survey has, since the start of the 1990s shown that about 60 per cent of all people over the age of 65 suffer from some form of chronic illness or disability (Walker et al., 2001). Yet, when asked in similar surveys how they rate their health, less than 25 per cent of people rate it as poor. One possible explanation is that they are using different accounts of health. When asked to define 'health', well over half talked in terms of psychological well-being or feeling good, another 12 per cent said that it was about having energy (Blaxter, 1990). Only about 12 per cent saw health as the absence of disease, with about a quarter defining health as the ability to function.

Accounts of health

Morbidity statistics which describe 60 per cent of the older population as diseased operate within a biomedical account of health. This is still the most influential of the health accounts of Western societies. It sees health as the absence of diagnosed disease. This view of health is both sanctioned and supported by the healthcare system. Biomedical explanations relate to the physical body, and health is explained in terms of biology. It is a mechanistic view which concentrates on the structure of the body, its anatomy, and the way it works, its physiology. This functional view of health sees the human being as a complex organism which can best be understood by breaking it into isolated parts, each with a

From: Sidell, M., Jones, L., Katz J., Peberdy, A. and Douglas, J. (eds) (2003) *Debates and Dilemmas in Promoting Health: A Reader* (2nd edn). Basingstoke: Palgrave Macmillan, Chapter 3, pp. 33–9. Reproduced with permission of Palgrave Macmillan.

'normal' way of working. Disease can then be narrowed down to the malfunction of a particular part of the body. Medical treatment focuses on the diseased part and the tendency is to concentrate on discrete parts or organs and pay less attention to the whole or the interaction of the parts.

The mechanistic and disease-orientated view of health inevitably paints a bleak and negative view of the prospects for health in old age. Later life is portrayed as a time of declining strength and increased frailty as organs and tissues wear out or succumb to disease and degeneration. It views individuals narrowly in terms of their bodies, which are in decline as the natural consequence of growing older. Hope for better health in old age will come from maintaining the body in better shape, eradicating the diseases to which the ageing body is prone, and replacing defective organs. Increasingly, medicine is accepting wider social and psychological influences on health and reflecting elements of other models of health, but most doctors and research scientists still believe that the way our bodies work can be understood within a biological framework and that a cause and therefore a treatment can be found for all disorders, whether physical or mental.

But biomedicine, with its emphasis on the functioning of individual bodies, has little to say about emotional and psychological health. Some strands of biomedicine have tended to see mental illness as some form of malfunctioning of the brain. Yet the separation of mind and body in explanations of health is a fairly recent phenomenon. In earlier historical periods in Western society and in some contemporary Eastern cultures mental and physical health are linked inseparably.

The humanistic psychology tradition developed the notion of a healthy personality with an ideal of health as a thinking, feeling and reflecting being, able to change and grow – a rounded, balanced personality (Stevens, 1990). A. Maslow and Carl Rogers have explored more positive aspects of psychological health, with an ideal of health moving from fulfilling basic human needs to reaching a state of 'self-actualisation' or 'becoming what one is capable of becoming' (Maslow, 1954). In this model, self-esteem and the ability to express one's emotions are important elements of healthy growth in people.

A holistic account of health is more concerned with the whole person as a unique individual. The older person is not seen as a collection of bodily ills but as a thinking, feeling, creative being who has strengths and weaknesses of body, mind and spirit. It is possible to be healthy in mind and spirit even though the body may be frail. Holism is often lined with equilibrium or a state in which body, mind and spirit are in balance. These are concepts drawn from ancient Eastern traditions and have become very popular in the West, particularly in the alternative health movement. But, as with biomedicine, the focus of attention is on the individual. Critics of a holistic account of health argue that this ignores the impact on the individual of the wider physical and social environment.

There is now widespread support for a more overarching social model of health which extends the medical model and draws attention to the adverse effects on health in the physical and social environment, such as poor housing, poverty, pollution, unemployment and poor working conditions (Heller et al., 2001). This represents a challenge to orthodox medical views and puts health concerns on wider agendas, emphasising the link between the economic, political and social environment and health.

The social mould of health puts less emphasis on decline and decay of the organism and more on the interactions with the physical and social environment. So disease and decline are not inevitable in old age and not attributable to age *per se*, but to the conditions in which people age and in which they have lived their lives. Disease is never just 'due to your age' but to hostile forces in the environment, such as poverty and poor housing.

All the accounts of health explored so far see the normal state of affairs to be one of homoeostasis. Any disruption of this homoeostasis is considered to be abnormal, and if homoeostasis is not restored then the organism is said to be in a state of pathology or disease. Aaron Antonovsky (1984) has called this 'the pathogenic paradigm' and he claims that all our models of health, even the biopsychosocial models, are dominated by this paradigm.

Moving to a salutogenic paradigm

Antonovosky (1984) points out some of the consequences of the domination of the pathogenic paradigm. The first is that 'we have come to think dichotomously about people, classifying them as either healthy or diseased' (p. 115). Those categorised as 'healthy' are normal, while those categorised as non-healthy or diseased are deviant. If 60 per cent of older people have some form of chronic illness or disability then the majority of older people are not healthy. There is no place in this dichotomy for those who have a chronic illness yet are able to function perfectly well or for those who have a handicap yet are well satisfied with life. Second – and this echoes the holistic account – we have come to think of specific diseases such as cancer or heart disease instead of being in a state of disease. We have become obsessed with morphology instead of relating to generalised dis-ease and its prevention. This leads to Antonovosky's third concern, which is that we look for specific causes for these specific diseases so that the causes can be eradicated instead of accepting that 'pathogens are endemic in human existence' (p. 115). He believes that we need to explore the capacity of human beings to cope with pathogens. Fourth, the pathogenic paradigm deludes us into thinking that if we can eliminate 'disease' we will have health. This 'mirage of health' (Dubos, 1961) has been the driving force behind the 'technological fix' and 'magic bullet' attitude to eradicating disease. This attitude leads to the fifth consequence that Antonovsky identified, which is that the pathogenic paradigm concentrates on 'the case' and identifies high-risk groups instead of studying the 'symptoms of wellness' (1984, p. 116). Adopting this approach would entail studying the smokers who do not get lung cancer, or the 'fat eaters' who do not have heart trouble.

Antonovsky believes that we should think 'salutogenically'. He claims that instead of assuming that the normal state of the human organism is one of homoeostasis, balance and equilibrium, it makes more sense to acknowledge that the 'normal state of affairs for the human organism is one of entropy, of disorder, and of disruption of homoeostasis' (1984, p. 116). He suggests that none of us can be categorised as being either healthy or diseased, but that we all can be located somewhere along a continuum which he calls 'health-ease-dis-ease'. He explains:

> We are all somewhere between the imaginary poles of total wellness and total illness. Even the fully robust, energetic, symptom-free, richly functioning person has the mark of mortality: he or she wears glasses, has moments of depression, comes down with flu, and may well have as yet non-detectable malignant cells. Even the terminal patient's brain and emotions may be fully functional. (p. 116)

This way of thinking would have profound effects on the way we view health in old age. It would discourage a percentage approach to assessing the health of older people. Instead of assuming that because 60 per cent have a chronic illness or disability they are therefore in poor health, while the other 40 per cent are in good health, we would need to look behind those figures to ask how those 60 per cent are actually affected by their chronic illness or disability, and to explore their wellness. We would have to ask questions such as why do some people cope while others do not, and why some consider themselves to be healthy in spite of their chronic illness while others do not. We would also need to ask about the dis-ease of the 40 per cent without chronic illness or disability. Do they have non-classifiable aches and pains, discomforts and feelings of unwellness?

Antonovsky is anxious that this reorientation towards health does not minimise the achievements of medical science, nor would he wish to impede the progress of technological change. Rather, his purpose is to redress an imbalance inherent in the way we view health; not to abandon the struggle against disease but to widen the armoury and explore other ways of achieving health. We need the availability of hip replacement surgery but we also need to understand why one person copes well with the operation and regains full mobility while another does not. We need to identify all the factors that might help us move along the continuum, and not just focus on the disease. We ask not so much how we can eradicate certain stressors but how we can learn to live with them, concentrating on the ability to adapt. This very much resonates with the empowerment approach of Keith Tones (2001), who states:

> (A)lthough we must acknowledge the specific illnesses and diseases to which older people are prey, it is both more ethical and more efficient to develop a positive approach and seek to enhance well-being of older people. The most useful way of encapsulating such an approach is in terms of empowerment. (p. xvi)

Antonovsky's salutogenic paradigm helps in our understanding of health in later life in that it turns on its head the notion that older people are a high risk group in terms of disease. As Antonovsky says, all of us 'by virtue of being human are in a high risk group' (1984, p. 177). If we locate people dynamically along a continuum of health we are less likely to stereotype 'the elderly' as being diseased. By adopting a salutogenic paradigm we can reconceptualise questions about health in later life to concentrate on why and how people cope well with chronic illness and disability. The questions change from what stops people becoming sick to what helps them to become healthy in spite of disease.

In an attempt to define the mechanisms that help people to cope with adverse health conditions, Antonovsky developed a construct that he calls a *Sense of Coherence*, and abbreviates to SOC. He describes it as follows:

> The sense of coherence is a global orientation that expresses the extent to which one had a pervasive, enduring though dynamic feeling of confidence that one's internal and external environments are predictable and that there is a high probability that things will work out as well as can reasonably be expected. (Antonovsky, 1979, p. 123)

In a later refinement he identified three main components – comprehensibility, manageability and meaningfulness. Comprehensibility is the ability to see one's own world as understandable, to 'have confidence that sense and order can be made of situations' (1984,

p. 118). One views the future as being reasonably predictable rather than chaotic, disordered or unpredictable. Meaningfulness is the 'emotional counterpart of comprehensibility … life makes sense emotionally' (p. 119). Life is worth living for those who see their lives as comprehensible and meaningful. Manageability reflects the extent to which people feel that they have adequate resources, mental, physical, emotional, social and material to meet whatever demands are put upon them. He believes that wherever a person is located on the health-ease-dis-ease continuum at any particular time, those with a stronger SOC are more likely to move towards the health end of the continuum.

A person's SOC is built up from a range of experiences and sources through the life course and should be well developed by adulthood. Antonovsky sees the SOC developing from the degree to which our life experiences provide 'consistency', an 'underload/overload balance' and provide for participation in decision making. We experience consistency when a given behaviour results in the same consequences whenever we exhibit it, and when people respond to us in consistent ways. This allows us to predict the outcome of behaviour and therefore our lives seem reasonably predictable. Underload/overload balance is achieved when the demands made upon us are appropriate to our capacities. Underused capacity due to lack of challenges can be as harmful as not having sufficient capacity to meet the challenges with which we are faced. The extent to which we participate in decision making is important to the emergence of a strong SOC and is the basis of the meaningfulness component. When everything is decided for us and we have no say in the matter, when the rules are set by others without consultation, then the experience is alien to us. The issue is not so much having control over the events in our lives but in having some part in the decision-making process.

Antonovsky's theory provides a useful framework for analysing the health status of older people, both collectively and individually. The health-ease-dis-ease continuum allows us to locate older people along the continuum rather than categorising them in terms of either health or disease. It allows us to explore how people move along the continuum towards the health end in spite of chronic illness disability.

It is possible that Antonovsky's theory of SOC could be interpreted in a very individualistic way and thus be 'victim blaming': if only those older people with chronic illness had developed a strong SOC they would cope better with their lot. This was clearly not Antonovsky's intention, and in a paper presented at the WHO seminar on 'Theory in Health Promotion: Research and Practice' held in September 1992, he makes a case for seeing the SOC as a theoretical basis for health promotion. He asks, 'Can it be contended that strengthening the SOC of people would be a major contributor to their move toward health?' (1996, p. 16). He goes on to make it clear that this strengthening of the SOC is not aimed at individuals but at a given population, and frames the question for health promotion programmes:

What can be done in this 'community' – factory, geographic community, age or ethnic or gender group, chronic or even acute hospital population, those who suffer from a particular disability, etc. – to strengthen the sense of comprehensibility, manageability and meaningfulness of the persons who constitute it?

It is important to remember that older people are a very diverse group, each with a unique biography and different life experiences and access to social and economic resources. But old age is a time when the threat to a sense of coherence can be great. Manageability, comprehensibility and meaningfulness can be hard to maintain in the face of much loss and change. This is particularly true of those old people who spend their last years in institutions, where it is likely to be even more difficult to maintain any sense of coherence.

Antonovsky's theory presents ways of both understanding health in old age and of helping older people to move towards the health end of the continuum whatever their circumstances. In order to do this they require ageing-friendly environments which must be both prosthetic and stimulating at the same time. Unfortunately, many older people experience extremely ageing-unfriendly or ageist environments which are a threat to any sense of coherence.

References

Antonovsky, A. (1979) *Health, Stress and Coping: new perspectives on mental and physical well-being.* San Francisco: Jossey-Bass.

Antonovsky, A. (1984) The sense of coherence as a determinant of health. In Matarazzo, J.P. (ed.), *Behavioral Health.* New York: Wiley.

Antonovsky, A. (1996) The salutogenic model as a theory to guide health promotion, *Health Promotion International,* 11 (1), 11–18.

Blaxter, M. (1990) *Health and Lifestyles.* London: Routledge.

Dubos, R. (1961) *Mirage of Health.* New York: Andor Books.

Heller, T., Lloyd, C. and Sidell, M. (2001). *Working for Health,* Level 2 distance learning course K203. Milton Keynes: The Open University.

Maslow, A. (1954) *Motivation and Personality.* New York: Harper & Row.

Stevens, R. (1990) Humanistic psychology. In Roth, I. (ed.), *Introduction to Psychology.* Milton Keynes: The Open University and Lawrence Erlbaum Associates.

Tones, K. (2001) Foreword. In Chiva, A. and Stears, D. (eds), *Promoting the Health of Older People: the next step in health generation.* Buckingham: Open University Press.

Walker, A., Maber, J., Coulthard, M., Goddard, E. and Thomas, M. (2001) *Living in Britain: results from the 2000 General Household Survey.* London: The Stationery Office.

Chapter 6

Emerging Theories into the Social Determinants of Health: Implications for Oral Health Promotion

Richard Geddie Watt

Health promotion practice and policy is currently undergoing a process of radical change. For many years, a health education model has been the dominant approach in prevention. This approach placed the emphasis on lifestyle and behavioural change through education and awareness raising programmes. The focus of many health education interventions has been on defined diseases, targeted at changing the behaviours of high-risk individuals. Health professionals have dominated this approach in terms of the programme development, implementation and evaluation. This health education model has been very popular with the dental profession as it fits the clinical approach to care and treatment of individual patients. Recent effectiveness reviews of the oral health education and promotion literature have, however, identified the limitations of many educational interventions to produce sustained improvements in oral health. Another common finding of the reviews was the lack of theory underpinning many interventions.[1-5]

In recent years a shift has taken place in public health and health promotion policy. The emphasis is increasingly now on reducing health inequalities through action on changing the determinants of health.[6-9] In the UK the Acheson Review highlighted the importance of the socioeconomic determinants of health inequalities and identified a range of social and welfare policies to promote the health and well-being of the population.[10] In the USA the Institute of Medicine has reviewed the evidence base for public health interventions and has recommended a change in approach is required.[11] The report stresses the importance of focusing on the social determinants of disease, injury and disability, and of adopting a complementary range of different interventions to promote health. The World Health Organisation global strategy for the prevention and control of noncommunicable diseases also places emphasis on developing interventions which address the environmental, economic, social and behavioural determinants of chronic disease.[12] In addition, the recently

Edited from: Geddie Watt, Richard (2002) Emerging theories into the social determinants of health: implications for oral health promotion, *Community Dentistry and Oral Epidemiology*, 30: 241–7. Reproduced with Permission from Blackwell Publishing Ltd.

published US Surgeon General's Report on Oral Health has highlighted the importance of social and environmental determinants of oral health and the need to adopt a more holistic approach to oral health promotion activities.[13]

This chapter aims to review and highlight the potential value to oral health promotion of emerging theories in public health research into the social determinants of health. The implications for the development of more innovative and effective approaches in oral health promotion policy and practice will also be discussed. First, the limitations of the traditional theory base of dental health education will be reviewed.

Limitations of psychological theoretical base

Dental health education has been heavily influenced by health behaviour research based upon psychological theories developed to explain individual lifestyle.[14] The health behaviour literature has been dominated by theoretical approaches which stress cognitive processes as determinants of behaviour. This is despite the findings of many studies which reveal a weak relationship between psychological concepts such as motivations, beliefs, attitudes and opinions with actual behaviour.[15] The shortcomings of the knowledge-attitude-behaviour (KAB) model have been highlighted for many years[16,17] but this is still being used as the theoretical framework for many dental health education interventions.[4] More elaborate and complex psychological models also have limited value. In a recent meta analysis of studies using the well-known models of Theory of Reasoned Action and Theory of Planned Behaviour, only 40–50 per cent of variance of intention and 20–40 per cent variance of behaviour were explained by the models.[18]

Many psychological theories, such as the Health Belief Model, are based on the hypothesis that a sense of susceptibility to disease induces behaviour change.[19] This view has been challenged on two counts. First, such a hypothesis is based upon the assumption that direct health concerns are the underlying reasons for change. Evidence from many studies have, however, revealed the importance of social or other motivating factors rather than health concerns as driving behaviour change.[20] Secondly, the psychological analysis largely assumes a rational and logical basis of human behaviour, which is not a true reflection of human experience in the real world where social, environmental and political factors greatly determine behaviour.[6] Psychological theories of health behaviour largely ignore the fundamental importance of the social, environmental and political determinants of health.[21]

As Bunton and colleagues have stated, 'failure to include social, economic, environmental and political factors in any analysis of health behaviours ultimately results in a very negative and victim blaming understanding which can lead to the development of potentially harmful and largely ineffective health policies'.[22]

In search of a contemporary theory base for oral health promotion

An alternative theory base is needed to support the development of effective oral health promotion policy and practice, and which acknowledges the importance of the wider social determinants of oral health. Interventions to reduce oral health inequalities need to be guided by theoretical frameworks that are developed from an analysis of the origins and processes underlying health disparities.

Three emerging theoretical approaches will now be described and their potential value to the development of oral health promotion highlighted. The theoretical approaches selected all focus upon exploring the basis for health inequalities and recognise the importance of the social and enviromental determinants of health. The theories reviewed below have provoked considerable debate and controversy within the public health research community over their relevance and salience. It is important that within the field of oral health promotion an informed debate also takes place on the potential value of these theories.

Life-course analysis

This theory is based upon an analysis of the complex ways in which biological risk interacts with economic, social and psychological factors in the devlopment of chronic disease throughout the whole life course.[23,24] A life-course perspective considers an individual's disease status as a marker of their past social position. As Blane powerfully states, 'A person's past social experiences become written into the physiology and pathology of their body. The social is, literally, embodied; and the body records the past, whether as an ex-officer's duelling scars or an ex-miner's emphysema'.[25]

A wealth of epidemiological data supports this approach. The importance of early life circumstances on health in adulthood have been highlighted in birth cohort studies.[26,27] For example, a relationship between low birth weight and later socioeconomic circumstance has been demonstrated.[28] Indeed, birth weight can be considered as a marker of social conditions in later life. The idea of biological programming in which intrauterine and infant circumstances are associated with the prevalence of chronic diseases in middle age and later life is also supportive of the life-course perspective.[29]

The life-course perspective places particular emphasis upon the social context and the interaction between people and their environments in the passage through life. This approach is of value in assessing how advantage and disadvantage may cluster cross-sectionally and accumulate longitudinally, thus contributing to the creation of health and social inequalities in society. A person who is long-term unemployed is likely to live in relatively poor quality accommodation, have restricted access to a healthy diet and smoke as a means of coping with stress and boredom. This is an example of how disadvantage may cluster cross-sectionally. In contrast, a child born into a middle-class family is likely to acquire the necessary educational requirements to enter a relatively stable professional position in the labour market. On retirement this individual will have access to an occupational pension which will provide financial security in later life, an example of the accumulation of advantage longitudinally.[25]

It has been proposed that there are socially critical periods in development which can have profound long-term effects.[24] A range of critical periods in human development which may have particular importance in dertermining health status of individuals and levels of health inequalities within populations are listed below.[24]

- transition from primary to secondary school;
- school examinations;
- entry to labour market;

- leaving parental home;
- establishing own residence;
- transition to parenthood;
- job insecurity, change or loss;
- exit from labour market.

Salutogenic model

Rather than focus attention understanding the nature of disease and its associated risk behaviours, this approach considers the factors responsible for creating and maintaining good health, in other words the origins of health or salutogenesis.[30,31] The model's central construct, sense of coherence, seeks to explain the relationship between life stressors and individuals' and communities' health status. The central hypothesis of the salutogenic model is that stressors are a standard feature of human existence and that individuals and communities with a stronger sense of coherence are better equipped to deal with them and therefore maintain good health and well-being. Researchers have investigated the value of the model in relation to an individual's adjustement to the impacts of chronic diseases, including diabetes, AIDS and arthritis.[32–34] As yet very little research has been undertaken in relation to oral health. Two studies produced conflicting results in relation to patients' coping strategies in response to oral cancer.[35,36] In a more recent study with young people, sense of coherence was identified as a psychosocial determinant of adolescents' patterns of dental attendance.[37]

The salutogenic model has been futher developed recently into a framework that is termed 'a salutogenic setting'.[38] This development focuses attention on identifying and modifying the socio-structural factors that influence the health status of populations. By promoting salutary factors within communities this approach would aim to move the population more towards the health end of the health–disease continuum. Such an approach is very much in line with a whole population strategy.[39] Examples of population salutery factors include levels of education, safe working and housing conditions and supportive public policies. These factors have a positive influence on a range of diverse health outcomes, including oral health.

Social capital

In recent years a great deal of interest and debate within the international public health research community has focused upon the concept of social capital. One of the criticisms of social capital is the lack of clarity over the exact meaning of the concept.[40,41] Within the field of public health, interest in social capital has largely been stimulated by Putnam's work on civic participation and the impact of this on local governance.[42] Putnam defines social capital as 'features of social organisation, such as civic participation, norms of reciprocity, and trust in others, that facilitate co-operation for mutual benefit'.[42] It is essentially assessing the level of social trust that operates within a community, how safe people feel together, how much help people give each other for their own and collective benefit and the degree of involvement in social and community issues, such as voting and participation in community groups. In sociology and devlopment economics the value and relevance of social capital has also been explored, with greater emphasis being placed in these displines on the material and political aspects of the concept.[43,44]

Varying levels of social capital have been used as an explanation for differing life expectancy rates between different countries. Based upon Wilkinson's work on the importance of relative poverty, research has demonstrated a consistent and strong relationship between income distribution and life expectancy in a selection of developed countries.[45–50] In egalitarian countries which have a narrower wealth gap separating the rich from the poor, life expectancy was shown to be much higher than in countries with greater economic inequalities. The research identifies the extent of inequality, or relative poverty as the critical factor determining differences in life expectancy. In the richest countries in the world, but which have a very unequal distribution of wealth, life expectancy was shown to be less than relatively poorer countries with more equitably distributed incomes.[46]

A research group from the Harvard School of Public Health have published results from a study in which data from the US General Social Survey was assessed to measure the relationship between measures of social capital, income inequality and mortality in 39 states across the USA.[49] The results indicated that income inequality was strongly associated with lack of social trust and that states with high levels of social mistrust had higher age-adjusted mortality rates from a range of conditions, including coronary heart disease, maligant neoplasms, cerebrovascular disease, unintentional injury and infant mortality. Kawachi and colleagues concluded that 'the growing gap between the rich and the poor affects the social organisation of communities and that the resulting damage to the social fabric may have profound implications for the public's health'.[49]

The findings of research studies exploring the psychosocial basis of health inequalities based upon the concept of social capital have been challenged by critics who instead stress the available evidence on the importance of absolute poverty and the material and structural basis for health inequalities.[40,41,48]

The findings from studies assessing the relationship between social capital and health are, however, in accordance with previous research which has highlighted the impact of social support and social networks on mortality and morbidity.[51–53]

A recent ecological study in Brazil has assessed the relationship between income inequality, social cohesion and dental caries levels in 12-year old schoolchildren.[54] The study demonstrated that income inequality, expressed by the GINI coefficient, was significantly associated with the percentage of children free of caries and mean DMF. Social cohesion was significantly inversely associated with the percentage of caries-free children.

Implications for oral health promotion

What implications can be drawn from these theoretical approaches for the development of more effective oral health promotion policies and practices? it is certainly very clear that many of the elements in these interesting and challenging theories have some salience to the promotion of oral health. The list below shows the potential implications of these theories for oral health promotion. Although none of these points is new or especially radical in nature, they are supportive of the continuing development of oral health promotion:

- focus of interventions: determinants of oral health;
- strategies adopted: complementary range of actions;
- community empowerment and involvement: active participation of target populations;
- timing of interventions: window of opportunity to maximise health gain;
- partnership working: multidisciplinary collaboration.

The theories reviewed have highlighted the need to focus action on the underlying social, economic and environmental determinants of oral health. It is very apparent that conditions largely determine behaviour and therefore the focus of interventions should be on changing the health-damaging conditions. Actions on improving the environment to create a more health-promoting setting where the healthier choices are the easier choices has enormous potential in oral health promotion. At a local level, oral health input into initiatives such as the Health Promoting School network can produce sustainable improvements in oral health outcomes.[55] Action through advocacy and lobbying is also required at a national and international level to protect and maintain a safe environment.[20]

The limitations of health education in effecting sustained improvements in oral health are even more apparent when one considers the theories reviewed. A comprehensive range of complementary strategies, including healthy public policies, are required to effectively promote oral health and reduce inequalities. The actions outlined in the Ottawa Charter, although first published in the 1980s, are more relevant now than ever.[56] Dental health education programmes alone will have only a marginal impact and can indeed increase oral health inequalities.[57] Policies that provide health, social and welfare support can act as a springboard to assist the most vulnerable groups to achieve their full potential in society.[25]

The active participation of local communities in the development, planning and implementation of interventions is critical. Community development approaches to health promotion in which empowerment, ownership and participation of local people in the projects are central, have not been utilised fully in oral health promotion.[58] Active involvement in local health issues can stimulate a sense of belonging and community spirit and therefore increase social capital within a community.

The importance of timing and identifying 'windows of opportunity' when interventions may have the greatest long-term benefits in promoting oral health and reducing inequalities is an issue that needs to be explored further. Developing and implementing interventions that offer appropriate support at critical periods has enormous potential. For example, supporting mothers and young children with a range of complementary measures should have many longer-term benefits.[10] Oral health promotion interventions which seek to create a health promoting environment in nurseries offer great potential.[59]

Oral health professionals working in isolation are unlikely to achieve sustained long-term improvements in oral health.[4] Working in collaborative partnerships with other relevant professionals and agencies is more likely to produce desired results. Successful collaborative working requires a shared agenda for action in which common risks/health factors are identified.[60]

Conclusion

Oral health promotion as an emerging discipline needs to be based upon appropriate, rigorous, high-quality theory if it is to develop and mature. Within public health, discussion and debate are focusing on the value of new theories and concepts. It is important that oral health promoters engage in an informed debate over the theoretical nature of their work. As Hochbaum and colleagues have stated, 'Any profession that is not based on sound and continuously evolving theories that yield new understanding of its problems and yields new methods, is bound to stagnate and fall behind in the face of changing challenges'.[61]

References

1. Brown, L. (1994) Research in dental health education and health promotion: a review of the literature. *Health Education Quarterly*, 21: 83–102.
2. Schou, L., Locker, D. (1994) *Oral Health: a Review of the Effectiveness of Health Education and Health Promotion*. Amsterdam: Dutch Centre for Health Promotion and Health Education.
3. Kay, L., Locker, D. (1996) Is dental health education effective? A systematic review of current evidence. *Community Dentistry and Oral Epidemiology*, 24: 231–5.
4. Sprod, A., Anderson, R., Treasure, E. (1996) *Effective Oral Health Promotion. Literature Review*. Cardiff: Health Promotion Wales.
5. Kay, L., Locker, D. (1998) *A Systematic Review of the Effectiveness of Health Promotion Aimed at Promoting Oral Health*. London: Health Education Authority.
6. Syme, L. (1986) Strategies for health promotion. *Preventative Medicine*, 15: 492–507.
7. Dahlgren, G., Whitehead, M. (1991) *Policies and Strategies to Promote Social Equity in Health*. Stockholm: Institute of Futures Studies.
8. Marmot, M., Wilkinson, R. (1999) *Social Determinants of Health*. Oxford: Oxford University Press.
9. Ziglio, E., Hagard, S., Griffiths, J. (2000) Health promotion development in Europe: achievements and challenges. *Health Promotion International*, 15: 143–54.
10. Acheson, D. (1998) *Independent Inquiry into Inequalities in Health*. London: Stationery Office.
11. Smedley, B., Syme, L. (2000) *Promoting Health: Intervention Strategies from Social and Behavioral Research*. Washington, DC: Institute of Medicine.
12. World Health Organisation (2000) *Global Strategy for the Prevention and Control of Noncommunicable Diseases*. Geneva: World Health Organisation.
13. Oral health in America (2000) *A Report of the Surgeon General*. Washington, DC: Department of Health and Human Services.
14. Sogaard, A. (1996) Theories and models of health behaviour. In: Schou, L., Blinkhorn, A. (eds), *Oral Health Promotion*. Oxford: Oxford Medical Publications pp. 25–57.
15. McQueen, D. (1996) The search for theory in health behaviour and health promotion. *Health Promotion International*, 11: 27–32.
16. Young, M. (1970) Dental health education – an overview of selected concepts and principles relevant to programme planning. *International Journal of Health Education*, 13: 2–7.
17. Haefner, D. (1974) School dental health programmes. *Health Education Management*, 2: 212–18.
18. Sutton, S. (1998) Predicting and explaining intentions and behaviour: How well are we doing? *Journal of Applied Social Psychology*, 28: 1317–38.
19. Rosenstock, I. (1974) The health belief model and preventive health behaviour. *Health Education Monographs*, 2: 354–86.
20. Hunt, S., Macleod, M. (1987) Health and behavioural change: some lay perspectives. *Community Medicine*, 9: 68–76.
21. Labonte, R. (1999) Health promotion in the near future: remembrances of activism past. *Health Education Journal*, 58: 365–77.
22. Bunton, R., Murphy, S., Bennett, P. (1991) Theories of behavioural change and their use in health promotion: some neglected areas. *Health Education Research*, 6: 153–62.

23. Kuh, D., Ben Shlomo, Y. (eds) (1997) *A Life Course Approach to Adult Disease*. Oxford: Oxford University Press.
24. Bartley, M., Blane, D., Montgomery, S. (1997) Health and the life course: why safety nets matter. *British Medical Journal*, 314: 1194–6.
25. Blane, D. (1999) The life course, the social gradient, and health. In: Marmot, M., Wilkinson, R. (eds), *Social Determinants of Health*. Oxford: Oxford University Press, pp. 64–80.
26. Kuh, D. Wadsworth, M. (1993) Physical health status at 36 years in a British national birth cohort. *Social Science & Medicine*, 37: 905–16.
27. Power, C., Matthews, S., Manor, O. (1998) Inequalities in self rated health: explanations from different stages of life. *Lancet*, 351: 1009–14.
28. Bartley, M., Power, C., Blane, D., Davey Smith, G., Shipley, M. (1994) Birth weight and later socioeconomic disadvantage: evidence from the 1958 British cohort study. *British Medical Journal*, 309: 1475–8.
29. Barker, D. (1994) *Mothers, Babies and Disease in Later Life*. London: British Medical Journal Publishing.
30. Antonovsky, A. (1979) *Health, Stress and Coping*. San Francisco: Jossey-Bass.
31. Antonovsky, A. (1996) The salutogenic model as a theory to guide health promotion. *Health Promotion International*, 11: 11–18.
32. Lundman, B., Norberg, A. (1993) The significance of a sense of coherence for subjective health in persons with insulin-dependent diabetes. *Journal of Advanced Nursing*, 18: 381–6.
33. Linn, J., Monnig, R., Cain, W., Usoh, D. (1993) Stage of illness, level of HIV symptoms, sense of coherence and psychological functioning in clients of community-based AIDS counseling centres. *Journal of Associated Nurses AIDS Care*, 4: 24–32.
34. Buchi, S., Sensky, T., Allard, S., Stoll, T., Schnyder, U. (1998) Sense of coherence: a protective factor for depression in rheumatoid arthritis. *Journal of Rheumatology*, 25: 869–75.
35. Sinclair-Cohen, J. (1993) An investigation into sense of coherence and health locus of control in patients with oral cancer. Masters Thesis. University College London.
36. Langius, A., Bjorvell, H., Lind, M. (1994) Functional staus and coping in patients with oral and pharyngeal cancer before and after surgery. *Head and Neck*, 16: 559–68.
37. Freire, M., Sheiham, A., Hardy, R. (2001) Adolescents' sense of coherence, oral health status and oral health-related behaviours. *Community Dentistry and Oral Epidemiology*, 29: 204–12.
38. Frohlich, K., Potvin, L. (1999) Health promotion through the lens of population health: toward a salutogenic setting. *Critical Public Health*, 9: 211–22.
39. Rose, G. (1992) *The Strategy of Preventive Medicine*. Oxford: Oxford University Press.
40. Lynch, J., Due, P., Muntaner, C., Davey Smith, G. (2000) Social capital – is it a good investment strategy for public health? *Journal of Epidemiology and Community Health*, 54: 404–8.
41. Muntaner, C., Lynch, J., Davey Smith, G. (2000) Social capital and the third way in public health. *Critical Public Health*, 10: 107–24.
42. Putnam, R. (1993) *Making Democracy Work*. Princeton, NJ: Princeton University Press.
43. Portes, A. (1998) Social capital: its origins and applications in modern sociology. *Annual Review of Sociology*, 29: 1–24.
44. Woolcock, M. (1998) Social capital and economic development: Toward a theoretical synthesis and policy framework. *Theory and Society*, 27: 151–208.
45. Wilkinson, R. (1992) Income distribution and life expectancy. *British Medical Journal*, 304: 165–8.
46. Wilkinson, R. (1996) *Unhealthy Societies: the Afflictions on Inequality*. London: Routledge.
47. Kaplan, G., Pamuk, E., Lynch, J., Cohen, R., Balfour, J. (1996) Inequality in income and mortality in the United States: analysis of mortality and potential pathways. *British Medical Journal*, 312: 999–1003.
48. Muntaner, C., Lynch, J. (1998) Income inequality and social coherence versus class relations: a critique of Wilkinson's neo-Durkheimian research program. *International Journal of Health Services*, 24: 59–81.

49. Kawachi, I., Kennedy, B., Lochner, K., Prothrow-Stith, D. (1997) Social capital, income inequality and mortality. *American Journal of Public Health*, 87: 1491–8.

50. Kennedy, B., Kawachi, I., Prothrow-Stith, D. (1996) Income distribution and mortality: cross sectional ecological study of the Robin Hood index in the United States. *British Medical Journal*, 312: 1004–7.

51. Berkman, L., Syme, S. (1979) Social networks, host resistance and mortality: a nine-year follow-up study of Alameda County residents. *American Journal of Epidemiology*, 109: 186–203.

52. Reynolds, P., Kaplan, G. (1990) Social connections and risk for cancer: prospective evidence from the Alameda County study. *Behavioral Medicine*, 16: 101–10.

53. Stansfeld, S. (1999) Social support and social cohesion. In: Marmot, M. Wilkinson, R. (eds), *Social Determinants of Health*. Oxford: Oxford University Press, pp. 155–78.

54. Pattuss, M.P., Marcenes, W., Croucher, R. and Sheiham, A. (2001) Social deprivation, income inequality, social cohesion and dental caries in Brazilian school children, *Social Science and Medicine*, 53 (7): 915–25.

55. Moyses, S. (2000) The impact of health promotion policies in schools on oral health in Curitiba, Brasil. PhD Thesis. University College London.

56. World Health Organisation (1986) *The Ottawa Charter for Health Promotion: Health Promotion 1*: i–v. Geneva: World Health Organisation.

57. Schou, L., Wight, C. (1994) Does dental health education affect inequalities in dental health? *Community Dentistry & Health*, 11: 97–100.

58. Watt, R., Sheiham, A. (1999) Inequalities in oral health: a review of the evidence and recommendations for action. *British Dentistry Journal*, 187: 2–8.

59. Watt, R. (1999) *Oral & Health Promotion: a Guide to Effective Working in Pre-School Settings*. London: Health Education Authority.

60. Sheiham, A., Watt, R. (2000) The common risk factor approach – a rational basis for promoting oral health. *Community Dentistry and Oral Epidemiology*, 28: 399–406.

61. Hochbaum, G., Sorenson, S., James, R., Lorig, K. (1992) Theory in health education practice. *Health Education Quarterly*, 19: 295–313.

Chapter 7

Towards a Politics of Health

Clare Bambra, Debbie Fox and Alex Scott-Samuel[1]

Introduction

It is profoundly paradoxical that, in a period when the importance of public policy as a determinant of health is routinely acknowledged, there remains a continuing absence of mainstream debate about the ways in which the politics, power and ideology, which underpin it influence people's health. For a rare example see Navarro and Shi (2001). While to some extent the unhealthy policies of the Reagan and Thatcher governments of 20 years ago acted as a stimulus to such debate, as early as the mid-1980s, the introduction of the World Health Organization's Health For All strategy (World Health Organization, 1985) created the illusion that these issues had finally – and adequately – been acknowledged. Experience since then suggests that such views can and very clearly should be challenged.

In this chapter we argue that health, and its promotion, are profoundly political. We explore the possible reasons behind the absence of a 'politics of health' in mainstream debate and demonstrate how an awareness of the political nature of health will lead to a more effective health promotion strategy and more evidence-based health promotion practice.

The political nature of health

It is time that the implicit, and sometimes explicit but unstated, politics within and surrounding health were more widely acknowledged. Health, like almost all other aspects of human life, is political in numerous ways:

- Health is political because, like any other resource or commodity under a neo-liberal economic system, some social groups have more of it than others.
- Health is political because its social determinants are amenable to political interventions and are thereby dependent on political action (or more usually, inaction).

Edited from: Bambra, C., Fox, D. and Scott-Samuel, A. (2005) Towards a politics of health, *Health Promotion International*, 20 (2): 187–93. By permission of Oxford University Press.

- Health is political because the right to 'a standard of living adequate for health and well-being' (United Nations, 1948) is, or should be, an aspect of citizenship and a human right.

Ultimately, health is political because power is exercised over it as part of a wider economic, social and political system. Changing this system requires political awareness and political struggle.

Health inequalities

Evidence that the most powerful determinants of health in modern populations are social, economic and cultural (Doyal and Pennell, 1979; Townsend and Davidson, 1992; Whitehead, 1992; Blane et al., 1996; Acheson, 1998) comes from a wide range of sources and is also, to some extent, acknowledged by governments and international agencies (Townsend and Davidson, 1992; Acheson, 1998; Department of Health, 1998; Social Exclusion Unit, 1998). Yet inequalities in health continue, within countries (on the basis of socio-economic class, gender or ethnicity) and between them (in terms of wealth and resources) (Davey Smith et al., 2002; Donkn et al., 2002).

How these inequalities in health are approached by society is highly political: are health inequalities to be accepted as 'natural' and inevitable results of individual differences both in respect of genetics and the silent hand of the economic market, or are they social and economic abhorrences that need to be tackled by a modern state and a humane society (Adams et al., 2002)? Underpinning these different approaches to health inequalities are not only divergent views of what is scientifically or economically possible, but also differing political and ideological opinions about what is desirable.

Health determinants

Causes of, and genetic predispositions to ill-health are becoming increasingly well understood. However, it is evident that in most cases, environmental triggers are equally if not more important and that the major determinants of health or ill-health are inextricably linked to social and economic context (Acheson, 1998; Marmot and Wilkinson, 2001). Factors such as housing, income and employment – indeed many of the issues that dominate political life – are key determinants of our health and well-being. Similarly, many of the major determinants of health inequalities lie outside the health sector and therefore require non-health sector policies to tackle them (Townsend and Davidson, 1992; Acheson, 1998; Whitehead et al., 2000). Recent acknowledgements of the importance of the social determinants of health are welcome but fail to seriously address the underlying political determinants of health and health inequity.

Citizenship

Citizenship is 'a status bestowed on those who are full members of a community. All who possess the status are equal with respect to the rights and duties with which the status is endowed' (Marshall, 1963). There are three types of citizenship rights: civil, political and social. Health, or the 'right to a standard of living adequate for health and well-being' (United Nations, 1948; International Forum for the Defense of the Health of People, 2002), is an important social citizenship right. These citizenship rights were only gained as a result of extensive political and social struggle during Western industrialization and the development of capitalism (Marshall, 1963). However, despite their parallel development, the relationship between capitalism and citizenship is not an easy or 'natural' one (Marshall, 1963). Health is a strong example of this tense relationship as under a capitalist economic system health is, like everything else, commodified. Commodification is 'the process whereby everything becomes identifiable and valued according to its relative desirability within the economic market (of production and consumption)' (de Viggiani, 1997). Health became extensively commodified during the industrial revolution as workers became entirely dependent upon the market for their survival (Esping-Andersen, 1990). In the 20th century, the introduction of social citizenship, which entailed an entitlement to health and social welfare, brought about a 'loosening' of the pure commodity status of health. The welfare state decommodified health because certain health services and a certain standard of living became a right of citizenship.

In short, capitalism and citizenship represent very different values: the former, inequality and the latter, equality. This tension means that the implementation of the right to health, despite its position in social citizenship and in the UN Universal Declaration of Human Rights, will for the foreseeable future require continuing political struggle.

Why has health been apolitical?

It is perhaps puzzling that despite its evident political nature, the politics of health has been underdeveloped and marginalized: it has not been widely considered or discussed as a political entity within academic debates or, more importantly, broader societal ones. There is no simple explanation for this omission; the treatment of health as apolitical is almost certainly the result of a complex interaction of issues. We describe some of these below, though we would not claim that our list is exhaustive.

Health = health care

Health is often reduced and misrepresented as health care (or, in the UK, as the National Health Service). Consequently, the politics of health becomes significantly misconstructed as the politics of health care – see for example Freeman (Freeman, 2000). As an illustration, the majority of popular UK political discussions about health concern issues such as the 'state or the market?' debate about National Health Service (NHS) funding, organization and delivery, or the demographic pressures on the future provision of health-care facilities (Rhodes, 1997). The same applies in most other – especially 'developed' – countries.

The limited, one-dimensional (Carpenter, 1980) nature of this political discourse surrounding health can be traced back to two ideological issues: the definition of health and the definition of politics. The definition of health that has conventionally been operationalized under Western capitalism has two interrelated aspects to it: health is both considered as the absence of disease (biomedical definition) and as a commodity (economic definition). These both focus on individuals, as opposed to society, as the basis of health: health is seen as a product of individual factors such as genetic heritage or lifestyle choices, and as a commodity that individuals can access either via the market or the health system

(Scott-Samuel, 1979). This remains the case despite our sophisticated understanding of health promotion – as is evident if one ignores the rhetoric of the governments of 'developed' nations and looks instead at their health policies.

Health in this sense is an individualized commodity that is produced and delivered by the market or the health service. Inequalities in the distribution of health are therefore either a result of the failings of individuals through, for example, their lifestyle choices; or of the way in which health care products are produced, distributed and delivered. In order to tackle these inequalities, political attention is directed towards the variable that is most amenable to manipulation – the health-care system.

It is important to note that this limiting, one-dimensional view of health is common across the ideological spectrum, with left-wing versus right-wing health debates usually consisting of a more versus less state intervention dichotomy. Orthodox UK left-wing politics is guilty of placing health care and the NHS at the centre of its discussions and struggles about health. This 'NHS illusion' has resulted in the naive perspective among health activists that societal ill-health can be cured by more and better NHS services. At best, this perspective is slowly changing, as is shown by the enthusiasm of some in the UK for New Labour's emphasis on tackling health inequalities through the NHS – while it simultaneously widens them through its neo-liberal macroeconomic, trade and foreign policies (Bambra et al., 2003).

Health and politics

Figure 7.1 outlines four broad definitions of politics. The first concept, which is the most prevalent definition within mainstream political discourse, places very restrictive boundaries around what politics is – the activities of governments, elites and state agencies – and therefore also restricts who is political and who can engage in politics (i.e. the members of governments, state agencies and other elite organizations). It is a 'top-down' approach that essentially separates politics from the community. This should be contrasted with the last definition, which offers a much more encompassing view of politics: politics is everything; it is a term that can be used to describe any 'power-structured relationship' (Millett, 1969). This is a 'bottom-up' approach as any and every issue is political and likewise anyone and everyone can engage in a political act.

The dominance of the first conceptualization of politics, as the art of government and the activities of the state, influences which aspects of health are considered to be political. Health care, especially in countries like the UK where the state's role is significant, is an immediate subject for political discussion. Other aspects of health, such as health inequalities or health and citizenship, are excluded from this narrow popular definition of politics and are thereby seen as non-political. In order to increase which aspects of health are regarded as political, our understanding of politics needs to be contested and redefined.

Responsibility and authority

The conceptualization of health as non-political is also in part due to medicalization – the transfer of power over and responsibility for health from individuals, the public and therefore political life, to powerful elites, namely the medical and health professions and the multinational pharmaceutical companies.

The definition of politics is in itself a political act (Leftwich, 1984). This is evident in the divergent conceptualizations of the political that are utilized both by different political ideologies (Heywood, 2000) and schools of thought in political science (Marsh and Stoker, 2002):

- *Politics as government* – Politics is primarily associated with the art of government and the activities of the state. Associated with Behaviouralist and Institutionalist political science.
- *Politics as public life* – Politics is primarily concerned with the conduct and management of community affairs. Associated with Rational Choice Theory.
- *Politics as conflict resolution* – Politics is concerned with the expression and resolution of conflicts through compromise, conciliation, negotiation and other strategies. Associated with International Relations theorists.
- *Politics as power* – Politics is the process through which desired outcomes are achieved in the production, distribution and use of scarce resources in all areas of social existence. Associated with Feminist and Marxist political science.

Figure 7.1   Definitions of politics

When we conceive of ill-health as episodes of disease manageable by the delivery of healthcare, we are ... transferring the responsibility for health from society as a whole to an elite possessing what we define as the necessary professional and technical expertise for the management of disease. (Scott-Samuel, 1979)

However, unlike the impression given in the above quote, this transfer of responsibility is not always voluntary. Drug companies and the medical profession have taken the power and responsibility for health for themselves (Illich, 1977). They have thus been able to determine what health is and, therefore, how political it is (or, more usually, is not).

Their historic power over the definition and management of health has contributed substantially to its depoliticization: health is something that doctors are responsible for, they are the providers, and we are the recipients. Their authority and responsibility over health has further emphasized its commodity status – when ill, an individual visits a doctor and/or purchases drugs (commodity) to regain health (another, albeit less obvious commodity). Ill-health is a transient state caused by the presence of disease. It can be ended by the appropriate application of medical technology. This depoliticization of health, via the transfer of power and responsibility to these professional and/or commercial groups, means that we do not acknowledge our power over our own health or our autonomy over our own bodies.

Health policy

Health policy, as currently popularly conceptualized, is usually synonymous with policy content. Certainly, it is relatively unusual to find discussions of health policy that are not focused on the pros and cons of particular courses of action in relation to particular political parties. In reality, however, health policy is part of a broader public policy agenda, whose practical aspects are inextricably linked with power and politics. Given this, the reduction of 'health policy' to 'the content of health policies' diverts attention from, and renders invisible the political nature of the policy process. Policy is formulated within certain preset political parameters, which define what is, and what is not, possible or acceptable. For example, the fundamental requirement within Western neo-liberal economies for inequality (between those who labour and those who profit) makes the meaning of UK government policies to 'tackle inequalities' at best highly questionable – no modern government will support a policy process that permits the full implementation of radical equity policy. Government policy in this area therefore consists of (loudly trumpeted) minor reform; no policy connections are ever made with the macro-political causes of the major economic, social and health inequalities, such as macroeconomic policy, trade policy, defence policy, foreign policy and international development. For example, none of these featured in the UK Treasury's Cross Cutting Spending Review on Health Inequalities (HM Treasury and Department of Health, 2002), which was intended to examine the impact on health inequalities of the expenditure programmes of all government departments. Nor are the actions of the World Trade Organization, of trans-national corporations, or of the World Bank usually taken into account. One conclusion regarding this failure to see the wood for the trees is that there is an important need for awareness of how the political context limits how health policy is formulated. Another is that this failure does not occur by chance: both the masking of the political nature of health, and the forms of the social structures and processes that create, maintain and undermine health, are determined by the individuals and groups that wield the greatest political power.

Towards a politics of health

What this all adds up to is nothing less than a challenge to a wide range of actors – health promotion and public health specialists, policy makers, politicians, health and political scientists – to emerge from the closet and to begin the long-overdue task of elaborating the practice, policy and theory of a newly identified discipline – health politics, the political science of health. We believe that we have more than adequately justified the need for health politics to emerge as a discipline and field of practice no less important than medical sociology or health economics on the one hand, or than political sociology or political psychology on the other. We are confident that the practice of health promotion and public health will gain immeasurably from the explicit recognition of this key determinant of health and its incorporation into evidence-based strategies, policies and interventions.

Note

1. Clare Bambra works in the Centre for Public Policy and Health, University of Durham. Debbie Fox and Alex Scott-Samuel both work in the Division of Public Health, University of Liverpool.

References

Acheson, D. (Chairman) (1998) *Independent Inquiry into Inequalities in Health*. The Stationery Office, London.

Adams, L., Amos, M. and Munro, J. (eds) (2002) *Promoting Health: Politics and Practice*. Sage, London.

Bambra, C., Fox, D. and Scott-Samuel, A. (2003) *A New Politics of Health*. Politics of Health Group, Liverpool http://www.liv.ac.uk/PublicHealth/Publications/publications01.html (last accessed 7 August 2004).

Blane, D., Brunner, E. and Wilkinson, R. (eds) (1996) *Health and Social Organization: Towards a Health Policy for the Twenty-First Century*. Routledge, London.

Carpenter, M. (1980) Left orthodoxy and the politics of health. *Capital and Class*, 11: 73–98.

Davey Smith, G., Dorling, D., Mitchell, R. and Shaw, M.(2002) Health inequalities in Britain: continuing increases up to the end of the 20th century. *Journal of Epidemiology and Community Health*, 56: 434–435.

Department of Health (1998) *Saving Lives: Our Healthier Nation*. The Stationery Office, London.

de Viggiani, N. (1997) *A basis for health promotion*. Southbank University, London.

Donkn, A., Goldblatt, P. and Lynch, K. (2002) Inequalities in life expectancy by social class 1977–1999. *Health Statistics Quarterly*, 15: 5–15.

Doyal, L. and Pennell, I. (1979) *The Political Economy of Health*. Pluto Press, London.

Esping-Andersen, G. (1990) *The Three Worlds of Welfare Capitalism*. Polity Press, Cambridge.

Freeman, R. (2000) *The Politics of Health in Europe*. University of Manchester Press, Manchester.

Heywood, A. (2000) *Key Concepts in Politics*. Macmillan, London.

HM Treasury and Department of Health (2002) *Tackling Health Inequalities: Summary of the 2002 Cross-cutting Review*. Department of Health Publications, London.

Illich, I. (1977) *Limits to Medicine*. Penguin, Harmondsworth, UK.

International Forum for the Defense of the Health of People (2002) Health as an essential human need, a right of citizenship, and a public good: health for all is possible and necessary. *International Journal of Health Sevices*, 32: 601–606.

Leftwich, A. (1984) *What is Politics? The Activity and its Study*. Blackwell, Oxford.

Marmot, M. and Wilkinson, R. (2001) Psychosocial and material pathways in the relation between income and health: a response to Lynch et al. *British Medical Journal*, 322: 1233–1236.

Marsh, D. and Stoker, G. (eds) (2002) *Theory and Methods in Political Science*. Palgrave Macmillan, Basingstoke, UK.

Marshall, T.H. (1963) *Sociology at the Crossroads*. Hutchinson, London. See also Marsh, D. and Stoker, G. (eds) (2002) *Theory and Methods in Political Science*. Palgrave Macmillan, Basingstoke, UK.

Millett, K. (1969) *Sexual Politics*. Virago, London.

Navarro, V. and Shi, L. (2001) The political context of social inequalities and health. *International Journal of Health Services*, 31: 1–21.

Rhodes, M. (1997) The welfare state: internal challenges, external constraints. In Rhodes, M., Heywood, P. and Wright, V. (eds), *Developments in West European Politics*. Palgrave Macmillan, London.

Scott-Samuel, A. (1979) The politics of health. *Community Medicine*, 1: 123–126.

Social Exclusion Unit (1998) *Bringing Britain Together: A National Strategy for Neighbourhood Renewal*. Cabinet Office, London.

Townsend, P. and Davidson, N. (1992) The Black Report. In Townsend, P. and Davidson, N. (eds), *Inequalities in Health*. Penguin, London.

United Nations (1948) *Universal Declaration of Human Rights*. General Assembly Resolution 217A (III), UN Doc. A/810 at 71. United Nations, New York.

Whitehead, M. (1992) The health divide. In Townsend, P. and Davidson, N. (eds), *Inequalities in Health*. Penguin, London.

Whitehead, M., Diderichsen, F. and Burstrom, B. (2000) Researching the impact of public policy on inequalities in health. In Graham, H. (ed.), *Understanding Health Inequalities*. Open University Press, Buckingham.

World Health Organization (1985) *Targets for Health For All*. WHO Regional Office for Europe, Copenhagen.

Part II
Deconstructing and Reconstructing Public Health

Introduction

Sarah Earle

As some of the chapters in Part I of this Reader have shown, modern multi-disciplinary public health is constantly evolving in that it has been, and continues to be, shaped by the tensions and conflicts between health promotion and public health. As such, multidisciplinary public health embraces a vast range of ever-changing policy and practice, which includes a diversity of initiatives involving different people, at different levels, and in a whole range of settings. Historically, health has been equated with health care but it is now increasingly recognised that this is not so and that successful efforts to promote public health must adopt a multidisciplinary approach. In Part II of the Reader, the chapters explore an eclectic range of cutting-edge issues which serve to deconstruct and reconstruct public health in the 21st century.

Chapter 8 focuses on substance use and harm minimisation in nightclubs. In this chapter Mark Bellis, Karen Hughes and Helen Lowey argue that, in order to protect young people's health, strategies must necessarily focus on reducing harm, while taking good care not to minimise all the fun. They adopt a healthy settings approach to club health, suggesting that the risk to health posed by substance use is related to the nightlife environment in which they are used. Thus, they argue that at both national and international levels, a healthy settings approach to nightclubs allows environmental issues and substance use to be tackled effectively together.

In Chapter 9, Sue Spurr presents an interesting personal account of her journey into yoga, exploring the relationship between yoga and modern multidisciplinary public health. She begins by contextualising yoga within the increasing popularity of complementary and alternative medicine (CAM), drawing on her own experiences and the experiences of those with whom she practises yoga. Following on from this, Sue Spurr reflects on some of the themes developed in Part I, and considers whether participating in yoga (or other CAMs) reflects an ethos of individual responsibility for health within an increasingly consumer-driven health market. In this chapter Sue Spurr also considers issues of difference and diversity, and questions whether such a choice is equally available to all.

In Chapter 10, disability activist Bill Albert explores the relationship between disability rights, genetics and public health. Like other disability activists and writers, Bill Albert believes that the science of genetics is little more than a modern form of eugenics that determines who will, or will not, be born. He notes that since the 19th century, the core goal of public health has been the prevention of disease and the promotion of good health. Modern public health, he argues, perpetuates these ideals while concealing a more sinister desire. He concludes by asserting that modern approaches to reproductive choice – in particular the practice of prenatal screening – are little more than a convenient mantra for eugenic policies to limit the births of disabled children.

Controversially, in Chapter 11, Sarah Earle and Keith Sharp argue against the disability rights perspective, in defence of a woman's 'right to choose'. They point out that although disability activists are correct to be concerned by the geneticisation of everyday life, only a very tiny proportion of abortions are actually carried out under Section 1(1)(d) of the 1967 Abortion Act, which permits abortion after 24 weeks of gestation in the case of severe foetal abnormality. While expressing some sympathy for the disability rights perspective, Sarah Earle and Keith Sharp draw on feminist politics to show that assuring women's full participation in society requires respect for their physical autonomy. They argue that aborting a foetus on the grounds of impairment does not mean that the lives of disabled people are any less valuable than those of non-disabled people but, simply, that a woman should have the right to choose whether to carry, bear and nurture a child, or not.

In Chapter 12, Stephen Handsley and Carol Komaromy consider the threat of contagion to public health by exploring media accounts of disasters, in particular the hurricane that devastated New Orleans, Louisiana in 2005. In this chapter, they cogently argue that while the sight of mass death instils horror and provokes a fear of contagion, the greatest threat to the public health arises not from the infectious contamination of putrefying flesh but from the culturally insensitive and disrespectful treatment of dead bodies. They argue that whereas the actual risk of contagion from dead bodies is comparatively low, the sight and disposal of the dead is a symbolic contamination of life itself.

Lastly, and in their second of two contributions to this Reader, Sarah Earle and Keith Sharp examine the relationship between sex work and the public health. By exploring the regulation of sexuality, they argue that it is the female sex worker who has been the most visible within lay, medical, legal and religious discourses and that it is she who, subsequently, has been the greatest focus of public health intervention. In Chapter 13 Sarah Earle and Keith Sharp argue that while female sex workers have taken centre-stage, the men who pay for sex have been, until quite recently, curiously absent from public health research, policy and practice. Like Stephen Handsley and Carol Komaromy, this chapter explores perceptions of contagion and the way in which the bodies of female sex workers have been positioned as contagious to the men who pay for sex. This chapter considers the methodological problems of bringing these invisible men into view to enable more effective safe sex promotion.

Chapter 8

Healthy Nightclubs and Recreational Substance Use: From a Harm Minimisation to a Healthy Settings Approach

Mark A. Bellis, Karen Hughes and Helen Lowey

1. Introduction

In the UK alone, approximately 3.5 million individuals go to nightclubs each week (Mintel International Group, 2000). Most of these are younger people and a large proportion of them consume illegal drugs often in combination with alcohol (Measham et al., 2001). The relationship between recreational drug use and dance music events is now well established (Release, 1997; Winstock et al., 2001). In the UK, for instance, estimates of ecstasy, amphetamine, and cocaine use in regular clubbers (i.e. attendees at nightclubs) or those travelling abroad to visit international nightclub resorts (e.g. Ibiza) far exceed average levels of consumption by individuals in the general population (Bellis et al., 2000) (Table 8.1).

The acute and long-term problems relating to *recreational* (i.e. ecstasy, amphetamine, and cocaine) drug use are the subject of a wide range of studies (Parrott et al., 2001; Reneman et al., 2001) and form the rationale for a variety of health interventions (Niesnk et al., 2000; Page, 2000). Thus, ecstasy use has been linked to short-term health effects such as hyperthermia (Henry et al., 1992) as well as long-term effects such as memory problems (Reneman et al., 2001). Interventions addressing recreational drug use have often been outreach based (Crew 2000, 2001) and focused on disseminating information on adverse effects of drugs and how to avoid them, problems around combining substances (often drugs and alcohol), and courses of action necessary when acute adverse effects are experienced. However, there is now a growing recognition that the adverse effects of club drugs

Edited from: Bellis, M.A., Hughes, K. and Lowey, H. (2002) Healthy nightclubs and recreational substance use: from a harm minimisation to a healthy settings approach, *Addictive Behaviors*, 27: 1025–35.

Table 8.1   Levels of drug use in three UK surveys

	British Crime Survey[a] (%)	Ibiza Uncovered Survey[b] (%)	Dancing on Drugs Survey[c] (%)
Cannabis	22	51	69.5
Ecstasy	5	39	51.4
Amphetamine	5	27	53.5
Cocaine	5	26	27.1

[a]16–29 year-olds in the general population; drugs used in last 12 months (Ramsay et al., 2001).
[b]16–29 year-olds who visited Ibiza during Summer 2000; drugs used in last 6 months (Bellis et al., 2000).
[c]15–57 year-olds attending dance events; drugs used in last 3 months (Measham et al., 2001).

are strongly related to the environment in which they are used rather than resulting solely from the toxic properties of substances themselves (Calafat et al., 2001). Often, reports of ecstasy-related deaths refer to the temperature of the environment – the most likely cause of death is heatstroke; the temperature inside the club had reached 40°C (Burke, 2001) – or in other instances the lack of basic facilities to redress the effects of dancing and substance use – a number of people complained about lack of water (Bowcott, 2001).

   In this chapter, we argue that the relationship between the health effects of substance use and the environment in which they are used is much wider than temperature control and access to water, and extends across the entire nightlife setting. We explore the wide range of factors that contribute to risk in night-time environments and describe initiatives that effectively address these issues without curtailing fun. Consequently, we argue that by adopting a broad settings approach (World Health Organisation, 1997) to nightclubs, inclusive solutions to reducing harm in clubs (including that caused by drugs) can be better developed and disseminated. Furthermore, the same approach can also facilitate multidisciplinary involvement in nightlife health, taking health issues solely from health departments and placing the responsibility also in the hands of organisations such as local authorities, police, voluntary organisations, club owners and managers, door staff, and clubbers themselves. Finally, we suggest that with worldwide growth in dance music tourism, this multidisciplinary approach needs to be extended to include travel and tourism organisations and requires collaboration on an international level.

2. Healthy settings and nightclubs

A healthy settings approach (World Health Organisation, 1997) recognises that the effects of any particular setting on an individual's health are related to the general conditions within that setting, perhaps more than they are to provision of health or other care facilities. The nightclub setting at its most basic is a building that provides loud music, often with a repetitive beat, a dance area that usually has low background light and intermittent bright lighting effects and a licensed bar. Developing this environment as a healthy setting must recognise that large numbers of clubbers regularly consume substances such as alcohol, drugs, and tobacco (often in combination) and consequently experience a variety of psychological and physiological effects. Furthermore, the criminal nature of some drug use and environmental factors such as poor ventilation mean substance consumption can directly affect staff, for example, pressure on door staff to allow drugs into clubs (Morris, 1998) and passive smoking affecting bar staff, respectively (Jones et al., 2001).

Some settings approaches to club health are well established. Harm minimisation messages advising sipping water, avoiding mixing alcohol with ecstasy, and taking periods of rest provide the essential information for individuals to protect their health (London Drug Policy Forum, 1996). However, without cool areas within the club, often referred to as chill out areas (London Drug Policy Forum, 1996) and access to free cold water, such advice cannot be implemented. Equally, when adverse reactions to drugs are experienced, a separate appropriately stocked first-aid room, trained staff, and access for emergency services are all required to allow the best chance of recovery. However, other often more deleterious effects on health are also related to nightlife and substance use. In the UK in 1999, 19 per cent of all violent acts ($n = 3,246,000$) occurred outside a pub or club. Overall, 40 per cent of violent incidents were related to alcohol use and 18 per cent to drugs (Kershaw et al., 2000). The paraphernalia of alcohol use also contributes to harm, with 5,000 people being attacked with pint glasses every year, of whom many are scarred for life (Deehan, 1999). Thus, both the promotion of aggression by, for instance, alcohol (Institute of Alcohol Studies, 2001) and the paraphernalia of substance use play parts in the harm caused by violence.

Less frequently addressed issues, which are important to a settings approach to club health, include the risk of smoking and in particular fire, large amounts of electrical equipment, the use of old converted premises, low lighting, and a high proportion of smokers (Measham et al., 2001) all contribute to making nightclubs high-risk environments. Additionally, substance use can mean that patrons can be disorientated, leading to further implications, particularly if an emergency evacuation of the building is required. A healthy setting should promote well marked fire exits (some have been known to be camouflaged to fit in with club décor), crowd control training (Newcombe, 1994), and strict compliance with fire limits on the building's capacity (Ministry of Health, 1999). The effects of fires in clubs can be horrific, as graphically illustrated by the loss of life associated with recent incidents (BBC News, 2000; CNN, 2000; The Guardian, 2001). However, the effects of smoking alone may also be significant. Dancing while holding a cigarette can result in damage to eyes of those nearby (Luke, 1999), while non-smoking bar staff are subject to heavy exposure to environmental tobacco smoke while at work (Jarvis et al.,1992).

Noise levels in clubs can also pose a substantial risk to health. UK guidance on protection at work suggests earplugs are used when levels regularly exceed 90 dB (Health and Safety Executive, 1999). However, noise levels in many nightclubs reach 120 dB (Royal National Institute for Deaf People, 1999) and at some points noise can approach the pain threshold (140 dB) (Walsh, 2000). However, those utilising the night-time environment in conjunction with substance use, distracts from concerns about health effects and in the case of some drugs (e.g. ketamine or cocaine) may even anaesthetise the user against pain (European Monitoring Centre for Drugs and Drug Addiction, 2000). As increasing numbers of young people are exposed to loud music in dance clubs, it would be expected that more young people would develop hearing problems. In fact, a survey by the Medical Research Council Institute of Hearing Research found that 66 per cent of club goers reported temporary hearing problems after attending a nightclub (Smith and Davis, 1999). Policies about maximum noise levels in clubs can address some of these issues. However, noise is not just a concern within the club but may also affect the surrounding environment, either through loud music contaminating nearby residential areas or through the noise of inebriated clubbers appearing on the street when clubs finally close (BBC Devon News, 2001). Such noise may also be associated with violence (often related to alcohol and drug use), lack of appropriate access to public transport (leaving long waits or drink/drug driving as the only alternatives), and difficulties in co-ordinating an adequate police presence when clubs close (Calafat et al., 2001).

Furthermore, any comprehensive approach to a healthy club setting should recognise the close relationship between substance use and sexual health. A variety of studies identify the relaxation of safe sex measures (particularly condom use) associated with alcohol and drug-taking (e.g. Poulin and Graham, 2001). One study has identified individuals using drugs, particularly GHB, specifically in order to temporarily forget safe sex messages they have previously heard (Clark et al., 2001). Addressing such issues means providing safe sex information within the club setting and combining this with easy access to condoms. Fire, noise, sex, and other areas for health promotion and protection in the night-time environment as well as their relationship with substance use are summarised in Table 8.2

3. Disseminating knowledge and developing solutions

The use of substances often contributes to the dangers presented within the night-time environment. Previously, harm minimisation has tended to focus on direct effects of drug use. However, basic measures to alter the environment can substantially reduce substance-related harm. Measures to reduce violence in and around clubs include training and registration of door staff, good lighting around the main entrance, and public transport integrated into the night-time environment so that individuals can quickly and easily leave city centres (Calafat et al., 2001; London Drug Policy Forum, 1996). Specific measures to reduce spillage of bottles from bars and clubs onto streets can also reduce the risk of glass-related injuries (The Kirklees Partnership, 1999). Inside, club design should anticipate and acknowledge the exuberant behaviour and intoxicated state of patrons by restricting access to any areas where falls are likely and ensuring exits are well lit and distinctive (London Drug Policy Forum, 1996).

Importantly, the process of tackling harm reduction across the entire nightlife setting legitimises the inclusion of a wide variety of organisations and individuals who may have felt that they could not engage in dialogue solely on a drug use agenda. These groups may include club and bar owners, club goers and club staff, event promoters, local authorities and politicians, environmental health officials, and travel and tour operators as well as youth services, health services, police, and other emergency services. Furthermore, sometimes, this mix of individuals produces novel solutions. For example, to reduce night crime and increase public safety, the owners of a number of neighbouring venues have supported the employment of a uniformed police officer dedicated to patrolling outside their premises (Greater Manchester Police, 2001). Also, in North Devon, a police initiative involved handing out free lollipops as clubbers left nightclubs in order to reduce noise in the surrounding areas (BBC Devon News, 2001).

Table 8.2   Some wider club health issues, their relationship with substance use, and developing a setting response

Health risk	Relationship to substance use	Setting response	Groups involved
Dehydration and hyperthermia	Ecstasy alters thermoregulation (McCann et al., 1996) Increased energetic dancing Alcohol consumption causes dehydration	Prevent overcrowding Well ventilation and temperature control Cool and quieter *chill outs* areas or ability to leave and re-enter Access to cool, free water Information on effects of taking drugs Pill testing First-aid room and staff training	Club owners/staff Drug outreach workers Health promotion groups Licensing authority Club goers Local A&E
Fire	High levels of smoking among club goers Intoxication leads to disorientation when exiting clubs Flammable clubbing clothes (e.g. PVC)	Prevent overcrowding High visibility and accessible emergency exits Availability and maintenance of all fire equipment Ensure electrical equipment is safe Encourage use of non-combustible material	Club owners/staff Fire authorities Building inspectors Licensing authority Club goers
Damage to hearing	Alcohol and drugs reduce awareness of potential hearing damage Greater exposure to noise due to prolonged dancing	Set maximum levels on systems Restricted areas around speakers Make earplugs available Information on the effects of excessive noise Information on signs of hearing damage	Club owners/staff Club goers Environmental inspectors Licensing authority Health promotion Club goers
STIs and unwanted pregnancies	Alcohol and drugs reduce inhibitions (Calafat et al., 2001) Substances help forget safe sex message (Clark et al., 2001)	Easy availability of condoms Information on safer sex	Health promotion Public health department Contraception services Club owners Club goers
Accident Glass Burns Falls General	Disorientation Anaesthetising effect of substances (European Monitoring Centre for Drugs and Drug Addiction, 2000)	Toughened glass or plastic bottles No drinking/smoking on dance floor Provide places to dispose of cigarettes	Club owners/staff Public health departments Health promotion groups Licensing authority Club goers

(Continued)

Table 8.2   (Continued)

Health risk	Relationship to substance use	Setting response	Groups involved
	Lack of fear and increased confidence Increased risk-taking	Well-lit and clear stairwells Restricted access to potentially dangerous areas Secure fixtures and fittings On-site first-aid	
Violence	Alcohol and drugs increase aggression Drug dealing (Morris, 1998) Steroid and cocaine use by door staff (Lenehan and McVeigh, 1998) Increased risk-taking, lower inhibitions	Stagger closing times Increase public transport availability throughout night Plastic/toughened glass Registration and training of door staff Complaints procedures and Policing	Club owners/staff Police Licensing authority Club goers Transport authority
Drink/drug driving	Increased confidence Lack of co-ordination Increased risk-taking, lower inhibitions (Crowley and Courney, 2000)	Provide cheap soft drinks Public transport: taxis, buses, and trains available Information on safety issues Special club buses provided by clubs	Club owners/staff Health promotion groups Club goers Police Transport authority
Passive smoking	Increased smoking when out Many 'occasional' smokers Link between smoking and other substance use (Lewinsohn et al., 1999)	Adequate ventilation (especially behind the bar) Adequate 'break areas' for staff No smoking areas Information on dangers of smoking	Club owners Outreach workers Smoking prevention groups Health promotion groups Licensing authority Club goers

4. International considerations

The recent clubbing phenomenon probably has its roots in Ibiza where the mix of music (known as the Balearic Beat) and concurrent use of ecstasy rose to popularity (Calafat et al., 1998). Today, travelling in the form of dance music tourism (individuals specifically travelling abroad to attend dance events or choosing to holiday in destinations renowned for their nightlife) is more popular than ever. Major international clubbing resorts include

Ibiza in Spain, Rimini in Italy, and Ayia Napa in Cyprus. Clubbing abroad is often unfamiliar, and combined with a different language, this can mean health services or other forms of help are difficult to locate and access. Furthermore, accessing items such as condoms or emergency contraception may also prove more difficult. Legislation can be different and poorly understood, leading to unexpected confrontations with judicial services. If drugs are purchased, the supplier will often be untested, raising the possibility of counterfeits. Equally, alcohol measures may vary in size and purity from standard measures within individuals' home countries. When alcohol and drugs are consumed, a combination of hotter climates, longer periods of dancing, and possible gastrointestinal infections increase the risk of severe dehydration. Importantly, however, along with environmental change, individuals abroad are often free from the social constraints of work and family that restrict their substance use and sexual behaviour (Ryan and Kinder, 1996). Thus, an individual may go clubbing one night per week while at home, whereas during a two-week trip abroad the same individual may visit a club every night. This in turn can significantly alter an individual's exposure to substances. For instance, around a third of all young people from the UK who visited Ibiza in 1999 used ecstasy while on the island. The vast majority of these also used ecstasy in the UK (Bellis et al., 2000). However, the way in which people used ecstasy while abroad was significantly different. Of ecstasy users, only 3 per cent used the drug five or more days a week in the UK while 45 per cent of the same group used the drug five or more days a week while in Ibiza. Similar trends in increased frequency of use were also seen for alcohol, amphetamine, and cocaine.

Little is currently known about the health effects of such periods of intense substance use. Clearly, the opportunities for adverse reactions are substantially increased where multiple drugs are being regularly consumed along with alcohol on a nightly basis. Furthermore, intense periods of consumption provide at least the possibility that more frequent drug use could continue when individuals return home, potentially moving individuals' habits further towards problematic use.

In order to address the health needs of the increasingly large numbers of young people who regularly travel to experience international nightlife, new approaches to health promotion and protection are required. New literature and campaigns are needed that provide international information on substance use and nightlife health for those travelling abroad. They should tackle the broad range of risks to health, including environmental considerations, but should also address the changes in substance use that occur while abroad (Bellis et al., 2000). Access to such information can utilise new technologies affiliated with club culture (e.g. the Internet) and popular with the major clubbing age groups (Hughes et al., 2002). Good examples of such sites are already available (www.dancesafe.org and www.ravesafe.org).

5. Conclusions

Around the world, clubbing is now well established as a major feature of the night-time environment. It provides a social outlet for millions of individuals every week and developing a popular club scene has reinvigorated many cities bringing money and employment. Substance use in clubs is strongly affiliated with relaxation, exercise (Gaule et al., 2001), and meeting new sexual partners. Whether these pastimes lead to increased well-being or ill health depends on the environment and the specific behaviour of individuals. Developing clubs as a healthy setting requires interventions that protect and promote health while retaining fun as a central feature. Where interventions or regulations substantially reduce fun, young people may look elsewhere for their entertainment (e.g. illegal parties). Consequently, organisations need to recognise the importance of involving young people in the development of night-time health interventions.

Substance use is one of the major risks to health in the night-time environment both through its direct effects on individuals' health and through the alterations in behaviour and perception that it causes. However, many organisations and individuals do not feel either comfortable or equipped to engage in drug-specific interventions or even discussions. By developing a healthy settings approach to clubs, the emphasis of health interventions can be diverted away from solely drug use to include a wider range of issues. This means key individuals and organisations (including club owners, staff, promoters, and major industries) can be engaged in a harm minimisation agenda that includes drug use along with alcohol, tobacco, transport, security, and other environmental issues. Furthermore, tackling a broad range of issues in the night-time environment reaches groups that are difficult to reach through education or occupational settings, such as those who play truant or are unemployed.

Some countries have already engaged in this more holistic approach to night-time health by generating broader guidelines on safer clubs and clubbing (e.g. London Drug Policy Forum, 1996; Ministry of Health, 1999; Newcombe, 1994). However, with cheaper air travel and young people having grater expendable income (Calafat et al., 2001) combined with the international nature of the clubbing phenomenon, a significant proportion of an individual's annual clubbing nights can be spent in nightclubs abroad where risks to health may be even greater. As a result, guidelines are required to provide basic standards for nightclubs on an international basis and different interventions need to be developed to address local and international needs. Efforts to develop international guidelines on club health are already underway (www.clubhealth.org.uk). However, empirical evidence on changes in individuals' behaviour when abroad (Bellis et al., 2001) and the resultant effects on health are both rare and urgently needed. Without such intelligence, the appropriate structure of health interventions to minimise harm for millions of dance music tourists remains unclear and the burden of ill health carried especially by younger people may unnecessarily be increasing.

References

BBC Devon News (2001). Lollipops gag late-night revellers. *BBC News* (online).

BBC News (2000). Mexico club blaze kills 19. *BBC News*, Friday, 20 October 2000.

Bellis, M.A., Hale, G., Bennett, A., Chaudry, M., and Kilfoyle, M. (2000). Ibiza uncovered: changes in substance use and sexual behaviour amongst young people visiting an international night-life resort. *International Journal on Drug Policy*, 11: 235–244.

Bellis, M.A., Hughes, K., Bennett, A., and Thomson, R. (2001). The role of an international nightlife resort in the proliferation of recreational drugs. *Addiction*, 98: 1713–21.

Bowcott, O. (2001). Ecstasy deaths may have been caused by heat, not a bad batch. *The Guardian*, Saturday, 30 June 2001.

Burke, J. (2001). Ecstasy's death toll 'set to go on rising'. *The Guardian*, Sunday, 1 July 2001.

Calafat, A., Fernandez, C., Juan, M., Bellis, M.A., Bohrn, K., Hakkarainen, P., Kilfoyle-Carrington, M., Kokkevi, A., Maalste, N., Mendes, F., Siamou, I., Simojn, J., Stocco, P., and Zavatti, P. (2001). *Risk and Control in the Recreational Drug Culture: SONAR Project*. Spain: IREFREA.

Calafat, A., Stocco, P., Mendes, F., Simon, J., van de Wijngaart, G., Sureda, M., Palmer, A., Maalste, N., and Zapatti, P. (1998). *Characteristics and Social Representation of Ecstasy in Europe.* Valencia: IREFREA and European Commission.

Clark, P., Cook, P.A., Syed, Q., Ashton, J.R., and Bellis, M.A. (2001). *Re-emerging Syphilis in the North West: Lessons from the Manchester Outbreak.* Liverpool: Public Health Sector, Liverpool John Moores University.

CNN (2000). Christmas fire kills at least 309 at China shopping centre. *CNN*, 27 December 2000.

Crew 2000 (2001). Development of strategies for secondary prevention in drug use. Patterns of drug use amongst young people at clubs and pre-club bars in Edinburgh. *Project Report.* Edinburgh: Crew 2000.

Crowley, J. & Courney, R. (2000). The relation between drug use, impaired driving and traffic accidents. *The Results of an Investigation Carried Out for the European Monitoring Centre on Drugs and Drug Addictions (EMCDDA), Lisbon.* Proceedings of Road Traffic and Drugs, Strasbourg, 19–21 April 1999. Council of Europe Publishing.

Deehan, A. (1999). *Alcohol and Crime: Taking Stock.* Policing and Reducing Crime Unit, Crime Reduction Research Series Paper 3. London: Home Office.

European Monitoring Centre for Drugs and Drug Addiction (2000). *Report on the Risk Assessment of Ketamine in the Framework of the Joint Action on New Synthetic Drugs.* Portugal: EMCDDA.

Gaule, S., Dugdill, L., Peiser, B., and Guppy, A. (2001). *Moving beyond the Drugs and Deviance Issues: Rave Dancing as a Health Promoting Alternative to Conventional Physical Activity.* Proceedings of club health 2002. Liverpool John Moores University and Trimbos Institute. Available at: www.clubhealth.org.uk.

Greater Manchester Police (2001). *Manchester City Centre Venues Team Up with Police to Reduce Night Crime.* Press release.

Health and Safety Executive (1999). *Introducing the Noise at Work Guidelines: a Brief Guide to the Guidelines Controlling Noise at Work.* INDG75 (rev) C150 11/99. Suffolk: HSE Books.

Henry, J.A., Jeffreys, K.J., and Dawling, S. (1992). Toxicity and deaths from 3, 4-methylene-dioxymethamphetamine ('Ecstasy'). *Lancet*, 340: 384–387.

Hughes, K., Bellis, M.A. and Tocque, K. (2002). *Public Health and Information and Communications Technologies: Tackling Health and Digital Inequalities in the Information Age.* Liverpool: North West Public Health Observatory.

Institute of Alcohol Studies (2001). *Alcohol and Crime: IAS Factsheet.* St Ives: Institute of Alcohol Studies.

Jarvis, M.J., Foulds, J., and Feyerabend, C. (1992). Exposure to passive smoking among bar staff. *British Journal of Addiction*, 87: 111–113.

Jones, S., Love, C., Thomson, G., Green, R., & Howden-Chapman, P. (2001). Second-hand smoke at work: the exposure, perceptions and attitudes of bar and restaurant workers to environmental tobacco smoke. *Australian and New Zealand Journal of Public Health*, 25: 90–93.

Kershaw, C., Budd, T., Kinshott, G., Mattinson, J., Mayhew, P., and Myhill, A. (2000). *The 2000 British Crime Survey.* Home Office Statistical Bulletin 18/00. London: Home Office.

Lenehan, P., & McVeigh, J. (1998). *Anabolic Steroids: a Guide for Professionls.* The Drugs and Sport Information Service, University of Liverpool.

Lewinsohn, P.M., Rohde, P., and Brown, R.A. (1999). Level of current and past adolescent cigarette smoking as predictors of future substance use disorders in young adulthood. *Addiction*, 94: 913–921.

London Drug Policy Forum (1996). *Dance till Dawn Safely: a Code of Practice on Health and Safety at Dance Venues.* London: Drug Policy Forum.

Luke, C. (1999). A little nightclub medicine. In M. Kilfoyle, & M.A. Bellis (eds), *Club Health: the Health of the Clubbing Nation.* Liverpool: Department of Public Health, Liverpool John Moores University.

McCann, U.D., Slate, S.O., and Ricaurte, G.A. (1996). Adverse reactions with 3,4-methylene-dioxymethamphetamine (MDMA: 'ecstasy'). *Drug Safety*, 15, 107.

Measham, F., Aldridge, J., and Parker, H. (2001). *Dancing on Drugs: Risk, Health and Hedonism in the British Club Scene*. London: Free Association Books.

Ministry of Health (1999). *Guideliness for SAFE Dance Parties: the Big Book*. New Zealand: Ministry of Health.

Mintel International Group (2000). *Nightclubs and Discotechques: Market Size and Trends*. Report Code 11/2000, London.

Morris, S. (1998). *Clubs, Drugs and Doormen*. Crime Detection and Prevention Series Paper 86, Police Research Group, London: Home Office.

Newcombe, R. (1994). *Safer Dancing: Guidelines for Good Practice at Dance Parties and Nightclubs*. Liverpool: 3D Pub.

Niesnk, R., Nikken, G., Jansen, F., and Spruit, I. (2000). *The Drug Information and Monitoring Service (DIMS) in the Netherlands: a Unique Tool for Monitoring Party Drugs*. Proceedings of Club Health 2002. Liverpool John Moores University and Trimbos Institute. Available at: www.clubhealth.org.uk.

Page, S. (2000). *Death on the Dancefloor*: Proceedings of Club Health 2002. Liverpool John Moores University and Trimbos Institute. Available at: www.clubhealth.org.uk.

Parrott, A.C., Milani, R.M., Parmer, R., and Turner, J.D. (2001). Recreational ecstasy/MDMA and other drug users from the UK and Italy: psychiatric problems and psychobiological problems. *Psychopharmacology*, 159: 77–82.

Poulin, C., & Graham, L. (2001). The association between substance use, unplanned sexual intercourse and other sexual behaviours among adolescent students. *Addiction*, 96: 607–621.

Ramsay, M., Baker, P., Goulden, C., Sharp, C., and Sondhi, A. (2001). *Drug Misuse Declared in 2000: Results from the British Crime Survey*. Home Office Research Study 224. London: Home Office.

Release (1997). *Drugs and Dance Survey: an Insight into the Culture*. London: Release.

Reneman, L., Lavalaye, J., Schmand, B., de Wolff, F.A., van den Brink, W., den Heeten, G.J., and Booij, J. (2001). Cortical serotonin transporter density and verbal memory in individuals who stopped using methylenedioxymethamphetamine (MDMA or 'ecstasy'): preliminary findings. *Archives of General Psychiatry*, 58: 901–906.

Royal National Institute for Deaf People (1999). *Safer sound: an analysis of musical noise and hearing damage*. London; RNID.

Ryan, C., and Kinder, R. (1996). Sex, tourism and sex tourism: fulfilling similar needs? *Tourist Management*, 17: 507–518.

Smith, P., & Davis, A. (1999). Social noise and hearing loss. *Lancet*, 353, 1185.

The Guardian (2001). Dutch fire toll climbs to 10 with 17 fighting for life. *The Guardian*, Wednesday, 3 January 2001.

The Kirklees Partnership (1999). *Boiling Point Preventer: a Code of Practice for Dealing with Drugs and Violence in Pubs and Clubs*. Huddersfield: The Kirklees Partnership.

Walsh, E. (2000). *Dangerous Decibels: Dancing until Deaf*. San Francisco: The Bay Area Reporter, Hearing Education and Awareness for Rockers.

Winstock, A.R., Griffiths, P., and Stewart, D. (2001). Drugs and the dance music scene; a survey of current drug use patterns among a sample of dance music enthusiasts in the UK. *Drug and Alcohol Dependence*, 64: 9–17.

World Health Organisation (1997). *The Jakarta Declaration on Leading Health Promotion into the 21st Century*. Fourth international conference on health promotion, Jakarta, 21–25 July 1997.

Chapter 9

Yoga and Promoting Public Health

Sue Spurr

This chapter is a personal exploration of how yoga, a complementary therapy, can promote public health in the UK. First, I will explore the benefits of practising yoga, drawing on my own perspective and those of other people in my yoga teacher's classes, as well as making reference to published research. I will then examine where yoga, as a complementary therapy, is situated in the complex spectrum of promoting public health and what are the implications of it being used to promote public health.

What is yoga?

The House of Lords Select Committee classifies yoga as a complementary therapy and as such it is most often used to complement conventional medicine and does not purport to embrace diagnostic skills. The Committee describes yoga as 'a system of adopting postures with related exercises designed to promote spiritual and physical well-being' (House of Lords, 2000: para 2.1).

Yoga is more than being about physical exercise. It is underpinned by or rooted in a philosophy and discipline – a way of life – that promotes well-being. The Sanskrit (Indo-European classical language of India) word 'yoga' is translated as union between mind, body and spirit (British Wheel of Yoga, 2006).

More than a million people in the UK practise yoga (Hanc, 2006) and, just as more and more people are turning to complementary and alternative medicine (CAM), its popularity is increasing. Estimates suggest that in the UK between 2 per cent and 6.6 per cent of the population use CAM (Ong and Banks, cited in Heller et al., 2005). The reasons why people are turning to CAM are complex and fluid and, as Cant (2005) suggests, reflect differing perceptions of health and illness. Furthermore, people are taking a more active and critical role as consumers of health care and are increasingly sceptical about the role of science (Giddens, cited in Heller et al., 2005) and orthodox medicine in particular (Gabe et al., cited in Heller et al., 2005).

There are many different forms of yoga and too many to detail within the scope of this chapter. At my yoga class, we practise 'hatha' yoga, which means 'physical', and is the most widely practised form of yoga in the UK, comprising breath and movement, relaxation and meditation.

What are the benefits from doing yoga?

The British Wheel of Yoga (2006) suggests that people 'may be drawn to yoga simply for health and fitness, or be seeking relief for a specific physical condition. You might want help with managing stress, or would like pregnancy yoga classes or exercises suitable for the less able-bodied. Whatever your objectives, there are yoga classes that can meet them.'

After a brief introduction to yoga as a student in the early 1970s, I returned to it eight years ago and since then have been going to a yoga class taught by Jean on Monday evenings. I go to yoga because I know that I benefit. I feel better in that I sleep well, and I feel calmer and more centred after yoga class. Each week is different. For me, it's like a journey where I discover more about myself and what I can do. I now know a lot more about yoga than I did a few years ago but I still consider myself to be a relative novice both in experience and knowledge.

Jean teaches several yoga classes and I asked people from her classes to suggest how they feel they benefit from participating in them. Of course, this personalised and small-scale investigation is limited and does not, for instance, include any conversations with 'drop outs' or 'non-enthusiasts'. Nevertheless, it does provide a vivid snapshot of how one teacher's group of students perceive the health benefits of yoga.

Many people talked about how yoga results in a sense of calm and feeling of well-being, helps them to feel more relaxed and to cope with the stresses and strains of modern living:

> Yoga has helped me to cope with the ups and downs of life. I have been practising for 30 years and I have reached a stable time in my life and yoga has helped me enormously. (Jane)

> I chose yoga originally to get away from the stress of teenage boys with their heavy metal music. … I benefit from yoga by relaxation and keeping my joints more supple. (Sheila)

> I always get a good night's sleep after a yoga class … poses can be easy or more difficult and makes it ideal for all, young or old, fit or infirm. It's also something that you can do at home, especially breathing exercises and relaxation. (Yvonne)

> I like yoga for the relaxation, breathing, focusing of the mind, also the 'sweet pain' you get from the exercises as some of the movements are quite challenging. (Patricia)

It is interesting to note that Dr Alan Breen, Director of the Institute for Musculoskeletal Research and Clinical Implementation, argues:

> Previous research had suggested that strengthening and stretching exercises were no more effective than other types of exercise for chronic back pain. … However, yoga requires learning about exercise as well as doing it, and active treatments, where patients take the initiative, are already recognised to be better than ones where they are just passive recipients. (BBC News, 2005).

Most people from Jean's classes mentioned how the gentle stretches – working with the breath – enable them to feel stronger, more flexible and supple in their joints and muscles, and to have a more positive attitude to looking after their body:

I chose to go to yoga on my wife's recommendation that it might help to alleviate the pain I get around my neck and increase my flexibility. ... The benefit was instantaneous and the pain that I used to feel had reduced considerably and I felt very relaxed. (Tim)

... yoga gives me a greater awareness of the mechanics of the body and breathing techniques. ... It gives me more flexibility and a more positive attitude in looking after my body. (Alan)

I'm sure I'm more supple physically and it's also 'food' for your mind. I like the stretching and feeling that you are using all the muscles from the eyes to the toes! (Angelina)

I'd seen the benefit in a friend. ... [It] keeps my joints moving ... better posture and therefore less aches ... Being in tune and in control of your body. (Kathy)

According to the British Wheel of Yoga (2006), 'yoga can also complement medical science and therapy for specific conditions'. In their study of people with chronic back pain, Sherman et al. (2005) concluded that yoga was more effective than a self-care book and other forms of exercise for improving function and reducing chronic lower back pain, and the benefits persisted for at least several months. DiBenedetto et al. (2005) suggest that yoga offers a cost-effective approach to age-related changes in gait function, improving hip extension and stride length and decreasing anterior pelvic tilt in healthy older adults.

Many people in Jean's classes talked about how yoga helps them with specific symptoms like back ache, arthritis or other chronic conditions:

I choose to go to yoga because I suffered back ache after the birth of my second child 30 years ago and thought yoga might be helpful. It is. (Bess)

I have a lung condition called sarcoidosis which also affects my muscles and joints. Yoga was recommended to me to try and strengthen my muscles and joints. It also helps me to stay positive. I can take the level of exercise to my ability. (Dawn)

I am partially disabled caused through a RTA 25 years ago and cannot do any strenuous exercise. Yoga is beneficial to me. I get professional advice on exercises I can do and it is also mentally stimulating. (Felix)

I used to do yoga before I got rheumatoid arthritis and enjoyed it very much. As the RA progressed I was unable to do many exercises. ... I was so glad to hear of Jean's class and get back to using all parts of using my body again. It is easy to do as much (or little) as is possible given restricted joints. (Lesley)

People in Jean's classes enjoy the social side of a friendly yoga class and how they can have a good laugh:

... meeting other people in our group we tend to encourage each other along and we also have good laugh which is also good for us all. (Olivia)

The best thing about doing yoga is the resultant feeling of well-being, friendship and total trust in a brilliant teacher. (Elizabeth)

I like the relaxation and the fact that the hour is totally mine to enjoy myself and meet others. (Lesley)

The British Wheel of Yoga (2006) suggests that:

Yoga offers us a holistic approach to body, mind and spirit, which can provide us with the 'tools' to cope with the challenges of daily life. … By making yoga a part of your daily routine, you may become aware of subtle changes in your approach to life. In your yoga class you may well begin to glimpse a state of inner peace … your true Nature.

A few people whom I spoke to from Jean's classes talked about an increased awareness of the body, mind and spirit and how yoga helps them in this respect:

I am learning to be more aware of my body and mind week by week, having more control over separating physical areas and relaxing them leading to de-stressing at will whereas before taking up yoga I was not able to 'listen to my body'. (Pauline)

I like the meditation which helps with relaxing my mind and also relieves stress. (Sandie)

It has increased my flexibility [but] has [also] proved to me that my mind can make my body do things I previously did not think were possible. It also gives me a tremendous sense of well-being. … I love the meditation aspect of it. (Pam)

Yoga and promoting public health

Organisations such as the British Wheel of Yoga clearly suggest that yoga can benefit people's health and my conversations with people from Jean's yoga classes would certainly support this view. However, what are the implications of yoga being used to promote public health?

For many people, practising yoga is a lifestyle choice and in this sense it can be argued that they are promoting their health. However, most multidisciplinary public health stems from the National Health Service so yoga, as a complementary therapy and like most CAMs, is therefore normally regarded as being outside orthodox health settings and services.

A core value underpinning promoting public health is how people, as individuals or groups, should have a choice and should play an active and participative role in promoting their own quality of life and health (World Health Organisation, 1986). In his foreword to the Government White Paper *Choosing Health*, the Prime Minister writes:

For each of us, one of the most important things in life is our own and our family's health. I believe that this concern, and the responsibility that we each take for our own health, should be the basis for improving the health of everyone across the nation. … We are clear that Government cannot – and should not – pretend it can 'make' the population healthy. But it can – and should – support people in making better choices for their health and the health of their families. It is for people to make the healthy choice if they wish to. *Choosing Health* sets out what this Government will do to help them. (Department of Health, 2004)

For many people, practising yoga is making a 'healthy choice' and is playing a definite role in promoting their own health. In order to access a yoga class, as with other forms of CAMs, people usually have to act as consumers in the sense that they need to purchase a place in a class. Yet this is not a choice that is accessible to all who would choose to practise yoga.

Accessibility is much broader than being solely about being able to pay. Other obstacles may include an inability to travel to the venue or to leave dependents unattended, and a lack of knowledge or understanding about yoga. In other words, there are currently significant barriers for certain sectors of the community in terms of gaining access to yoga.

What if yoga were available via the NHS? While this may go some way to addressing the issues of accessibility in terms of people possibly no longer having to pay, yoga would then be subject to much tighter regulation and in turn this might seriously impact on its availability. Apart from chiropractic and osteopathy (which are both statutorily regulated), CAMs are not subject to regulation. Regulation of CAMs is a much contested and complex field, although regulation would be welcomed by organisations such as the British Wheel of Yoga, as there are concerns about the link between the growth in the number of injuries sustained through people doing yoga and the number of poorly trained yoga teachers. The British Wheel of Yoga suggests that only half the estimated 10,000 people who now teach yoga in the UK are properly qualified (BBC News, 2002). Well trained practitioners such as Jean are greatly concerned about how it is possible for yoga to be taught by people who have not undergone rigorous training, who therefore could be teaching yoga unsafely, and for whom there is no accountability.

Keith Weldon, Vice Chair of the Society of Sports Therapists, told BBC News Online that 'yoga should be tightly regulated' (BBC News, 2002). However, Julie Stone and Geraldine Lee-Treweek (2005) argue that, although the orthodox medical profession has been statutorily regulated for over 150 years, regulation (especially in the form of statutory self-regulation) is not a panacea. Regulatory mechanisms are effective only if they are relevant and properly enforced. This would be costly for yoga and probably prohibitive under current NHS funding.

In conclusion, for a significant (and growing) number of people, yoga represents an active lifestyle choice with important and perceived health benefits. Yoga, a complementary therapy and therefore outside of orthodox health care systems, is not accessible in a way that is compatible with the core values of promoting public health. However, if a complementary therapy such as yoga were to be promoted via the NHS, this may go some way towards addressing the issues of accessibility and safety but would involve a huge and probably prohibitive cost.

Hill (2003) studied the professional interface between health promotion and complementary and alternative medicine. She identifies the 'potential for closer integration but also reports on substantial barriers to collaboration between these professional groups'. She suggests that 'health promoters committed to individual empowerment and community action are the most likely to support some form of involvement with complementary and alternative medicine'. Hill concludes that 'one thing appears to be certain – health promotion in the 21st century cannot afford to ignore developments in CAM'.

Grateful thanks to Jean Reid and her yoga students for their support in writing this chapter. Jean holds a Diploma in Yoga Teaching Training from the British Wheel of Yoga.

References

BBC News (2002) *Yoga Injuries Increasing.* Available at: http://news.bbc.co.uk/1/hi/health/2245807.stm (accessed 6 February 2006).

BBC News (2005) *Yoga Can Help to Cut Back Pain.* Available at: http://news.bbc.co.uk/1/hi/health/4541682.stm (accessed 6 February 2006).

British Wheel of Yoga (2006) website: http://www.bwy.org.uk/ (accessed 5 February 2006).

Cant, S. (2005) Understanding why people use complementary and alternative medicine, in Heller, T., Lee-Treweek, G., Katz, J., Stone, J. and Spurr, S. (eds), *Perspectives on Complementary and Alternative Medicine.* Abingdon: Routledge.

Department of Health (2004) *Choosing Health: Making Healthy Choices Easier.* London: The Stationery Office. Available at: http://wwwdh.gov.uk/PublicationsAndStatistics/Publications/PublicationsPolicyAndGuidance/PublicationsPolicyAndGuidanceArticle/fs/en?CONTENT_ID=4094550&chk=aN5Cor (accessed 5 February 2006).

DiBenedetto, M., Innes, K.E., and Taylor, A.G. (2005) Effect of a gentle lyengar yoga program on gait in the elderly: an exploratory study, *Archives of Physical Medicine and Rehabilitation*, 86 (9): 1830–7.

Hanc, J. (2006) Yoga party, *Runner's World*, 14 (4): 51.

Heller, T., Lee-Treweek, G., Katz, J. Stone, J. and Spurr, S. (eds) (2005) *Perspectives on Complementary and Alternative Medicine.* Abingdon: Routledge.

Hill, F. (2003) Complementary and alternative medicine: the next generation of health promotion? *Health Promotion International*, 18 (3): 265–72.

House of Lords (2000) *Complementary and Alternative Medicine. Sixth Report of the Select Committee on Science and Technology.* London: HMSO. The Stationery Office. Available at: http://www.parliament.the-stationery-office.co.uk/pa/1d199900/ldselect/1dsctech/123/12301.htm (accessed 5 February 2006).

Sherman, K. J., Cherkin, D.C., Enro, J., Miglioretti, D.L. and Richard, A. (2005) Comparing yoga, exercise, and a self-care book for chronic low back pain: a randomized, controlled trial, *Annals of International Medicine*, 143: 849–56.

Stone, J. and Lee-Treweek, G. (2005) Regulation and control, in Lee-Treweek, G., Heller, T., MacQueen, H., Stone, J. and Spurr, S. (eds), *Complementary and Alternative Medicine: Structures and Safeguards.* Abingdon: Routledge.

World Health Organisation (1986) *Ottawa Charter for Health Promotion.* Ottawa: WHO.

Chapter 10

Disability Rights, Genetics and Public Health

Bill Albert

Introduction

Disease prevention and the promotion of health have been the core goals of public health since the 19th century. Defining these goals and deciding how they should be addressed has changed over time and, along with what constitutes the realm of public health, continues to remain the subject of vigorous debates. Genetic concerns of one sort or another have always been part of these debates. Currently there are a wide range of issues around clinical genetics which are seen as being of interest to public health. One of the most important of these relates to ante-natal screening and testing, and it is here, most significantly, that questions of disability rights, genetics and public health intersect or, to be more precise, collide. Of course, at this particular intersection other social issues are caught in the pile-up, including 'race', ethnicity, gender, class and religion. But, while recognising this complexity and the problems of focusing on only one element, we concentrate here on disability rights.

Public health and pre-natal screening

In the UK, as in many other countries, prenatal screening is seen as a basic public health provision and a routine aspect of pre-natal care. It is carried out by ultrasound scanning and a blood test. The latter, called a triple test, measures levels of specific proteins in the blood, raised levels of which indicate an increased chance of Down's Syndrome or neural tube defects such as spina bifida or anencephaly. Screening for other conditions, for example, inherited blood disorders, such as sickle cell disorders and thalassaemias, are also offered to specific populations with a high probability of having these conditions (Godard et al., 2003).

Pre-natal diagnostic testing, DNA or chromosomal tests, is done when screening has identified a potential problem. Testing can also be undertaken when the family is known to have a genetic marker or predisposition for a certain condition. It is important to distinguish screening that is carried out on entire populations and testing which is targeted on individuals identified as being potentially at risk. The most common diagnostic tests are amniocentesis and chorionic villus sampling (CVS), done to identify Down's Syndrome and neural tube defects. If the test is positive, indicating that the foetus may have an impairment, then women and their partners can decide, after having counselling and the necessary information, whether to continue with the pregnancy. New tests are being introduced which will give earlier diagnoses.

The principal argument in favour of pre-natal screening for various conditions or foetal abnormalities is that it is the first stage of a process for facilitating reproductive choice. Screening provides vital health information, giving prospective parents the option of a diagnostic test and then, depending on the outcome of the test, the choice of whether to continue with the pregnancy. The case for pre-natal diagnostic testing offered outside screening programmes for families with a known risk of having a child with a particular condition is also one of offering reproductive choice. If it can be determined, families should not be denied vital medical information on which to base their decisions, as being without this information would seriously limit their autonomy. Being free to make informed choices, especially on such personal family issues, is a question of social justice and human rights.

While officially the main criteria for recommending screening has to do with facilitating informed reproductive choice, other, possibly less publicly acceptable, reasons for supporting these procedures are understood but rarely expressed. For example, Karl Atkin quotes a health commissioner saying that pre-natal counselling was about: 'Empowering [parents] to make their own decisions. And to prevent [the birth of disabled children] by giving people an informed choice' (Atkin, 2003: 93).

Disability, eugenics and public health

The last statements highlight one of the principal concerns of the disability movement in the UK (BCODP, 2000), that the oft-repeated mantra of 'reproductive choice' is little more than a cover for supporting what are essentially eugenic policies to limit the birth of disabled children. This does not mean that the medical profession has hatched a plot against disabled people, but rather that most of them are simply not aware of or do not accept that there is any connection between the discredited 'science' of eugenics and modern genetics and associated technologies and practices. A similar tension between cure and birth prevention and claims of eugenic intent is evident in the case of screening for sickle cell disorders and thalassaemias, especially as these conditions are most prevalent within ethnic minority communities (Anionwu and Atkin, 2001).

Eugenics is derived from the Greek meaning 'good in birth' and was concerned with promoting the biological improvement of humanity. The 'science' of eugenics was first proposed in 1883 by Francis Galton, who was interested in improving the human stock of the nation. This was to be done in a positive manner by encouraging the most able and healthy to produce more children, thereby passing down good 'genes' to future generations (Kevles, 1985). To get the least able to produce fewer children, or preferably none at all, 'negative eugenics' was developed later, primarily in the USA and Scandinavia, where, among other measures, laws were enacted to permit the compulsory sterilisation of 'degenerates', mainly disabled people. This strand of eugenics was taken to the extreme by the Nazis who, in the early 1940s, began the systematic 'mercy killing' of disabled children and later, with the first introduction of gas chambers, the systematic genocide of disabled adults.

Up until the 1930s eugenic ideas were championed across the political spectrum. It was only from about this time that their popularity began to wane and were finally discredited by their direct association with the Nazi Final Solution (Kerr and Shakespeare, 2002). In the years after 1945, geneticists, many of whom had been active in the eugenics movement, began to distance themselves from it. Various eugenics societies changed their names and explicit promotion of eugenic policies ceased. Nonetheless, many claim that the eugenic assumptions and the ideal of improving the gene pool continue to underpin current clinical practice in genetics.

Although historically there were differences between public health and eugenics, there were also some significant similarities, particularly in relation to disability. It has been observed (Pernick, 1997) that in the famous *Buck v. Bell* case in the USA, which gave the green light for enforced eugenic sterilisation, Chief Justice Oliver Wendell Holmes made a direct link between this and public health vaccination programmes. Pernick concludes that:

> historical similarities are not moral equivalents. Their intertwined past certainly does not mean that public health was 'as bad' as eugenics or that human genetics is 'as good' as public health today. Past similarities between eugenics and public health serve as an alarm clock for all health sciences, not as a lullaby for genetics. (Pernick, 1997: 1770)

A disability rights' critique of ante-natal screening and testing starts from this point. For example, rather than focusing on individual reproductive choice, which many support in any case, it sees the state's promotion of screening and testing as framing a social understanding of what kind of people should inhabit the world. In other words, hidden behind the popular rhetoric of choice a broader, implicit eugenic intention is perceived (Parens and Asch, 2000). Of course, this is vigorously denied by those who promote screening and testing. Not only do they see these as addressing basic health issues, but also have set out some strong arguments why the concerns of the disability movement are misguided and misplaced (Buchanan et al., 2000).

Eugenics? What eugenics?

The first point made against criticisms of there being a programme of eugenic cleansing of potentially disabled foetuses is simply that there is no evidence it has happened. For example, the rates of abortion for so-called foetal abnormalities, at least in the UK, have remained fairly steady (about 1,800 a year, or 1 per cent, of the total number of abortions, Office of National Statistics, various years). Some will say this is still too many, but the point is that the advances in screening and testing and other genetic and non-genetic reproductive interventions have not as yet led to a wholesale elimination of foetuses who might be disabled. Furthermore, only a tiny proportion of this total has anything to do with new techniques of DNA analysis. Ultrasound scanning, traditional blood-based testing, and chromosomal analysis remain overwhelmingly the most common forms of detection. Finally, despite genetic hype, approved ante-natal population screening remains limited to a small handful of conditions.

Also, while alarms have been raised about the impact on disabled people of the use of IVF and pre-implantation genetic diagnosis (PGD), and of the related spectre of designer babies, the latter is still science fiction and the numbers of the former successfully conceived remain extremely small (something like 1,000 worldwide since 1990). Unless we see major changes in techniques and clinical practice, together with changes in attitudes towards the more traditional ways of reproduction, PGD is unlikely to become anything more than a fringe reproductive choice. Also it is important to remember that more than 90 per cent of disabled people acquire their impairment and of those born with one, many of these, for example most cases of cerebral palsy or, even technically, Down's Syndrome and other chromosome-derived conditions will not be genetic in origin.

At the same time as all that is *not* happening, improved neo-natal medical procedures mean more premature and very premature babies, and those with formerly life-threatening conditions, are surviving and many of these children will have impairments. Between the 1970s and the 1990s the survival rates of premature babies in the UK (those less than 32 weeks) has tripled, while the proportion of those surviving with impairment (about 50 per cent) has remained the same.

At the same time, and possibly partly because of this, governments are becoming more sensitive, at least on paper, to the fact that disability is a human rights issue. The Americans with Disabilities Act in the USA, the Disability Discrimination Act in the UK and similar legislation in other countries, and the United Nations' current work on developing an international convention on human rights for disabled people, all attest to the beginning of an important sea change in thinking about disability.

So what is the problem? Why are disabled people, at least those in the disability movement, so upset about the new genetics, most importantly about pre-natal testing and screening, and its impact on their human rights? More to the point, what is the problem with genetic advances *per se* when it seems that they have had little discernible impact at all?

Screening and disability: the social context

It must be remembered that throughout the world, even in those countries with effective anti-discrimination legislation and where social provision is comprehensive, albeit rarely adequate, disabled people remain an extremely disadvantaged minority. Disabled people are still routinely discriminated against in education, employment, access to all kinds of social and cultural activities as well as access to health care. Disability is stigmatised, which not only means disabled people may be seen as lesser beings by others, but worse, many disabled people internalise this and see themselves as inferior. They also remain the poorest of the poor, in every country in the world. For example, even in the UK most disabled people live near or below the poverty line. And in many countries disabled people find their basic human rights, often their right to life itself, violated as a matter of course. For example, in many countries, including the UK, the so-called 'mercy killing' of disabled people goes either lightly punished or unpunished (Dyer, 2005).

All of these broader social considerations become somehow amplified when we look at disability from a medical perspective. And it is, of course, from here that many of the negative social attitudes are derived and/or confirmed. The massive increase in social authority that the human genetic project has bestowed on medicine is also worrying, and more than bears out Irving Zola's warning:

> Medicine is becoming a major institution of social control, nudging aside, if not incorporating, the more traditional institutions of religion and law. It is becoming the new repository of truth, the place where absolute and often final judgements are made by supposedly neutral and objective experts. (Zola, 1972: 489)

In this arena the focus tends to be, some would say naturally, on abnormality and cure. Medical information given to potential parents, even if presented in a non-directive manner (and it often isn't), cannot help but be directive – medical conditions are, after all, problems. Attention given to probable symptoms or management cannot help but offer, or at least be interpreted as, a negative assessment. And why is screening being offered in the first place? Do we screen for what is desirable? If 95 per cent of people who had a positive test for Down's Syndrome decided to continue with their pregnancies, would Down's screening continue in order that people could have reproductive choice?

With respect to the more immediate socio-economic context, this too is far from neutral. A disabled friend of mine recently felt compelled to have an abortion not only because of directive prodding from the hospital, but also because she was advised that the social support she would need might not be available. Parents who have to do endless battle to get proper health or social care or a decent education for their disabled children would attest to the same disabling environment. What is the message here about bringing a child with an impairment into the world? What kind of reproductive choice does this allow? In a study on genetics and the National Health Service, published by the Institute for Public Policy Research in the UK, Lenaghan (1998) suggests that genetic testing should be about giving individuals real choices. In order that such choice is genuinely available, 'a greater emphasis on positively welcoming children and adults affected by genetic conditions into our society and de-emphasising the link between genetic tests and abortions would be the best way of ensuring the genetic services genuinely facilitate informed choices' (Lenaghan, 1998: 50.)

But even if this did happen, who, looking out at the disablist world we live in, would choose to bring a disabled child into it? This is one reason why, for the disability movement, disability is seen overwhelmingly as an issue of systematic discrimination and social exclusion; it is a human rights issue. The new human genetic discourse as well as that around reproductive choice frames it very powerfully as a medical issue. Popular genetic understanding, which promotes the social desirability of testing and screening, PGD and selective termination, adds another powerfully sinister layer of prejudice upon a group which is already socially disadvantaged and excluded.

Many people have said that there is no contradiction between supporting the abortion of disabled foetuses and advocating for the full civil rights of disabled people. Perhaps not, but it is to be questioned whether such fine distinctions will counter the powerful social message conveyed by both popular genetic ideas and the state promotion of screening for foetal abnormality. Although most in the disability movement would not equate the new genetics with the Nazi atrocities against disabled people, it is still possible to hear the echoes and feel the icy touch of eugenic elimination in this latest, ostensibly softer, public health-promoted, consumer-driven phase. And it is not difficult to find statements from some of the leading proponents of the new genetics which serve to reinforce this impression. For example, Dr Bob Edwards, who with Patrick Steptoe, was the pioneer of IVF treatment in Britain, speaking at a recent international conference said: 'Soon it will be a sin for parents to have a child which carries the heavy burden of genetic disease. We are entering a world where we have to consider the quality of our children.' He went on to welcome the beginning of a new age when, 'every child would be wanted and genetically acceptable' (Rogers, 1999).

Why do calls for this new form of 'population improvement', this new form of eugenics, seem to be so readily accepted, or at least not condemned out of hand for what they are? Is it because in this consumer age disabled people are seen as defective products? Perhaps. But what is really happening now, has been happening and will become more prevalent as the genetic project becomes stronger and more pervasive is that medical conditions will increasingly be equated with the prospective child. All the many other things which make us who we are will be ignored, lost in these genetically targeted medical conditions. A Down's child, cystic fibrosis child, a deaf child – not a son or daughter, not a brother or sister, not a friend or lover, not a joy to the world or a pain in the ass – all of those rich possibilities, too, come sliced away by a cruel genetic logic which leads to such a convenient, socially efficient equation.

Rather more prosaically, remember one of the first questions you've heard a friend or relative say to someone who has had a baby: 'And, how's the baby?' Clearly too simple, but the easy acceptance of such a loaded question provides us with one key to understanding the deep-seated, very profound social assumptions about disability. It is the continuing power of these assumptions which allow society to hold at the same time the apparently contradictory views, which I have mentioned before, that disabled people should be granted full rights while at the same time leading us to embrace a social discourse allied to clinical genetic structures which promote the elimination of certain disabled people.

As suggested before, the data indicates that, at least in the UK, there has not been a wave of genetic cleansing. However, this situation could soon begin to change with the development of a whole range of new pre-natal screening techniques (DNA analysis of foetal cells in maternal blood, DNA chips, improved ultrasound scanning). Will this increased choice improve public health or simply further medicalise pregnancy while increasing anxiety among women and their partners? At the same time the popular determinist concept of geneticisation ('our future is in our genes') allied to big business and floating on the ethical solvent of individual choice has begun to stigmatise and, through this, threatens to reduce the social acceptance of human genetic diversity. By doing so it will make those of us who are left all the poorer.

References

Anionwu, E.N. and Atkin, K. (2001) *The Politics of Sickle Cell and Thalassaemia*. The Open University, Buckingham.

Atkin, K. (2003) Ethnicity and the politics of the new genetics: principles and engagement, *Ethnicity & Health*, 8 (2): 91–109.

BCODP [British Council of Disabled People] (2000) *The New Genetics and Disabled People*. Available at: http://www.bcodp.org.uk/about/genetics.shtml.

Buchanan, A., Brock, D., Daniels, N. and Wikler, D. (2000) *From Chance to Choice: Genetics and Social Justice*. Cambridge University Press, Cambridge.

Dyer, C. (2005) Legal review will mean fewer murder charges, *The Guardian*, 19 December. Available at: http://www.guardian.co.uk/crime/article/0,,1670390,00.html#article_continue.

Godard, B., ten Kate, L., Evers-Kiebooms, G. and Aymé, S. (2003) Population genetic screening programmes: principles, techniques, practices and policies, *European Journal of Human Genetics*, 11 (2): S49–S87. Available at: http://www.nature.com/ejhg/journal/v11/n2s/.

Kerr, A. and Shakespeare, T. (2002) *Genetic Politics: From Eugenics to Genome*. New Clarion Press, Cheltenham.

Kevles, D.J. (1985) *In the Name of Eugenics: Genetics and the Uses of Human Heredity*. Knopf, New York.

Lenaghan, J. (1998) *Brave New NHS? The Impact of the New Genetics on the Health Service*. Institute for Public Policy Research, London.

Office of National Statistics (various years) *Abortion Statistics England and Wales*. Available at: http://www.statistics.gov.uk/statbase/Product.asp?vlnk=68.

Parens, E. and Asch, A. (eds) (2000) *Prenatal Testing and Disability Rights*. Georgetown University Press, Washington, DC.

Pernick, M.S. (1997) Eugenics and public health in American history, *American Journal of Public Health*, 87 (11): 1767–72.

Rogers, L. (1999) Having disabled babies will be a 'sin', says scientist, *Sunday Times*, 4 July.

Zola, I. (1972) Medicine as an institution of social control, *Sociological Review*, 20 (November): 487–503.

Chapter 11

In Defence of Women's Right to Choose: Abortion, Disability and Feminist Politics

Sarah Earle and Keith Sharp

Introduction

Having a baby is an important life event but it carries a physical, emotional, social and financial toll – especially for women. Women are solely capable of carrying and bearing children, and are often wholly, or mostly, responsible for their own children throughout childhood, and beyond. In England, Scotland and Wales, and in most other countries across the world, women do not have the right to choose abortion on demand. Indeed, legislation in the UK is more restrictive than in other European countries and in Northern Ireland abortion is only permitted in extreme circumstances. It is for these reasons that we write in defence of a woman's right to choose. However, in recent years this right has been challenged by those who believe that the right to choose perpetuates a eugenic approach to public health. This idea has been promoted, disingenuously, by anti-choice organisations such as LIFE, and the Society for the Protection of Unborn Children, and is also promoted by some watchdog groups, such as Human Genetics Alert. More worryingly, the idea has also been put forward by the disability movement (e.g. see Chapter 10 in this volume) and even the Disability Rights Commission has stated that Section 1(1)(d) of the 1967 Abortion Act, which permits abortion after 24 weeks of gestation in the case of severe foetal abnormality, is offensive and incompatible with valuing disability.

Elsewhere, we (Sharp and Earle, 2002), and others (Hampton, 2005; Pritchard, 2005), have drawn attention to the conflict which exists between the feminist principle of the right to choose and the concerns of the disability movement that to permit abortion on the grounds of impairment is tantamount to endorsing an anti-disability eugenics. Many authors have sought to show that this conflict is illusory and that, with careful reasoning, the feminist and disability movements do not necessarily have to be at odds on this important issue (Shakespeare, 1998; Sheldon, 1999; McLaughlin, 2003; Pritchard, 2005).

It is the aim of this chapter to explore these claims in some detail, and to show that while there might be general points of ideological agreement between the two movements, on the issue of abortion, a fundamental and irreconcilable conflict inevitably remains. Consequently, while we accept many of the concerns reflected in the position endorsed by the disability movement, we argue in defence of woman's right to choose, whatever the circumstances.

Abortion, disability and feminist politics

It is useful to begin by setting out what we see as the defining features of the two positions on abortion. Of course to write of either the feminist movement or the disability movement is to invite the criticism that neither is homogeneous. However, while we acknowledge this, we also believe that it is reasonable to use these terms in relation to the issue of abortion and disability because in so far as either the feminist or disability movements represent coherent intellectual and ethical positions, they can be defined by their opposing stances on the issue of abortion.

The crux of the feminist position, as we see it, is that women have a fundamental right to physical autonomy, including the right to terminate a pregnancy. Petchesky (1986) argues that this is one of the principal tenets of feminist thought and that women's need for physical autonomy is an indispensable condition of their full participation in society. Arguably, since women carry, bear and nurture children, the right to choose how, when and in what circumstances to have a baby is the only way that women can be freed from the bind of their biology.

Any assertion of a right invites a consideration of how the exercise of this right might interfere with the putative rights of others, and, in this regard, the feminist position is quite clear. Any rights which may be accorded either to the foetus, the father, or any general other, are subordinate to the right to choose. Either these rights simply do not exist, or they are trumped by the rights of the mother. Within feminist politics, since a woman's entitlement to obtain an abortion is derived from her *right* to do so, it follows that there can be no differentiation between women who seek an abortion for one reason, and those who do so for another. If reasons for the abortion were held to be relevant in determining whether or not she should be permitted one, then we could not say that she had a *right* to obtain one (nor is this right conferred by the 1967 Abortion Act). This is an important point to which we return below, since it establishes one very important point of agreement between the feminist and disability positions, but is also at the heart of the conflict between the two.

Disability activists begin from a quite different position. Although on many issues one will find advocates of the disability movement talking about rights, the position on abortion does not arise from a concern with individual rights. Instead the concern is essentially about the eugenic implications of aborting impaired foetuses and, in particular, Section 1(1)(d) of the 1967 Abortion Act. However, it is worth noting here that of all abortions performed in the UK, very few indeed are carried out under Section 1(1(d). For example, in England and Wales only 1 per cent of all abortions were on the grounds of foetal abnormality in 2004 (Department of Health, 2005). In the same year, less than 0.1 per cent of such abortions were performed over 24 weeks' gestation.

The objection of the disability movement to abortion stems from a wider concern with attitudes towards, and treatment of, disabled people in society. For such writers, their quarrel is not with abortion *per se*, but with the specific case of abortion on the grounds of impairment. Disability activists need not, therefore, align themselves with anti-choice campaigners (as suggested by Davis, 1987), who generally base their objection to abortion either on abstract ethical principles concerning the sanctity of life, or on the specific assertion of foetal rights (although anti-choice campaigners have strategically aligned themselves with the disability movement). Consequently, much disability writing focuses on the issue of pre-natal screening, and the advice – both explicit and tacit – which surrounds this (Crow, 1996; Kallianes and Rubenfeld, 1997; Drake, 1998; Pritchard, 2005). Indeed, the medicalisation of pregnancy and childbirth in the modern western world and the routinisation of pre-natal screening and diagnosis is widely documented (Green and Statham, 1996; Press and Browner, 1997; Press et al., 1998; Kerr and Shakespeare, 2003).

The fact that the disability rights objection to abortion is so specifically directed at abortion on the grounds of foetal impairment means that it is not as straightforwardly translated into policy as the feminist objection to abortion on the grounds of women's rights. The principal difficulty is this: since there is no objection to abortion *per se*, but only to abortion on the grounds of suspected or proven impairment, it would seem to follow that policies should be directed at preventing abortion on these grounds while permitting it on every other. While this appears to be the logical consequence of the disability equality position, the practical difficulties it raises are very obvious, and are well documented by disability equality writers themselves (e.g. Morris, 1991; Shakespeare, 1998). Notwithstanding ethical difficulties, which we shall explore further below, it is far from clear that such an arrangement could work in practice. Presumably, the only person who could have access to the true grounds on which an abortion is being sought is the pregnant woman herself. Therefore, a policy which sought to deny abortion on the grounds of impairment, but permit it on any other, would be so easy to circumvent as to be effectively pointless.

Whatever the practical implications of these two positions, it is clear that feminist and disability equality approaches to abortion begin from very different assumptions.

Freedom, rights and the social context

The tension between the feminist and disability positions on abortion has been acknowledged by disability equality writers themselves. There seems to have been reluctance, however, to acknowledge just how fundamental this tension is. For example, Shakespeare (1998) has suggested that it is possible to retain a feminist emphasis on women's right to choose, while still critiquing the eugenic ways in which medical discourse and practice prioritises and justifies the abortion of impaired foetuses. He argues, for example, that pre-natal screening is biased towards the termination of impaired foetuses and that these underwrite a professional – and societal – discourse which systematically undervalues disabled lives. In this way, he suggests that the individual choices which women make to abort impaired foetuses cannot be considered free choices; instead, they are heavily influenced by wider cultural and economic forces.

This position thus simultaneously accepts the ethical legitimacy of women's right to choose, while claiming that prevailing social circumstances undermine this right. Arguably, it would seem to follow from this position that while in principle women have the right to choose, they should only be allowed to exercise this right once the discriminatory culture and its supporting structures have been eradicated. However, we have a problem with this. In a nutshell, if it can be shown that individual actions result from, or are in large measure influenced by, wider social, cultural and economic forces, then it is difficult to conclude that they also reflect the individual's true interests. If it can be shown, for instance, that a woman's desire to abort an impaired foetus results not from her own genuine interests, but instead from the distorting influences of a eugenic society, then it seems difficult to accept. Fundamentally, the termination would not be in her interests, but in those of a eugenic ideology. Indeed, it seems difficult to see how one could, in practice, distinguish between a legitimate expression of a woman's 'true' interests and the illegitimately held prejudices of society.

More generally, it is difficult to challenge the legitimacy of individual choices on the grounds that they emanate from wider beliefs and values. It seems to us to be self-evident that all human beliefs, attitudes and preferences are unavoidably bound up in the particular social, political, economic and cultural circumstances in which they are found, and therefore that it simply makes no sense to distinguish between those which are the product of wider influences and those which are not. Equally, it seems rather dangerous to imply that because one's beliefs, attitudes and preferences are influenced by wider social factors, one's entitlement to hold them and act upon them should be undermined.

The fundamental point is that none of this carries any weight at all as far as the feminist position on abortion is concerned. While we accept that, in practice, the realisation of any right is based on the existence of realisable conditions, for example legislation, the right to abortion 'on demand' is grounded in the assertion of women's inviolable right to choose.

The right to choose: a eugenic approach to public health?

We now turn to consider what is, for some, one of the fundamental questions in this debate: Is the 'right to choose' simply a guise for a eugenic approach to public health? Originally, the term 'eugenic' implied being from 'good stock': in short, it meant 'health'. It later came to refer to the prediction and control over who should and should not be born (Galton, 1979). Although the precise contemporary meaning of this term is still debated, most disability writers would agree that pre-natal screening and the selective abortion of disabled foetuses is a form of eugenics. For example, McLaughlin (2003: 308) argues:

> Antenatal screening policy in the UK has the potential to further a dangerous moral order in the network of decisions, actors and technology it represents and keeps together. Screening is part of a series of networks that construct disability as removable and marginal, and the categories of the non-disabled as central.

Other disability writers point to the 'unreasonable' desire for a healthy child, suggesting that this, in itself, is tantamount to a eugenic approach to public health. For example, Hampton

(2005) refers to the concept of 'family eugenics' to describe the way in which medicine and the state pass on the decision to prospective parents of who is to be born, or not. He argues: 'I am of the view that the wish for a healthy baby is the soil in which family eugenics is growing' (Hampton, 2005: 558).

It is our view that, taken to this extreme, the disability position on abortion moves even further away from feminist politics and from the principle of a woman's right to choose. The selective abortion of disabled foetuses does not automatically imply that disabled lives are not, or should not, be valued. Surely, health should be valued above ill-health? And, surely, the pursuit of health is a rational choice for both individuals and the state?

Of course, this does not mean that we cannot examine the underlying social and cultural mores which underpin the pursuit of health; on this matter, we agree with McLaughlin (2003), who argues that there are some points of agreement between the disability and feminist movements. As we have already stated above, all human actions and beliefs are unavoidably bound up in the social, political, economic and cultural circumstances in which they are found. While we do not necessarily subscribe to the interpretation of public health as neither deliberately nor incidentally eugenic, we acknowledge the concerns of the disability movement. However, the right to choose is based on the inviolable principle of physical autonomy, the exercise of which should not rest on the particular social circumstances in which decisions are made.

Conclusion

We have argued that the feminist position on abortion rests on the fundamental assertion of a woman's right to choose. While rights are often enacted and ensured via legislation, the assertion of this right is otherwise unconditional; it cannot be undermined by the grounds on which abortion is sought, nor the wider social, cultural, economic or political origins of the woman's desire to terminate the pregnancy. We conclude from this, therefore, that attempts to reconcile the feminist position with that of the disability movement must fail. We have some sympathy with the concerns expressed by the disability movement. However, we support women's right to choose because they have a right to physical autonomy, not because we value the lives of disabled people any less.

In this chapter we have sought to demonstrate that, whatever ideological allegiances between the feminist and disability movements may exist, on the issue of abortion, the two positions remain in fundamental opposition. We have also sought to show that a woman's full participation in society is dependent upon respect for her physical autonomy and that, because of this, we defend her right to choose. Abortion is no picnic and women are unlikely to terminate a pregnancy on whim, but having a baby bears a substantial toll. Aborting a foetus on the grounds of impairment does not mean that the lives of disabled people are any less valuable than those of non-disabled people but, simply, that women demand the right to choose whether to carry, bear and nurture a child who will be impaired, or not. Finally:

> A woman whose attitude to her pregnancy changes when she finds it is affected by an abnormality is not making a social or political statement about the abnormality, or about born people with that disability. She is making a statement about herself; what

she feels she can cope with and what she wants. Society should accept women's autonomy in decision making. Since women have to live with the consequences of those decisions they must be able to make the decisions they perceive to be moral. Abortion on grounds of fetal abnormality is not a matter of eugenics, it is a means to extend women's control over their lives and futures. (Furedi, 1998)

References

Crow, L. (1996) Including all of our lives: renewing the social model of disability, in C. Barnes and G. Mercer (eds), *Exploring the Divide: Illness and Disability*. Leeds: The Disability Press.

Davis, A. (1987) Women with disabilities: abortion and liberation, *Disability, Handicap and Society*, 2 (3): 276–84.

Davis, K. (1997) Embody-ing theory: beyond modernist and postmodernist readings of the body, in K. Davis (ed.), *Embodied Practices: Feminist Perspectives on the Body*. London: Sage.

Department of Health (2005) *Abortion Statistics, England and Wales: 2004. Bulletin 2005/11*. London: The Stationery Office.

Drake, R.F. (1998) *Understanding Disability Policies*. London: Macmillan.

Furedi, A. (1998) *Abortion for Foetal Abnormality: Ethical Issues*. Available at: http://prochoiceforum. org.uk.

Galton, F. (1979) *Hereditary Genius: an Inquiry into its Laws and Consequences*. London: Julian Freedman.

Green, J. and Statham, H. (1996) Psychosocial aspects of prenatal screening and diagnosis, in T. Marteau and M. Richards (eds), *The Troubled Helix: Social and Psychological Implications of the New Human Genetics*. Cambridge: Cambridge University Press.

Hampton, S.J. (2005) Family eugenics, *Disability & Society*, 20 (5): 553–61.

Kallianes, V. and Rubenfeld, P. (1997) Disabled women and reproductive rights, *Disability & Society*, 12 (2): 203–21.

Kerr, A. and Shakespeare, T. (2003) *Genetic Politics: From Eugenics to Genome*. Cheltenham: New Clarion.

McLaughlin, J. (2003) Screening networks: shared agendas in feminist and disability movement challenges to antenatal screening and abortion, *Disability & Society*, 18 (3): 297–310.

Morris, J. (1991) *Pride Against Prejudice*. London: Women's Press.

Petchesky, R. (1986) *Abortion and Woman's Choice: the State, Sexuality, and Reproductive Freedom*. London: Verso.

Press, N. and Browner, C.H. (1997) Why women say yes to prenatal diagnosis, *Social Science and Medicine*, 45 (7): 979–89.

Press, N., Browner, C.H., Tyran, D., Mortan, C. and Le Master, B. (1998) Provisional normalcy and 'perfect babies': pregnant women's attitudes toward disability in the context of prenatal testing, in S. Franklin and H. Ragoné (eds), *Reproducing Reproduction: Kinship, Power and Technological Innovation*. Philadelphia: University of Pennsylvania Press.

Pritchard, M. (2005) Can there be such a thing as a 'wrongful birth'?, *Disability & Society*, 20 (1): 81–93.

Shakespeare, T. (1998) Choices and rights: eugenics, genetics and disability equality, *Disability and Society*, 13 (5): 665–81.

Sharp, K. and Earle, S. (2002) Feminism, abortion and disability: irreconcilable differences?, *Disability & Society*, 17 (2): 137–45.

Sheldon, A. (1999) Personal and perplexing: feminist disability politics evaluated, *Disability & Society*, 14 (5): 643–57.

Chapter 12

Death and Contagion: Contaminating Bodies

Stephen Handsley and Carol Komaromy

The sight of death

This chapter considers the risk that is posed by dead bodies following mass death. It begins with recent examples of media representations of dead bodies following the 2005 hurricane disaster in Louisiana in the USA. The chapter then moves on to discuss the extent to which the risk of contagion is based on evidence and explores the underpinning reasons for these perceived threats, before concluding that the most significant threats are those which arise from the culturally insensitive and disrespectful treatment of dead bodies.

The following extract from the *Independent Online* (Andrew Buncombe, 2005) illustrates some of the outrage which was provoked by the sight of neglected dead bodies:

> In a makeshift grave on the streets of New Orleans lies the body of Vera Smith. She was an ordinary woman who, like thousands of her neighbours, died because she was poor. Abandoned to her fate as the waters rose around her, Vera's tragedy symbolises the great divide in America today.
>
> However Vera Smith may have lived her life, one thing was certain. In death, she had no dignity. Killed in the chaotic aftermath of Hurricane Katrina, her body lay under a tarpaulin at the junction of Magazine Street and Jackson Avenue for five full days. Not her friends, her grieving husband, not her neighbours could persuade the authorities to take her corpse away.

In the last two decades since 1990, media images of dead bodies following disasters in which hundreds and thousands of people die in a short space of time have served to remind everyone that death can happen without warning. In other words, death is not confined to 'other' vulnerable groups of society; neither can it easily be prevented. The psychic investment that many people share in keeping death at a distance is threatened by this form of reality, which is brought home to people either by the experience of being a survivor, someone bereaved by the death(s) or by the images of death to those not directly involved.

In New Orleans in September 2005, the media images of neglected dead bodies caused great distress and offence. These images of bodies lying on the road or floating in water, such as that of Vera Smith cited above, seemed to signify a lack of care about the whole situation of this particular disaster. If it is the case that the way in which dead bodies are treated serves to represent the value that societies place upon their members, these corpses became representative of the neglect associated with this particular disaster. In other words, it posed the question: if dead bodies could be ignored in this way, what did this say about the way that the government cared about the people of Louisiana?

This expression of neglect and lack of dignity was just *one* of the dominant discourses at this time. The article about Vera Smith went on to suggest a physical risk to the survivors from her remains:

> Finally, disgusted by the way she had been abandoned – and concerned, too, about the health implications of advancing decomposition – her friends buried her in a makeshift grave. A local man fashioned a simple cross, and on top of the soil that was shovelled over her body he placed a white plastic sheet and wrote 'Here Lies Vera. God Help Us.' (Buncombe, 2005)

More starkly, in an article from the *Manchester Evening News*, another discourse of the danger of contamination quoted Matthias Schmale, International Director of the British Red Cross:

> Clearly, where there are dead bodies in fairly stagnant water it creates a breeding ground for disease. A priority must be recovering those bodies, for health reasons and for their loved ones. He said: 'Even though there hasn't been a major outbreak of disease in the tsunami area, it is absolutely critical we are not complacent.' (Schmale, 2005)

Despite the claims by highly regarded authorities such as the World Health Organization (WHO, 2005) that dead bodies pose limited risk to the public's health, for many, the dead body has associations with contamination and continues to be viewed as a threat to public health (de Ville de Goyet, 2004; Morgan, 2004). De Ville points out that it can often be difficult to distinguish between respect for the dead and the fear of the cadaver. This symbolic–reality dyad forms part of the sociological debate about whether or not we are a death-denying society.

In this chapter we argue that the 'contagion' of dead bodies is more symbolic than real, rooted as it is in the investment that is made in keeping the boundary between life and death intact.

Threats and precautions

Protocols around handling dead bodies, such as those devised by the World Health Organization (WHO, 2005) and which include wearing gloves to protect against body-fluids and the handler covering any exposed wounds, suggest that the risks to those people who directly handle dead bodies following disasters are no greater than those posed by the handling of any corpse (Morgan, 2004; PAHO, 2004). It is possible that a population of people in any society killed by natural or deliberate means will share a profile of risk with any similar living group.

In a review of the literature on the risks of infection following natural disaster, Morgan (2004) provides a more realistic picture of the reality of this risk. From reading his litera-ture review and both the Pan American Health Organization (PAHO, 2004) and the World Health Organization (WHO, 2005) manuals on the management of dead bodies following disasters, it soon becomes clear that the risk of infection is only as great as any risk from living or deceased persons. Unsurprisingly, it is also apparent that some people who handle exposed body parts and fluids soon after death are more at risk than people who do not. However, by taking relatively simple precautions this risk is significantly reduced. Morgan (2004) argues that the combination of a 'natural' instinct for survivors to protect themselves against disease is compounded by a lack of clear information and guidance to all rescuers and body handlers about the level of risk. We would disagree that this is suffi-cient reason to explain the fear of the contaminated corpse and its potential to infect living people. Even in circumstances where universal precautions are clearly communicated and understood, this is not the case.

That aside, Morgan's review (2004) and the PAHO (2004) manual make clear that for cross-infection from a dead to a living person to take place requires the presence of an infectious agent. Even then, the level of risk is dependent upon the type of infectious agent and the level of exposure. Furthermore, it is the case that when the host dies, so does the environment that sustains those pathogenic and non-pathogenic organisms that live within it. The length of existence after the host dies varies between these organisms – for example, HIV can survive for up to 16 days following the death of the host (Demiryurek et al., 2002) – so that contamination can occur via blood, faeces, residual air from the lungs of people who have infectious tuberculosis and, occasionally, putrefying organs and tissue. Morgan (2004) makes the further point that the storage of bodies following disasters lengthens the time that the body is exposed and increases the number of people who might handle the body. This latter point includes problems with the lack of awareness of the pre-cautions needed in this situation for everyone involved in any rescue. While this 'expert', scientific analysis relays the reality of the disposal of the potentially contaminated dead body, the symbolic threat of contamination to the public's health is constructed in the moral panic and collective insecurity which surrounds the disposal of bodies such as those of people with HIV/AIDS.

What is common to all of the literature is the need to handle bodies in ways which show respect for the customs and cultures of the affected groups. This need for awareness of the psycho-social risks associated with the disposal of bodies is the focus of the next section.

Grief and disposal

While environmental factors associated with disposal may threaten health and well-being, for some, disposing of the body is bound up with religious or cultural factors. For exam-ple, cremation is an integral part of the death and bereavement practices of Hindus in India. Hindu social life, to a large extent, revolves around the notions of pollution and purifica-tion and as such the dead body represents a site of impurity. For Douglas (1984), the human body is a symbolic medium which is used to express particular patterns of social relationship. She argues that the corpses may be seen as polluting. Such contamination, she suggests, is symbolic rather than a reality.

While mass fatality incidents involve the physical management of dead bodies, several authors have described the survivors' fears and feelings (Calhoun and Tedeschi, 1999; Kaufmann, 2002). They argue that the grief and trauma associated with such public tragedies can shatter the basic assumptions we live by and impact especially upon those responsible for managing dead bodies. For example, Galea et al. (2002) have reported the complications faced by first responders to events such as the World Trade Center collapse. These complications include dismembered bodies and body parts, personal risk, the isolation of those injured in rescue efforts from their colleagues, multiple deaths of colleagues, failure to rescue more of their colleagues and others, and the focus of the public on those who died rather than those who survived. Thus, management of the bereaved is an important element in trauma care (Klein and Alexander, 2003).

For some, these types of response represent a pattern of behaviour which is seen as either normal or pathological (Stroebe and Stroebe, 1987). Whatever the behaviour, clinicians need to be familiar with the features of normal and pathological grief reactions. For example, normal grief is simply seen as an affective response to loss which, if it remains uncomplicated, does not require therapeutic intervention. The course of normal grief, it is argued, includes a series of systematic stages which the bereaved must go through before they enter a phase of recovery and restitution (see, for example, Stroebe and Stroebe, 1987). So, dealing with dead bodies and mass fatalities using this model would see someone progressing through these stages in a largely uncomplicated way, picking up the pieces of their lives once they have come to terms with what might potentially be loss on a grand scale.

Pathological grief, on the other hand, occurs when 'the grief reaction has gone wrong' (Stroebe and Stroebe, 1987). Here, grievers become 'stuck' in the process of suffering adverse reactions following bereavement caused mainly by less than normal circumstances of death. Mass public health disasters fall into such a classification, although Myers, Zunin and Zunin (1990) point out that non-pathological grief reaction is a normal part of recovery from disaster. Not only may individuals lose loved ones, homes and treasured possessions, but hopes, dreams and assumptions about life and its meaning may be shattered. Zunin and Zunin (1991) emphasize that the grief responses to such losses are common and are not pathological (warranting therapy or counselling), unless the grief is an intensification, a prolongation, or an inhibition of normal grief.

This has important implications for the physical and mental welfare of those managing dead bodies, many of whom are described by Raphael (1986) as 'third level victims' in that they too were traumatized by the work they undertook. For example, in a study exploring the psychosocial impact on four groups of professionals involved as helpers in the aftermath of two major disasters, Gibson and Iwaniec (2003) found evidence of severe post-trauma syndrome – acute traumatic stress experienced by people witnessing a traumatic event – in many of the professionals present.

While some argue that such responses are grounded in 'reality', others have begun to embrace the concept of 'meaning making' as an important process for grieving persons (Stroebe and Schut, 2001), one which resonates strongly with the notion of symbolic contamination. Here, grieving is seen as a process of meaning construction in which '[b]ereaved people develop "narratives" about the nature of the deceased's life and death, and these "social constructions" themselves can affect the outcome of grief' (Stroebe and Schut, 2001: 392). In other words, how bereaved individuals construe their loss experiences may affect subsequent adaptation during their grief trajectories.

Whether the risk of the dead body to the public's health is viewed as 'real' or symbolic, there is often considerable concern about its disposal (Morgan, 2004). While these risks include cross-infection, they are not, however, confined to the physical factors associated with disposing of the corpse, but also include risks to the mental health and well-being of survivors. Indeed, research into post-death contact found that trauma, ethnicity, gender and religiosity are all significant predictors of psycho-physiological harm (MacDonald, 1996). For example, as the World Health Organization note:

> The psychological trauma of losing loved ones and witnessing death on a large scale is the greatest cause for concern. It is, therefore, important to collect corpses as quickly as possible to minimize this distress. (WHO, 2005)

Symbolic contamination and the 'risk' to survivors

The conclusion from the evidence of experts shows that the risk from contagion of dead bodies is comparatively low – indeed no more than that from living infected bodies. The body as a container of contagion is certainly one of the powerful discourses on the dead body, as the quotes on page 88 illustrate. This begs the question of why this contagion is such a powerful myth. Sociological literature on the body helps to explain society's reactions to the corpse and challenges these myths. Sociologists would argue that both the living and dead body is invested with a diverse range of meanings. Synott (1993) argues that even after death, in every culture the body remains the symbol of the self. In his essays on 'bodies', Turner (1992) argues that the human body is subject to regulation and control and this has become the preoccupation of western societies. Part of this regulation and control derives from medical power as the body increasingly has been defined in medical terms. These essays build on the ideas of the French philosopher Foucault (1977), who argued that investing the body with types of social significance has served to legitimate the intervention of different forms of regulation and control.

In terms of further understanding social attitudes to the dead body, Douglas's (1984) anthropological account of 'dirt' explains aspects of the need to keep the body intact and the preoccupation of death workers with the integrity of the physical dead body. In her seminal work on the concepts of pollution and taboo, Douglas argued that rules of hygiene are only partially concerned with the biomedical dangers associated with dirt and, more significantly, that dirt and defilement carry *symbolic* meanings which are rooted in the religious order. Therefore, responses to dirt are more likely to be ritualistic. Douglas (1984) argues that the human body is a symbol of boundaries in society.

Since she claims death has long been perceived as a dirty and polluting thing, it follows that the dead body, as a container of death, is not just a potentially polluting object, it also symbolizes the fragility of the boundary between life and death. Such margins are invested with power yet are potentially dangerous (Douglas, 1984: 35) and require management in some way. For example, the handling of dead bodies is 'pulled off' by an appropriate performance which at the same time serves to 'mask' or create distance from the death (Komaromy, 2005). Certainly it would appear that the tasks of decontaminating the body (discussed in the previous section) are, indeed, more symbolic than instrumental. As Lock suggests, '[w]hatever form death takes, it conjures up that margin between culture and nature where mortality must be confronted' (Lock, 1996: 576).

Yet Douglas (1984) argues further that things are not of themselves intrinsically 'dirty' or 'polluted'. Rather, it depends on where objects are placed. It is this which dictates the extent to which they become 'dirt', which in her account become 'matter out of place'. What Douglas (1984) means by this is that 'pattern-making' tendencies in us all mean that we 'construct stable worlds' (or schema) which makes us locate objects within a 'system of labels', so that the objects which do not fit create discomfort. This is an iterative process and these individual constructs are mediated by the cultural values and categories and form a rigid pattern.

According to Douglas (1984), dirt is both a dangerous pollutant and 'matter out of place', and responses to 'dirt' are ritualistic. Therefore, providing an order to cope with 'dirt' – in this case dead bodies following disasters – can be interpreted as one way of sustaining the system; or what she would call the 'order of things'. From her argument, we would claim that when dead bodies unexpectedly occupy spaces reserved for living, this contravention of a rigid pattern threatens to contaminate the otherwise 'clean' space of 'living'. The outcome is that the suddenly-dead body reveals the arbitrariness of the 'living' and 'dying' categories and this resonates with the reality of the imminence of death (Page and Komaromy, 2005). In this chapter we argue that at the time of sudden mass death it is as if all of the systems that we have drawn on to keep death at a distance from life and provide a particular meaning to life have been thrown into chaos, and thus threaten the security of life and run the risk of making life seem meaningless.

In conclusion, we argue that the perceived risks that are associated with contamination from dead bodies are not supported by current evidence and that dead bodies following mass death do not pose a risk, both to physical and public health, any more than is present in gatherings of living people. Indeed, the work that is done to decontaminate the dead body following disaster is more symbolic than instrumental. Rather, if anything, the risk is more likely to be to the mental health of those affected as survivors, rescuers and bereaved people. Part of this effect is from the sight and disposal of a large population of dead bodies.

As sociologists working in the area of death, dying and bereavement, we have asked 'what is really going on here?' One suggestion is that the body is a site at which practices are articulated (Foucault, 1977; Synott, 1993; Turner, 1992). Therefore, rather than protecting themselves from the intrinsic dirtiness of the dead body, survivors enact symbolic rituals which keep death itself at a distance at a time when it has catastrophically and without warning 'contaminated' life itself by occupying the space reserved for life and living. This ontological insecurity is expressed through fears that can be located in activities performed to keep survivors safe. The tension between grief as 'normal' and grief as 'pathological', fits into this need to separate extraordinary events from the security of everyday life and everyday grief.

References

Buncombe, A. (2005) The city where the dead are left lying on the streets, *The Independent Online*, 6 September. www.independent.co.uk (accessed 14/06/06).

Calhoun, L.G. and Tedeschi, R.G. (1999) *Facilitating Post-traumatic Growth: a Clinician's Guide.* Mahwah, NJ: Erlbaum.

Demiryurek, D., Bayramoglu, A. and Ustacelebi, S. (2002) Infective agents in fixed human cadavers: a brief review and suggested guidelines, *Anatomical Record*, 269 (4): 194–7.

de Ville de Goyet, C. (2004) Epidemics caused by dead bodies: a disaster myth that does not want to die, *Pan American Journal of Public Health/Revista Panamerica de Salud Pública*, 15 (5): 297–9.

Douglas, M. (1984) *Purity and Danger: an Analysis of the Concepts of Pollution and Taboo.* London: Routledge and Kegan Paul.

Foucault M. (1977) *Discipline and Punish: the Birth of the Prison.* London: Penguin.

Galea, S., Ahern, J., Resnick, H., Kilpatrick, D., Bucuvalas, M. and Gold, J. (2002) Psychological sequelae of the September 11 terrorist attacks in New York City, *The New England Journal of Medicine*, 346: 982–7.

Gibson, M. and Iwaniec, D. (2003) An empirical study into the psychosocial reactions of staff working as helpers to those affected in the aftermath of two traumatic incidents, *British Journal of Social Work*, 33: 851–70.

Kaufmann, J. (ed.) (2002) *Loss of the Assumptive World: a Theory of Traumatic Loss.* New York: Brunner-Routledge.

Klein, S. and Alexander, D.A. (2003) Good grief: a medical challenge, *Trauma*, 5: 261–71.

Komaromy, C. (2005) The production of death and dying in care homes for older people: an ethnographic account. Unpublished thesis, Open University, Milton Keynes, UK.

Lock, M. (1996) Death in technological time: locating the end of meaningful life, *Medical Anthropology Quarterly*, 10 (4): 575–600.

MacDonald, W.L. (1996) Idionecrophonies: the social construction of perceived contact with the dead, *Journal for the Scientific Study of Religion*, 31 (2): 215–23.

Morgan O. (2004) Infectious disease risks from dead bodies following natural disasters, *Pan American Journal of Public Health/Revista Panamerica de Salud Pública*, 15 (5): 307–12.

Myers, D., Zunin, H.S. and Zunin, L.M. (1990) Grief: the art of coping with tragedy, *Today's Supervisor*, 6 (11): 14–15.

Page, S. and Komaromy, C. (2005) Professional performance: the case of expected and unexpected deaths, *Mortality*, 10 (4): 294–307.

(PAHO) (2004) *Management of Dead Bodies in Disaster Situations.* Disaster Manuals and Guidelines Series, No. 5. Washington, DC: Pan American Health Organization and World Health Organization.

Raphael, B. (1986) *When Disaster Strikes: a Handbook for Caring Professions.* London: Hutchinson.

Schmale, M. (2005) 10,000 dead in hurricane hell, *Manchester Evening News*, 6 September 2005. Available at: www.manchesteronline.co.uk/men/news/s/172/172814 (accessed 17/02/06).

Stroebe, M.S. and Schut, H. (2001) Models of coping with bereavement: a review, in Stroebe, M.S., Hansoon, R.O., Stroebe, W. and Schut, H. (eds), *Handbook of Bereavement Research: Consequences, Coping, and Care.* Washington, DC: American Psychological Association, pp. 375–403.

Stroebe, W. and Stroebe, M.S. (1987) *Bereavement and Health: the Psychological and Physical Consequences of Partner Loss.* Cambridge: Cambridge University Press.

Synott, A. (1993) *The Body Social: Symbolism, Self and Society.* London: Routledge.

Turner, B.S. (1992) *Regulating Bodies.* London: Sage.

WHO (2005) Disposal of dead bodies in emergency conditions. WHO Technical Note 8. Available at: http://www.who.int/water_sanitation_health/hygiene/emergencies/deadbodies.pdf (accessed 15/02/06).

Zunin, L.M. and Zunin, H.S. (1991) *The Art of Condolence: What to Write, What to Say, What to do at a Time of Loss.* New York: Harper Collins.

Chapter 13

Dirty Whores and Invisible Men: Sex Work and the Public Health

Sarah Earle and Keith Sharp

Introduction

Sex work transcends gendered and sexual boundaries in that both men *and* women sell and pay for sex. There are many different forms of 'sex work', ranging from sex chat-lines, stripping, table dancing, pornography, indoor and outdoor sex work, and all other forms of sexual exchange. There is also a growing volume of literature on other forms of sex work, including that which is coerced or involving children. For example, Brown's (2000) harrowing account of trafficking in Asia depicts stories of sexual slavery in which girls and young women are bought, sold and kept prisoner, often until such time as they die of HIV/AIDS, drug addiction, alcoholism or other diseases of poverty. Malarek's (2003) text also describes the experiences of the nameless 'Natashas': young women smuggled out of Eastern Europe under false promises of employment as nannies, models or domestics in other countries, only to find, however, that they have been trafficked for prostitution and that they 'owe' money which they are unlikely ever to be able to repay.

However, in spite of the varied nature of sex work, it is the female sex worker who has been the most visible within lay, medical, legal and religious discourses, and it is she, on the whole, who has been considered deviant. The men who pay for sex – the punters – have largely remained invisible. This chapter considers the regulation of female sexuality and the visibility of female sex workers within some of these discourses. It also considers the absence of punters from social research and reflects on the consequences of this imbalance for the public health.

Dirty whores: the regulation of female sexuality

Historically, and to date, sex work has been associated with the transmission of illness and disease. Sex workers have been seen as the harbingers of disease and the spreaders of contagion. They have been held responsible for everything 'from the fall of empires to the spread of venereal disease' (Wilton, 1999: 189). They have been placed in the category of 'contaminated other'; dirty whores who contaminate but are never contaminable. This is in stark contrast to the images of men who sell sex, who are variously described as 'hustlers', 'beach boys', 'rent boys' and 'gigolos' (for example, see Aggleton, 1998). However, female sex work is unique in that it has been seen both to constitute a social problem and to be the solution to a social problem. It has been regarded, for example, as a utilitarian outlet for men's sexual frustrations, without which such 'frustrations' would otherwise lead to sexual crimes. The regulation of women's sexuality, particularly the regulation of the bodies of female sex workers is long-standing (O'Neill, 2001). There are many examples of this in recorded history, some of them in the distant past, such as the regulation of medieval broth-els (Mazo-Karras, 1989), others more recent, for example, the regulation of women in tolerance zones in the Netherlands (see, for example, Drobler, 1991).

Henderson's (1999) account of London in the 18th century details the relentless policing and regulation of female sex workers, both on the streets and in brothels. In the 1730s, local watch committees were established to help regulate street sex work. Henderson's work provides evi-dence of different views at this time, but one view depicted the female sex worker as an agent of destruction who, through her actions, was able to foul society, 'spreading physical ruin and moral disintegration' (Henderson, 1999: 166–7). Acton's (1972/1870) work on prostitution in the late 19th century also urged the prevention, amelioration and regulation of prostitution – or sex work. As part of this prevention and regulation, the Contagious Diseases Act, operat-ing in garrison towns, allowed a Justice of the Peace to detain a 'common prostitute' (the sdefinition of which was much debated) and subject her to periodical medical examination for the purpose of ascertaining whether she was affected by a contagious disease. Beds were secured at the Victorian Lock Hospitals with the object of treatment, as well as moral and religious instruction. In a visit to one such hospital, Acton concludes that: 'Their disease appears to be entirely local, both in origin and character. It arises, as I believe, in the great majority of cases, simply from the continual irritation and excitement of the generative organs consequent upon their mode of life, although it may be caused, no doubt, occasionally by direct contagion from urethral discharges in the male' (Acton, 1972/1870: 86).

Sex work has been understood as a 'necessary evil' and a social, legal and medical prob-lem. Public concerns have centred on the regulation of women and women's sexuality, rather than on male desire and demand. Thus, the men who pay for sex have remained largely invisible within the literature and within the history of sex work.

Invisible men: a methodological conundrum

While there is a considerable body of literature dealing with the experiences of both female and male sex workers, there exists comparatively little research on the men who pay for sex. Perkins (1991) estimates that less than 1 per cent of all research in this area focuses on the punter. Some of the reasons for this anomaly are clearly apparent.

First, and as outlined above, it is the sex worker who has been traditionally perceived as 'the problem', rather than the pimp or punter. As such, female sex workers are the most 'visible' within both lay and professional discourses on sex work and social research (and, subsequently, within public health practice). Secondly, and with notably few exceptions, paying for sex remains among the most discreditable and potentially stigmatising of activities in which men can engage. Also, although sex workers are easily located – on the streets, in parlours or walk ups, via calling cards left in telephone booths and, more recently, on the net – punters are less readily located and it has been difficult for researchers to find men willing to participate in social research.

One commonly used method has been to approach clients directly in situations where they are thought to be purchasing sexual services. This has mainly entailed approaching men who are soliciting the services of street workers. Leaving aside the probably unrepresentative nature of street work, the main and, indeed, obvious, drawback of such an approach is that the majority of men will refuse to participate in the research. This was one of the approaches employed by McKeganey and Barnard (1996) in their study of sex workers and their clients in Glasgow. It is not surprising that, despite the sensitive nature of the approach made by the researchers, '[t]he response was almost always the same, a more or less polite "get lost"' (McKeganey and Barnard, 1996: 14).

McKeganey (1994) also found that men approached in the street would lie about the purpose for them being there, claiming that they had just stopped to 'catch up on some paperwork'; these men were often seen hours later with a sex worker in their car. Other studies have approached men who visit massage parlours (for example, see Plumridge and Chetwynd's (1996) study of commercial sex in New Zealand). However, these studies are limited in so far as they are reporting on only one form of indoor sex work.

A related avenue, also adopted by McKeganey and Barnard among others (see, also, Campbell, 1998), is to approach attendees at genito-urinary clinics and interrogate them on their contacts with female sex workers. McKeganey and Barnard report obtaining information from 68 men in this way. However, a number of points need to be made about this approach. First, there is no reason to believe that typical clients of sex workers are significantly more likely than members of the general population to attend genito-urinary clinics. It follows that samples of men obtained in this way are not necessarily likely to be typical of the population of clients as a whole. Secondly, samples obtained in this way are still self-selecting: anyone is at liberty to decline the invitation to participate in the research and so we see no reason why this method should yield better results than any other which relies on self-selection.

Previous studies have also contacted men once they have entered the criminal justice system. Monto and Hotaling (2001), for example, administered a survey to 700 men who had been arrested for offences related to commercial sex. Faugier et al. (1992) identified their respondents via local police stations. An obvious limitation of this type of approach is that it only includes men who have been arrested for sex-related offences, which not only may be biased in itself, but may influence the kinds of response men give when questioned.

A further approach employed by a number of researchers is to advertise for volunteers to take part in research, either through the printed media (for example, Campbell, 1998; McKeganey and Barnard, 1996) or via radio (Gemme et al., 1984). While there is no doubt that this approach can yield samples of men, as we have already discussed above, the self-selecting nature of these samples should lead us to treat any data which result with caution. First, at a general level, it seems reasonable to treat *any* sample obtained in this way with caution, whatever the population concerned. In the case of punters, it seems even more reasonable to suppose that men who respond to such advertisements are not typical of the population of men who pay for sex. The fact that paying for sex is so discreditable an activity is alone enough to recommend caution.

Another approach is to utilise women who work in the sex industry to act as researchers and gather data on their clients. Vanwesenbeeck et al. (1993), for example, constructed a typology of men who pay for sex based on the accounts given by female sex workers. Wojcicki and Malala (2001: 99) carried out interviews with 50 female sex workers in Johannesburg, South Africa, claiming that on the basis of this they were able to 'explore sexual negotiations between men and women in the sex industry'. While such an approach does not suffer so obviously from the biases inherent in the methods so far discussed, it is not without difficulties. First, there is the not insignificant difficulty of recruiting willing individuals and of equipping them with sufficient skills to undertake the investigations required, although this is not insurmountable and is, in fact, becoming a widely adopted method of social research. Secondly, there is the problem of perspective. Data gathered in this way must be considered as 'filtered' by the perspective and interests of the sex worker; what these might be will vary, but it seems likely that such women will have an interest – like their clients – in presenting themselves in as creditable a light as possible. It is worth pausing here to reflect on the extent to which much of our knowledge and understanding of the men who pay for sex has been based on the accounts of female sex workers, rather than men themselves.

Recently, some other approaches have been documented. For example, Pitts et al. (2004) sampled men at a large commercial event in Melbourne, Australia – the *Sexpo* exhibition – which offered products and services concerning all aspects of sex and sexuality. Clearly, the men attending such an event are less likely to be those who, for whatever reason, wish to conceal their interest in all things sexual.

There is also some evidence of increasing use of the internet as a form of data collection, for example, the use of internet surveys (see Atchison et al., 1998) as well as use of the internet as a source of data collection (for example, see Sharp and Earle, 2003; Soothill and Sanders, 2005). Of course, internet methods of data collection raise the question of authenticity. For example, it could be argued that the use of the internet allows respondents to falsely represent themselves. However, in contrast, other researchers believe that individuals are more likely to represent themselves and their actions honestly online in comparison to more traditional forms of face-to-face contact (Mann and Stewart, 2000).

There is now a growing body of literature on what Campbell (1998) calls the 'invisible men'. Most of these studies are motivated by the desire to answer one seemingly simple question: why do men pay for sex? McKeganey and Barnard's (1996) Glasgow study found that punters reported a desire for specific sexual acts, as well as enjoying the clandestine and illicit nature of commercial encounters. Other researchers (for example, Monto, 2000; 2001) have also identified a desire for specific sexual acts, particularly fellatio, and cite this as one of the fundamental reasons for visiting a sex worker. These studies support the idea that men pay for specific sexual acts that they are less likely to 'get at home'. However, a telephone survey carried out in Melbourne, Australia (Louie et al., 1998) found that 32 per cent of callers cited good sex as the major motivation of men who pay for sex, followed by convenience, which was mentioned by 20 per cent of callers. In another survey of 612 men in Victoria, Australia (Pitts et al., 2004), nearly 44 per cent of men felt that commercial sex offered them 'relief' – in some ways this reflects traditional, and popular, discourses of a male sex 'drive' and the idea that sex workers are performing a service within society.

Confidential questionnaires used in the National Survey of Sexual Attitudes and Lifestyles (Johnson and Mercer, 2001) reported that nearly 9 per cent of men in London had paid for sex and that these men were aged between 16 and 44 years; nationwide, the figure was 4.3 per cent. Wellings et al. (1994) have argued that men are more likely to visit a sex worker as they get older and state that over 10 per cent of the male population aged 45–59 years old admit to buying sex. It would also appear that many punters have wives, partners, or girl-friends and would not wish their activities to become known to them (McKeganey and Barnard, 1996; Hester and Westmarland, 2004).

Beyond this, we know very little about the men who pay for sex.

The implications for public health: concluding thoughts

The purpose of this chapter has been to stimulate critical reflection on the subject of research-ing paid-for sex by exploring the visibility of female sex workers in contrast to the invisibil-ity of the men who pay for sex. Most notable is the regulation of female sexuality within medico-legal discourses, the central role of women as spreaders of contagion, and the over-whelming involvement of the female sex worker within research. However, what can we con-clude from all this, and what are the implications for public health?

First, it is important to recognise that public health has played a role in reinforcing the notion that sex work is dirty and that sex workers are the source of disease and contagion. Public health practice has also reinforced the idea that sex workers (and women more generally) are responsible for safe sex and that they, rather than men themselves, are responsible for the actions of men.

Second, just as researching men who pay for sex poses a methodological conundrum, so too does promoting their sexual health. Paying for sex is a diverse activity located not only in the well-known red-light districts of cities such as London and Edinburgh, but on and off the streets, and in parlours and brothels, in private houses and hotel rooms. We know very little about the men who pay for sex, but we can reasonably assume that they have a lot to lose from being discredited. However, just as researchers have recognised that our knowledge of paid-for sex is limited, public health workers must also recognise that initiatives which target female sex workers are only partial. It is therefore important for public health workers to initiate or become involved in research on paid-for sex so that this might inform the planning, implementation and evaluation of public health practice.

Recognising the need to think creatively about how to promote sexual health within paid-for sex is the first step in making the invisible visible so as to bring men into view.

References

Acton, W. (1972/1870) *Prostitution Considered in its Moral, Social, and Sanitary Aspects in London and other Large Cities and Garrison Towns with Proposals for the Control and Prevention of its Attendant Evils*, Frank Cass & Co., London.

Aggleton, P. (ed.) (1998) *Men Who Sell Sex: International Perspectives on Male Prostitution and AIDS*, Taylor and Francis, Abingdon.

Atchison, A., Fraser, L. and Lowman, J. (1998) Men who buy sex: preliminary findings of an exploratory study. In J.E. Elias, V.L. Bullough, V. Elias and G. Brewer (eds), *Prostitution: on Whores, Hustlers and Johns*, Prometheus Books, New York.

Brown, L. (2000) *Sex Slaves: the Trafficking of Women in Asia*, Virago Press, London.

Campbell, R. (1998) Invisible men: making visible male clients of female prostitutes in Merseyside. In J.E. Elias, V.L. Bullough, V. Elias and G. Brewer (eds), *Prostitution: on Whores, Hustlers, and Johns*, Prometheus Books, New York.

Drobler, C. (1991) *Women at Work: Reader for the First European Prostitutes Conference*, Frankfurt, 16–18 October 1992, HWG., Frankfurt.

Faugier, J., Hayes, C. and Butterworth, C. (1992) *Drug Using Prostitutes: Their Health Care Needs and Their Clients*, University of Manchester, Manchester.

Gemme, R.A., Murphy, M., Bourque, M.A., Nemeh D. and Payment, N. (1984) A report on prostitution in Quebec, *Working Papers on Prostitution and Pornography, Report No. 11*, Ottawa, Department of Justice.

Henderson, T. (1999) *Disorderly Women in Eighteenth–century London: Prostitution and Control in the Metropolis, 1730–1830*, Longman, London.

Hester, N. and Westmarland, N. (2004) *Tackling Street Prostitution: Towards a Holistic Approach*, Home Office, London.

Johnson, A. and Mercer, C. (2001) Sexual behaviour in Britain: partnerships, practices and HIV risk behaviour, *Lancet*, 358: 1835–42.

Louie, R., Crofts, N., Pyett, P. and Snow, J. (1998) Project Client Call: Men Who Pay for Sex in Victoria, unpublished report, McFarlane Burnet Centre for Medical Research.

Malarek, V. (2003) *The Natashas: the New Global Sex Trade*, Viking, Ontario.

Mann, C. and Stewart, F. (2000) *Internet Communication and Qualitative Research: a Handbook for Researching Online*, Sage, London.

Mazo-Karras, R. (1989) The regulation of brothels in later Medieval England, *SIGNS: Journal of Women in Culture and Society*, 14 (3): 399–433.

McKeganey, N. (1994) Why do men buy sex and what are their assessments of the HIV-related risks when they do?, *AIDS Care*, 6 (3): 289–302.

McKeganey, N. and Barnard, M. (1996) *Sex Work on the Streets: Prostitutes and their Clients*, Open University Press, Buckingham.

Monto, M.A. (2000) Why men seek out prostitutes. In R. Weitzer (ed.), *Sex for Sale*, Routledge, London.

Monto, M.A. (2001) Prostitution and fellatio, *Journal of Sex Research*, 38: 140–5.

Monto, M. and Hotaling, N. (2001) Predictors of rape myth acceptance among male clients of female street prostitution, *Violence Against Women*, 7: 275–93.

O'Neill, M. (2001) *Prostitution & Feminism: Towards a Politics of Feeling*, Polity Press, Cambridge.

Perkins, R. (1991) *Working Girls: Prostitutes, their Life and Social Control*, Australian Institute of Criminology, Canberra.

Pitts, M.K., Smith, A.M.A., Grierson, J., O'Brien, M. and Misson, S. (2004) Who pays for sex and why? An analysis of social and motivational factors associated with male clients of sex workers', *Archives of Sexual Behavior*, 33 (4): 353–8.

Plumridge, E.W. and Chetwynd, S.J. (1996) Patrons of the sex industry: perceptions of risk, *AIDS Care*, 8 (4): 405–17.

Sharp, K. and Earle, S. (2003) Cyberpunters and cyberwhores. In Y. Jewkes (ed.), *Dot. Cons: Crime, Deviance and Identity on the Internet*, Willan Publishing, Devon.

Soothill, K. and Sanders, T. (2005) The geographical mobility, preferences and pleasures of prolific punters: a demonstration study of the activities of prostitutes' clients, *Sociological Research Online*, 10 (1), http:///www.socresonline.org.uk/10/1/soothill.html.

Vanwesenbeeck, I., de Graff, R., Van Zessen, G. and Straver, C. (1993) Protection styles of prostitutes' clients: intentions, behaviour and considerations in relation to AIDS, *Journal of Sex Education Theory*, 19: 79–92.

Wellings, K., Field, J., Johnson, A.M., Wadsworth, J. and Bradshaw, S. (1994) *Sexual Behaviour in Britain: The National Survey of Sexual Attitudes and Lifestyles*. Penguin: London.

Wilton, T. (1999) Selling sex, giving care: the construction of AIDS as a workplace hazard. In N. Daykin and L. Doyal (eds), *Health and Work: Critical Perspectives*, Macmillan, London, pp. 180–97.

Wojcicki, J.M. and Malala, J. (2001) Condom use, power and HIV/AIDS risk: sex-workers bargain for survival in Hillbrow/Joubert Park/Berea, Johannesburg, *Social Science & Medicine*, 53: 99–121.

Part III
Researching Health

Introduction

Cathy E. Lloyd

There are numerous ways in which the activities and experiences of all those involved in public health can be researched. Different professional groups, as well as the lay public, carry out research and develop their ideas around health using differing theoretical perspectives, and many different methods and underpinning methodologies. How research is conducted is informed by a range of knowledge and ideas, which impacts on the choice of methods to be employed. The third part of this Reader focuses on research, and how research can be carried out to inform the promotion of public health. The six chapters contained within Part III consider many of these issues from a range of standpoints and theoretical perspectives.

Part III of the Reader starts with a chapter written by Fran Baum, in which she sets out some of the key debates about the methods and methodologies that have been used by those carrying out research in field of public health. Increasingly, the terminology used in public health has been questioned and those people who are usually 'the researched' have begun to challenge how research is carried out and who is involved in that research process. Fran Baum identifies three main types of public health research activity and argues that both what she calls 'eclectic methods' as well as 'general quantitative methods' are appropriate for researching the new public health.

Notwithstanding the current debates around terminology and the overlapping but sometimes conflictual relationship between health promotion and public health, David McQueen, in Chapter 15, highlights one particular aspect of doing research – that of evaluation – and asks 'should health promotion look to classical scientific approaches for evaluation, or is it more appropriate to take a different approach?' He suggests that notions of 'evidence' are complicated by the multidisciplinary nature of health promotion and the current push to base practice on evidence. What that evidence consists of remains problematic but does include both quantitative and qualitative methodologies.

In Chapter 16 Jacqueline Urla and Alan Swedlund take a different aspect of research, that of measurement, and in particular anthropometry, to challenge some of the assumptions which underpin the use of numbers and statistics as 'objective' and hence 'scientific'. They use the 'Barbie' doll, characterised as the ideal of the female figure, to show that the way in which statistical averages can be used is often subjective and often biased. They suggest that Barbie makes a perfect icon of late capitalist constructions of femininity because she appears to achieve both the ideals of being feminine and the ideals of endless consumption. They discuss the way that the widespread use of anthropometry to develop 'average' body sizes for various purposes gradually moved towards the setting of 'desirable' or 'ideal' norms, which were far from being scientific and value-free.

Chapter 17 is by Gayle Letherby, who focuses on the politics and practice of feminist research in health and argues that it is not the methods but rather the way the methods are used which characterises them as feminist. Gayle Letherby highlights the different perspectives of men and women and how these impact on research, and acknowledges the importance of understanding not only the differences between men and women, but also the differences between women themselves. She comes to the conclusion that feminist-informed research is crucial if there is to be a better understanding of the gendered aspects of health.

Differences in health are also the focus of Cathy Lloyd's chapter, where she discusses her experiences of collecting the views of individuals whose main language is not English, and where there may not be a written form of the spoken language. Cathy Lloyd uses the increasing body of diabetes research to highlight the difficulties faced by researchers who want to find out the views of service users, but lack the appropriate tools to do so. Given the increasing prevalence of diabetes, particularly in minority ethnic groups in the UK, this issue has serious public health implications. She demonstrates the importance of involving both the researchers and the researched in the process of collecting data and suggests that this is the key to success in researching health.

Yasmin Gunaratnam's chapter completes Part III of the Reader, and takes the issue of researching ethnicity and health a step further. She questions how research is carried out and whether it is done so in a responsible manner, using three criteria: reinscription, micropolitics and difference. Yasmin Gunaratnam challenges the use of terminology, such as 'minority ethnic', because this ignores the differences of experience within groups. It also obscures the social positions of different groups and the power relationships therein. By problematising terminology such as this it is possible to disrupt and challenge existing social power relations. At the same time she notes how researchers are often caught up between questioning conceptual categories while having to work with these categories in order to secure research funding or engage with the wider debates in health research.

Chapter 14

Dilemmas in Public Health Research: Methodologies and Ethical Practice

Fran Baum

Introduction

This chapter considers recent debates about the nature of public health research. It does this in terms of the methodologies and methods used in public health research and through consideration of ethical issues that have become apparent as lay people have questioned the style and usefulness of public health research.

The term 'public health' can mean different things in different contexts. This chapter accepts a view of public health that has been described as the 'new public health' (Ashton and Seymour, 1988; Baum, 2002). It draws on the conceptualisation provided by a number of key international documents, including the World Health Organisation's series of documents and statements on health promotion (most importantly the *Ottawa Charter for Health Promotion* (WHO, 1986) and also *The People's Charter for Health* (People's Health Movement, 2000). On this basis the following definition of public health guides this chapter:

> The new public health is the totality of the activities organised by societies collectively (primarily led by governments) to protect people from diseases and to promote their health. It seeks to do this in a way that promotes equity between different groups in society. New public health activities occur in all sectors and will include the adoption of policies which support health. They will also ensure that social, physical, economic and natural environments promote health. The new public health is based on a belief that the participation of communities in activities to promote health is as essential to the success of those activities as is the participation of experts. (Baum, 2002: 531)

This broad definition of public health, which sees the associated activities as including sectors across government and society in general, made the need for broader methodological approaches very evident. The mandate to involve lay people in public health activities, including research, has offered a further ethical challenge to public health researchers.

These issues are explored in detail below and the discussion will emphasise that the debates about methodologies and ethics are ongoing and dynamic. Public health research is a rapidly evolving field which promises to continue to be so as the social and economic determinants of health and disease become more widely accepted as crucial in determining the health of populations.

Types of public health research

There are three main types of public health research activity:

1. Determining the causes, distributions, understandings and impact of diseases in populations (this may include immediate causes, such as individual risk factors, and more distal factors, such as environmental, social and economic factors, and cover a range of impacts). The impact and understanding of diseases is most likely to be based on qualitative research and the causes and distributions from quantitative research. These data and knowledge they generate may be used in needs assessment exercises that help determine what public health interventions should be planned and implemented.
2. Evaluations of public health interventions to determine what impact they have and why they have the impacts they do. The interventions may be those targeted at one disease or may be complex community-based initiatives or the evaluation of new policies designed to improve health.
3. Understanding factors that underpin the practice of public health, such as the role of the media, the impact of political economy on health or the impact of culture on public health.

Methodologies

For at least the past twenty years there have been debates within public health about the appropriateness or otherwise of the methods that are used. Up to the mid-1980s epidemiological methods were unquestioningly seen as the gold standard for studying public health problems, with the most robust of the methods in epidemiology's armoury seen as the randomised control trial. Public health research methods courses taught only epidemiology. In the past twenty years this dominance of epidemiological thinking has been increasingly questioned and the value of more diverse methodological approaches and the use of a range of methods have been more widely accepted, although it should be noted that the vast majority of articles in academic public health journals are based on epidemiological methods. This change has been accompanied by a fierce debate about the extent to which public health research should diversify and whether and how methodologies and methods can be mixed and used eclectically. Inevitably, the debates have involved both methodological and epistemological issues, as these are inevitably entwined. My own views on the issue were detailed a decade ago (Baum, 1995) and my view in that paper that good public health research seeks research approaches which will answer questions to guide practice and policy rather than seek methodological purity has stood the test of time. It will be helpful to lay out the features underlying these debates.

Table 14.1   Parameters of the debates over public health research methods

Practice or methodological issue	Traditional public health research	New public health
Underlying paradigm	Postivism	Interactionism/constructivism
Approach to values	Argues for value free	Is explicit about value base, especially pursuit of health equity and social justice
Primary discipline basis	Medical Science	Social Science
Focus of practice	Disease prevention	Health promotion
Understanding of causality	Mono-causation or web of causation, focus on immediate cause	Eco-social framework, including underlying factors
Focus of inquiry	Emphasis on outcome	Emphasis on processes and pathways
Approach to context	Context ignored, control for 'confounding' factors	Research conducted in context and tries to incorporate complexity of interactions within environments

Source: adapted from Baum (1995) & Vega (2005).

Defining the debate

The parameters of the debate over public health methods are shown in Table 14.1. In general, quantitative methods have been associated with the traditional public health approach and eclectic methods with the new public health. However, there is no reason why this should be the case, and this chapter argues that both types of method should be used to provide a research base for the new public health.

Positivism versus interactionism/ constructivism and role of values

... the characterisation of the debate as an irresolvable one between positivism and interpretivism is disingenuous in our view. It is a devise that obscures more than it reveals. (Kelly and Swann, 2004: v)

At least some researchers from both sides of the positivist versus constructivist debate argue that methods cannot be mixed and take a purist line in regard to methods. Epidemiologists tend not to make this argument explicit because their choice of methods has been dominant and they have not had to advocate for their approach. Qualitative researchers have been more prominent in making the argument. Chief among the advocates for a purist approach have been Lincoln and Guba (1985) and Denzin and Lincoln (2003), who see qualitative research as a distinct activity but acknowledge that there are competing paradigms within qualitative research.

Despite the perspectives of purists in this debate, more researchers appear to be accepting the value of mixing methods, selecting research approaches that will answer particular public health research questions (see, for example, Baum, 1995; Popay and Williams, 1996; Dixon-Woods et al., 2004). The chief advantage is that the use of multiple methods enables triangulations between methods (Burgess, 1984) and allows both measurement of the extent of a problem and detailed understanding of the issue. Adopting this eclectic view of methods does not mean ignoring the complex philosophical issues underpinning any research endeavour, whether it is using qualitative or quantitative methods. Rarely do any researchers reflect a consistent philosophical position. More typically, they will draw from a number and shift between perspectives over their career or depending on the task at hand. Given that new public health is grounded in social justice and seeks to change structures that create health inequities, new public health researchers are often most comfortable using a critical perspective. Crotty (1998), drawing on the work of others, summarises the key elements of critical inquiry as:

- recognition that all thought is mediated by power relations that are social and historically rooted
- facts are value laden and reflect ideologies
- the relationship between concept and object is inherently unstable and usually mediated by social relationships, especially those between production and consumption
- language is central to both conscious and unconscious awareness
- certain groups are privileged over others and this leads to oppression which is felt most forcefully when subordinates accept their social status as natural, necessary or inevitable
- research practices are often implicated, albeit unwittingly, in the reproduction of class, race and gender oppression.

These elements are relevant to research practice whether it is drawing on qualitative or quantitative methods. The critical perspective encourages researchers to be reflexive about the role of research in overcoming oppression and the ways in which research practices may be more or less helpful in pursuing a social justice agenda.

Medical and social science

Public health has historically been strongly associated with medicine. Many public health practitioners originally trained as medical doctors. With the advent of the new public health, social scientists have come to play a greater role in public health research. Sociologists, political scientists, economists, anthropologists and psychologists are all represented in public health research communities around the world. While there are still rifts between the medical and social science communities, the divides are less evident than in the past and collaborations more common, possibly driven by the requirements of funding bodies rather than necessarily through a greater understanding. Certainly there are real differences in perspectives between medicine and some social sciences, especially sociology. Sociology is concerned with people located in societies and with the ways in which structural factors affect the behaviours of individuals. Tesh (1988) has argued that biomedical research approaches both reflect and serve to reinforce individualism in public health research. In epidemiology this perspective is reflected by the fact that populations are conceptualised exclusively as groups of individuals who can be aggregated and subjected to analysis without considering the roles of these individuals within work places, communities, schools or other institutions. Tesh points out that epidemiologists are more likely to ask the question 'why do these particular people smoke?' than 'why do large numbers of people continue to smoke?' The first question directs research attention to the psychology and physiology of individual people; the second question to the tobacco culture in which we live. Similarly, Krieger (2000) asks whether we should see race or racism as the public health issue of concern, a distinction driven by a sociological rather than medical concern. A focus on race tends to focus on non-white people as a 'problem'. A focus on racism, by contrast, sees racist attitudes as the cause of health problems.

Focus on disease or health

Traditional public health research and practice focused on preventing particular diseases. Epidemiology was used to reveal patterns of disease and relationships with the immediate causes of the disease, and then public health would institute measures to prevent these causes. Classic examples are the link between polluted water and cholera, smoking tobacco and lung cancer, and between iodine deficiency and goitre. The new public health has argued that public health should be more proactive and also seek to create and promote the conditions that create health. Antonovsky (1996) argues that it is necessary to underpin both public health practice and research with a salutogenic orientation and ask the basic question 'How is health created?' This approach rejects the idea of public health as being about the minimisation of risk factors and sees it as having a wider role in shaping social institutions that affect health. For researchers, this salutogenic orientation issues the challenge of conducting research that moves beyond individuals to that on social constructs, social ecologies and a variety of community and institutional settings. Qualitative research is particularly useful for doing this. Recent developments in the field of social epidemiology (Kawachi and Berkman, 2000) promise to contribute more than traditional epidemiology as they focus on topics such as social and economic roots of health inequities, social capital and networks, and racism and health.

Focus on inquiry and understanding of causality

The metaphor and model for epidemiology has been the web of causation through which epidemiologists have become more and more concerned with modelling complex relationships among risk factors, but still largely ignoring the underlying social and economic factors (Krieger, 1994). More complex explanations of causality require methods that can reach an understanding of issues. Thus an epidemiological survey can demonstrate which groups in the population are most likely to smoke and how heavily they smoke. Qualitative research can then be used to conduct detailed research with the high-smoking groups to determine why they continue to smoke and what meaning smoking has in their lives. Similarly, survey research is able to demonstrate some of the effects of contingent forms of employment on people's health, but qualitative research is able to provide a detailed understanding of the ways in which people perceive the impact and why some people are more resilient to contingent employment than others.

Qualitative research should not only be seen as a means of enhancing epidemiological research. Popay and Williams (1997) distinguish between this use of qualitative research and what they term a 'difference' model, in which qualitative research can contribute to theory building and understanding public health independently of the research generated by other methods. This difference model is particularly useful when exploring complex relationships. Examples might be research which seeks to uncover how people understand the reasons for health inequities or that which is about understanding how Indigenous people interpret and understand health within their culture.

Approach to context

Epidemiological research most typically does not take account of social context. Shy (1997) points out that most epidemiological studies treat race, social class and economic status as potentially confounding factors rather than as potentially causative factors in their own right. He urges epidemiology to understand disease as a 'consequence of how society is organised and behaves, what impacts social and economic forces have on incidence rates, and what community actions will be effective in altering incidence rates' (Shy, 1997: 480). Such an approach requires far more attention to the interactions between individuals and the structures in which they lie. The recent research attention given to health inequities, and especially the questions of whether levels of income inequality within nations is, in and of itself, a determinant of population health, is a good example of the ways in which epidemiology can be used to examine structural factors (Wilkinson, 2005). At a broader level, Kickbusch (2004) has argued that the new global context poses significant challenges for public health research. These concern the need to address the distribution of wealth and power through governance and policy research questions. She comments: 'Public health research will increasingly need to incorporate not only epidemiological evidence but move into compiling new types of evidence related to policy and implementation. This inevitably relates to the analysis of the distribution of power and resources within and between countries and different actors' (Kickbusch, 2004). Obviously such research has to be centrally concerned with context and much of it will use policy analysis and qualitative methods (see Hahn, 1999; Castro and Singer, 2004, for many examples of the application of qualitative anthropological methods).

Ethical public health research practice

There has been increasing focus on ensuring that public health research is more ethical in terms of the ways in which it involves people and responds to the needs of less powerful groups in societies. A prime example of this has been the activities of the Global Forum for Health Research, which has consistently highlighted the 10:90 gap whereby only 10 per cent of worldwide health research funds are allocated to the problems responsible for 90 per cent of the world's burden of disease, which are mainly diseases prevalent in poor countries (Global Forum for Health Research, 2000). Marginalised groups have also argued that even when research has been conducted, it does not lead to health improvement because it ignores the social and economic position of poor people (see, for example, the advocacy of the People's Health Movement (McCoy et al., 2004). Australian Aboriginal people have made this claim very strongly and object to much traditional research on the following grounds:

1   Indigenous people are exploited and treated disrespectfully.
2   Research processes see non-Indigenous researchers and research bodies retain all the power and control.
3   The lack of specified short- and long-term benefits to Indigenous communities and individuals.
4   The misrepresentation of Indigenous societies, cultures and individuals by non-Indigenous academics and professionals.

Such objections led the Australian Health and Medical Health Council to work with Indigenous people to develop ethical guidelines for research (National Health and Medical Research Council, 2003). These guidelines stress the need for researchers to respect Indigenous cultures, to involve people in research and to conduct research that is likely to improve health status. Such an approach to research is reflected in the work of the Australian Co-operative Research Centre in Aboriginal Health (see Box 14.1), which is developing a partnership approach to research controlled by Aboriginal people.

Box 14.1   Australian Co-operative Research Centre in Aboriginal Health

The Co-operative Research Centre for Aboriginal Health (CRCAH) aims to achieve sustained improvement in Aboriginal health through strategic research and development. It is funded by the Australian government and brings together eight universities or research institutions, four industry partners and six associated partners. Aboriginal people control the organisation, with key positions such as CEO, Chair of the Board and Research Director all being filled by Aboriginal people. Australian Aboriginal people have a life expectancy 17 years lower than other Australians. The CRCAH has organised five programmes: comprehensive primary health care, health systems and workforce; chronic disease; healthy skin; social determinants of health; social and emotional well-being.

The CRCAH recognises that much research on Aboriginal health in the past was conducted without Aboriginal involvement and did not address issues that were identified by Aboriginal people as important. The CRCAH is very reflective about the need to develop research, commissioning and funding processes that involve Aboriginal communities and that will result in research that is directly related to improvement in health. This is done through industry and community representation on the Board, annual convocations (at which research priorities are debated and set) and a Research Development Group that includes both researchers and industry representatives. The limitations of traditional scientific peer review have been acknowledged and the CRCAH aims to develop research programmes that are of high quality but avoid undue competition between researchers (see rationale and background in Street, Baum and Anderson, 2006). Research transfer is also a crucial part of the CRCAH's activities (Henry et al., 2002).

For further details and the annual report, see: http://www.crcah.org.au/index.cfm.

Ethical issues have also been very prominent in the increasing moves to develop participatory research practices. These have taken many forms, including popular epidemiology, participatory action research, and the incorporation of lay perspectives into research.

Popular epidemiology

Popular epidemiology has evolved from the environmental justice movement (Novotny, 1994) and involves epidemiologists working with community people in social movements who want to research environmental threats to their health. Two examples highlight the type of work popular epidemiology gives rise to. Sebastian and Hurtig (2005) describe their work in the Ecuadorian Amazon where they worked with peasant movements and environment groups to research the impact of the oil industry on people's health. Local organisations set the agenda of the research, were involved in formulating an hypothesis, consulted during the study and then took responsibility for the dissemination of the findings and lobbying on the basis of them. Potts (2004) describes a similar experience in terms of the breast cancer movement, which has forced a focus on the potential environmental causes of breast cancer rather than individual risk and genetic susceptibility which have been the dominant discourse of breast cancer risk. She sees that the movement has forced attention on the role of factors outside the individual by examining patterns of cancer in relation to potential carcinogenic agents.

Thus popular epidemiology is responding to the criticism of epidemiology as having become divorced from public health practice and policy (Beaglehole and Bonita, 2004) and to the charges that epidemiology is only concerned with individual risk factors.

Participatory action research

Participatory action research (PAR) seeks to understand and improve the world by changing it so it is particularly suited to public health. It is also known as community-based participatory research (Minkler and Wallerstein, 2003). At its heart is collective, self-reflective inquiry that researchers and participants undertake, so they can understand and improve upon the practices in which they participate and the situations in which they find themselves. The reflective process is directly linked to action, influenced by an understanding of history, culture and local context, and is embedded in social relationships. The process of PAR should be empowering and lead to people having increased control over their lives (from Baum et al., 2006, adapted from Minkler and Wallerstein, 2003 and Grbich, 1999). PAR is not linked specifically to either qualitative or quantitative research and may involve both. It is an approach to research. PAR has been used in public health to tackle complex public health problems, including research with homeless people, drug users, exploited workers, environmental justice, minority groups such as migrants, and transgendered people (see Minkler and Wallerstein (2003) for preceding examples), work with an Aboriginal men's group and Aboriginal health workers (Hecker, 1997), and by the bus riders union in Vancouver, Canada (Chan et al., 2005). This latter report is an excellent example of research driven by bus users which considers racism, health and social justice in relation to transport, and which aims to protect and improve public transport systems based on focus-group and other qualitative methods.

Lay perspective in public health research

It is increasingly common to find lay perspectives incorporated into public health research. Popay and Williams (1996) argue strongly that both professional and lay knowledge can make contributions to understanding and that both are important to furthering public health. A good example of the value of lay knowledge comes from MacDougall and colleagues' (2004) research with children to discover their thoughts about exercise and fitness. Using focus groups, they found that children did not relate to the idea of exercise – it was seen as an adult concept. Children instead found the concept of play as more compelling. This insight was used to inform a health promotion campaign to encourage children to be active by focusing on play rather than exercise.

Conclusion

This chapter has described the changing nature of public health research, from an almost exclusive reliance on epidemiological methods to the contemporary situation where researchers are more reflective and eclectic in their choice of methods. A critical approach to research and research practice has been promoted in the chapter as most appropriate to a new public health that is concerned with both disease prevention and the positive promotion of health, and which recognises as central the environmental, social and economic determinants of health.

The chapter also examined the increasing tendency for public health research to be conducted in a participatory manner. This participation may result from the frustrations of groups such as Indigenous peoples or those active in social movements with the failure of traditional research approaches to respond to their health issues and concerns.

In the 21st century the public health challenges we face are perhaps the greatest ever. They include new infectious diseases, environmental degradation and a rapidly progressing economic globalisation that is increasing inequities (Baum, 2002; Beaglehole and Bonita, 2004). The public health research community needs to build upon the progress it has made in making its research effort more relevant to complex health problems, more able to deal with complex social and economic situations in which public health problems occur, and more open to involvement from people whose lives are most affected by public health problems. In this way public health research can contribute to a healthier and more socially just future.

References

Antonovsky, A. (1996) The Salutogenic model as a theory to guide health promotion, *Health Promotion International*, 11 (1): 11–18.

Ashton, J. and Seymour, H. (1988) *The New Public Health*. Milton Keynes: Open University Press.

Baum, F. (1995) Researching public health: behind the qualitative–quantitative methodological debate, *Social Science and Medicine*, 40 (4): 459–68.

Baum, F. (2002) *The New Public Health* (2nd edn). Melbourne: Oxford University Press.

Baum. F., MacDougall, C. and Smith, D. (2006) Participatatory action research glossary, *Journal of Epidemiology and Community Health*, forthcoming.

Beaglehole, R. and Bonita, R. (2004) *Public Health at the Crossroads* (2nd edn). Cambridge: Cambridge University Press.

Burgess, R.G. (1984) *In the Field: an Introduction to Field Research*. London: Allen & Unwin.

Castro, A. and Singer, M. (eds) (2004) *Unhealthy Health Policy: a Critical Anthropological Examination*. Walnut Creek, CA: Altamira Press.

Chan, Z., Grayer, B., Efting, J., Jones, H., Kaur, K. and Roberts, M. (2005) *Women in Transit: Organising Social Justice in our Communities*. (2nd edn). Vancouver: Bus Riders Union.

Crotty, M. (1998) *The Foundations of Social Research: Meaning and Perspective in the Research Process*. St Leonards, NSW: Allen & Unwin.

Denzin, N.K. and Lincoln, Y.S. (2003) *The Landscape of Qualitative Research*. Thousand Oaks, CA: Sage.

Dixon-Woods, M., Agarwal, S., Young, B., Jones, D. and Sutton, A. (2004) *Integrative Approaches to Qualitative and Quantitative Evidence*. London: Health Development Agency.

Global Forum for Health Research (2000) *The 10/90 Report on Health Research 2000*. Geneva: Global Forum for Health Research. Available at: http://www.globalforumhealth.ch/report.htm.

Grbich C. (1999) *Qualitative Research in Health: an Introduction.* St Leonards, NSW: Allen & Unwin.

Hahn, R.A. (1999) *Anthropology and Public Health: Bridging Difference in Culture and Society.* New York: Oxford University Press.

Hecker R.(1997) Participatory action research as a strategy for empowering Aboriginal health workers, *Australia and New Zealand Journal of Public Health*, 21 (7): 784–8.

Henry, J., Dunbar, T., Arnott, A., Scrimgeour, M., Matthews, S., Murakami-Gold, L. and Chamberlain, A. (2002) *Indigenous Research Reform Agenda: Rethinking Research Methodologies.* Darwin: Cooperative Research Centre for Aboriginal and Tropical Health.

Kawachi, I. and Berkman, L.F. (2000) *Social Epidemiology.* New York: Oxford Unviersity Press.

Kelly, M. and Swann, C. (2004) Foreword. In Dixon-Woods, M., Agarwal, S., Young, B., Jones, D. and Sutton, A. (eds), *Integrative Approaches to Qualitative and Quantitative Evidence.* London: Health Development Agency.

Kickbusch, I. (2004) Public health in the 21st century and the role of health research. Plenary Presentation presented at the Global Forum for Health Research, Mexico City, November 2004. Available at: http://www.globalforumhealth.org/Forum8/Forum8-CDROM/OralPresentations/Kickbusch%20I.doc (accessed 4 January 2006).

Krieger, N. (1994) Epidemiology and the web of causation: has anyone seen the spider?, *Social Science and Medicine*, 39 (7): 887–903.

Krieger, N. (2000) Passionate epistemology, critical advocacy and public health: doing our profession proud, *Critical Public Health*, 10 (3): 287–94.

Lincoln, Y.S. and Guba, E.G. (1985) *Naturalistic Inquiry.* Beverly Hills, CA: Sage.

McCoy, D., Sanders, D., Baum, F., Nararyan, T. and Legge, D. (2004) Pushing the international health research agenda towards equity and effectiveness, *The Lancet*, 364: 1630–1.

MacDougall, C., Schiller, W. and Darbyshire, P. (2004) We have to live in the future. In Schiller, W. (ed.), *Research at the Edge: Concepts and Challenges.* Special Issue: Early Child Development and Care, 174 (4): 369–88.

Minkler, M. and Wallerstein, N. (eds) (2003) *Community-based Participatory Research for Health.* San Francisco: Jossey-Bass.

National Health and Medical Research Council (2003) *Values and Ethics Guidelines for the Ethical Conduct in Aboriginal and Torres Strait Islander Research.* Canberra: NHMRC.

Novotny, P. (1994) Popular epidemiology and the struggle for community health: alternative perspectives from the environmental justice movement, *Capitalism, Nature and Socialism*, 5 (2): 29–42.

People's Health Movement (2000) *The People's Charter for Health.* Available at: http://phmovement.org/charter/pch-index.html (accessed 5 January 2006).

Popay, J. and Williams, G. (1996) Public health research and lay knowledge, *Social Science and Medicine*, 42 (5): 759–68.

Popay, J. and Williams, G. (1997) Qualitative research and evidence-based healthcare, *Journal of the Royal Society of Medicine*, 91 Supplement 35: 32–7.

Potts, L.K. (2004) An epidemiology of women's lives: the environmental risk of breast cancer, *Critical Public Health*, 14 (2): 133–47.

Sebastian, M.S. and Hurtig, A.K. (2005) Oil development and health in the Amazon basin of Ecuador: the popular epidemiology process, *Social Science and Medicine*, 60: 799–807.

Shy, C.M. (1997) The failure of academic epidemiology: witness for the prosecution, *American Journal of Epidemiology*, 145 (6): 479–84.

Street, J., Baum, F. and Anderson, I. (2006) *Quality Assessment of Research*, Research Monograph Series. Darwin: Co-operative Research Centre in Aboriginal Health.

Tesh, S. (1988) *Hidden Arguments: Political Ideology and Disease Prevention Policy.* New Brunswick, NJ: Rutgers University Press.

Vega, J. (2005) The Commission's focus: preliminary selection of scoial determinants to be examined. Presentaion made to Commision on Social Determinants of Health, Santiago, Chile, March 2005. Geneva: WHO.

Wilkinson, R. (2005) *The Impact of Inequality: How To Make Sick Societies Healthier.* London: Routledge.

World Health Organisation (1986) *Ottawa Charter for Health Promotion. Health Promotion*, 1 (4): i–v. Geneva: WHO.

Chapter 15

The Evaluation of Health Promotion Practice: 21st Century Debates on Evidence and Effectiveness

David V. McQueen

Introduction

The field of health promotion prides itself on being eclectic and multidisciplinary. It is the great strength of the field that it cuts across sectors, cuts across disciplines, and values pragmatism. Multiple approaches to improve health, re-orient healthcare systems, and empower people are welcomed (WHO, 1984). Many of the principal activities of health promotion pertain to advocacy, partnerships and coalition building, areas considered more an art than a science. Therefore, it may be asserted that health promotion is a field of action, highly applied, and having few characteristics of a discipline. Furthermore, it is relatively new as a concerted field of action, and is still defining its terms; for example, the word 'evidence' does not appear in the *WHO Health Promotion Glossary* (World Health Organization, 1998). Nevertheless, it may also be argued that the field is quite well established in some dimensions. There are foundations, centres, institutes, schools, departments, buildings, professorships and programmes named with the term 'health promotion'. Thus health promotion presents a dilemma with regard to the evidence debate. Should health promotion look to classical scientific approaches for evaluation or is it more appropriate to take a very different approach?

Recognizing this dilemma, one may consider the successful evaluation of health promotion practice on other terms, for example the terms of individual academic disciplines rather than on terms yet to be well articulated by the multidisciplinary field of health promotion practice. This is not necessarily a bad thing. Many people who work in health promotion, especially those who need to be convinced of its importance and effectiveness, are discipline based. Thus there is a good rationale for respecting the 'rules of evidence' put forward by scientists working in public health when making the case for the effectiveness of health promotion. At the same time, there is the need to respect and assist in the development of health promotion's own efforts to define the field of evaluation in health promotion.

The terms 'evidence' and 'evidence-based' are regularly invoked in health promotion discussions. Why should this be so? A partial answer may be that evidence has become common currency in population health discussions as well as in discussions of the evaluation of everyday medical practice, particularly preventive practice. Thus, in the West, a sociopolitical climate has permitted a discussion to flower, with emphasis on healthcare evaluation as one major element. Activity has been widespread.

Defining health promotion itself remains enigmatic, partly because of its historical development and close ties to the field of public health. Both public health and health promotion have been theoretically weak and practically strong. They share the constant challenges of whether they should focus on the individual or the social context or some combination of the two. They share the ongoing debate of how much they are rooted in the biomedical or in the social/behavioural sciences. The outstanding feature that would distinguish health promotion from public health is the stronger foundation of theory and practice based on the social sciences. Nevertheless, the development of health promotion is closely tied to the historical and theoretical development of public health.

As always, any attempt to provide a firm definition of a phenomenon such as health promotion is suspect and inadequate. As it developed in the last third of the 20th century health promotion took on different perspectives on the continent and in North America, notably the USA. On the continent, health promotion was largely framed by concerns with social, economic and political roots of health and offered a strong focus on the sociopolitical environment as the place for health promotion action. In the USA, health promotion was framed largely by the enlargement of the traditional scope of health education, an area of work that was quite well developed in the States and well established in the academic sector. Given its roots in education and educational psychology, it was no surprise that the primary focus of health promotion action should be on the individual and on changing attitudes, opinions, beliefs and behaviours. Whether or not modern health promotion, that is the health promotion practised now, has fully integrated these two traditions remains the subject of historical analysis and not of this chapter. Nonetheless, these two traditions will and do influence the meaning and scope of evaluation and evidence in health promotion. Thus any complete definition of health promotion must incorporate these diverse perspectives.

Defining health promotion precisely relates to the need for health promotion to prove its utility to both the sceptics and those who support the rhetoric of health promotion; thus the rise of the 'evidence' question, or what I have termed elsewhere the 'evidence debate' (McQueen, 2002). In the 1990s the evidence-based medicine discussion was extended to both health promotion and community-based public health interventions. The assumption is that this is a critical debate, that it is necessary to demonstrate what constitutes evidence and proof that actions are effective. Although the terms of the debate stem from clinical medicine rather than preventive medicine, the application of evidence criteria has taken evaluation down a path implying scientific rigour and justification.

Organized efforts to discover evidence of effectiveness

In the USA, the Centers for Disease Control and Prevention (CDC) has taken the lead in assisting an independent Task Force to produce a *Guide to Community Preventive Services* (see http://www.health.gov/communityguide for the Community Guide). The *Guide* defines, categorizes, summarizes, and rates the quality of evidence on the effectiveness of population-based interventions and their impact on specific outcomes. The *Guide* summarizes what is known about the effectiveness and cost-effectiveness of population-based interventions for prevention and control, provides recommendations on these interventions and methods for their delivery based on the evidence, and identifies a research agenda. This effort is an example of an approach that takes a strong biomedical/epidemiological definition of evidence (Zaza et al., 2005). The reader should note the introduction of the term 'effectiveness' at this point. This emerging vocabulary around what has been termed the 'evidence debate' will be discussed later.

What is noteworthy about the *Guide*'s work is the time and effort that have gone into defining evidence in terms of how interventions are designed (SAJPM, 2000). What this effort has revealed is that finding evidence of health promotion effectiveness is not an easy task. Indeed, the scope and size of the task taken on by the *Guide* are huge. There are some 20 members of the Task Force, chosen because of their broad knowledge of public health, preventive medicine, and health promotion. They are an independent body with representatives from local health departments, health care organizations, NGOs, and universities. In addition, five consultants are attached to the Task Force. The Task Force is supported at CDC by a staff of senior researchers, research assistants and administrative workers, 14 federal agency liaison members, 17 organization liaison members, and 14 liaison representatives of the CDC offices, institutes and centers. The author of this chapter has served as a senior adviser since its inception. The point is that to systematically explore and find evidence of effectiveness is a formidable task.

In the reviews of evidence regarding interventions, hundreds of studies are reviewed, evaluated and examined by a team of many abstractors using a lengthy, detailed and rigorous evaluation form. Even so, this search for evidence has been limited to published literature accessible to data retrieval systems such as MEDLINE, Embase, Psychlit, CAB Health, and Sociological Abstracts. Furthermore, generally only publications written in English, published since 1979, and conducted in industrialized countries, and studies that met the evidence criteria laid out by the *Guide* team (SAJPM, 2000) are considered. This is not to criticize the effort, but rather to emphasize that even a large-scale project has necessary limitations and has to define its parameters.

European efforts: the IUHPE report to the European Commission

An approach to evidence more rooted in health promotion was that taken by the International Union for Health Promotion and Education (IUHPE). An advisory group, consisting of 13 senior people in the health promotion field, 15 authors and a 'witness group' of some 25 'political experts', produced a report for the European Commission (EC) on the evidence of health promotion effectiveness (IUHPE, 1999). The great value of this report, which should be required reading for those interested in the field of health promotion, is that it identifies a considerable body of evidence pointing to the value of health promotion and attesting to its effectiveness. The report was also clear to map out those areas where more research was needed and areas that were open to debate about effectiveness, as well as those areas where health promotion actions have made a difference. Some areas of health promotion activity stand out as unquestionably of powerful value. For example, there is evidence of a strong inverse relationship between price and use of tobacco. Therefore, health promoting efforts that lead to price increases of tobacco should lead to less use of tobacco. This finding mirrors that from the CDC group working on tobacco for the community *Guide*. Thus there is an accumulating international evidence base for global efforts to reduce tobacco consumption through pricing.

Health promoting efforts with regard to tobacco control appear as the 'strong case' in the evidence debate. Other areas of health promotion activity, however, require careful thought and further analysis to reveal effectiveness. For example, transportation policies impact on health in many ways. However, demonstrating the efficacy of such policies is difficult. In this case complexity begins to play a major role. While many may believe that there is a highly probable association between transportation policy and the general health of a population, the evidence mechanisms to prove any scientific basis for this belief still need refinement. The derived standard is to develop as a first step a distinctive logic model or logic framework showing the causal links of each area of a health promotion intervention to an outcome. This logic model helps map out the links between social, environmental and biological determinants and related interventions. These models then serve as a guide for assessing where the evidence challenges are. The challenge is for the model to lead to an understanding of apparently true relationships, such as that between transport policy and health.

Despite all the difficulties with the notion of evidence, the writers of the EC report concluded that:

> ... evidence clearly indicates that: 1) comprehensive approaches using all five Ottawa strategies are the most effective; 2) certain 'settings' such as schools, workplaces, cities and local communities offer practical opportunities for effective health promotion; 3) people, including those most affected by health issues, need to be at the heart of health promotion action programmes and decision making processes to ensure real effectiveness; 4) real access to information and education, in appropriate language and styles, is vital; and 5) health promotion is a key 'investment' – an essential element of social and economic development. (IUHPE, 1999)

Other efforts: past and ongoing

The two concerted efforts to look at health promotion evidence and effectiveness highlighted above are exemplary, but they are hardly the whole picture. Other important contributions that have emerged are the Cochrane Collaboration on health promotion field work (Doyle et al., 2005), the EURO working group on health promotion evaluation (Rootman et al., 2000), and the ongoing work of the IUHPE Global Programme on Health Promotion Effectiveness (Jones and McQueen, 2005). And there are many other important efforts by Ministries of Health as well as private health promotion foundations. The reader who wishes a fuller understanding should look in detail at each of the efforts for further insight into the nature of the search for evidence of effectiveness in health promotion.

Issues arising in the 'evidence debate'

More than anything the evidence debate has served to illustrate the need for a stronger theoretical base for health promotion. The debate has made explicit theoretical notions such as contextualism. More than ever health promoters are aware of the social and cultural context in which they carry out their work. This awareness applies at all levels of society. At the local level they are sensitized to local needs and public understandings of health. At the global level they recognize the incredible diversity of nations in terms of development, cultural beliefs, and governance. Despite this accepted awareness of the great diversity in populations, some may still hold the belief that the evidence discussion is not affected by the contextual diversity.

Given the lack of a strong theoretical base, health promotion practice has been and remains difficult to define. The field of practice seems eclectic, encompassing many approaches from a wide range of research perspectives. Every approach seems relevant: policy research, evaluation research, survey research, action research, and social epidemiology. Many concerned with health promotion practice might disagree on the relative importance of the major areas for health promotion, but most would agree that there are critical issues with regard to the following areas:

1 theories and concepts in the field;
2 methodology and the whole issue of the 'style' of research which is appropriate to practice; and
3 issues of application of findings, with an emphasis on translation of research and practice into something useful and oftentimes for the formation of policy.

Methodology remains a critical issue for research and practice in health promotion and directly relates to the evaluation of evidence. Even as the methods used in health promotion have ranged from the qualitative to the quantitative, there is still unease as to what is appropriate. Despite its apparent implausibility as a methodological approach suitable to health promotion, the RCT, or randomized clinical trial, remains for many who would term themselves health promoters as an ideal to which health promotion research should aspire because it is seen as the most powerful method to use in evaluating interventions. The lingering power of the RCT is witnessed in numerous debates at health promotion meetings for its application. Despite forceful arguments to the contrary by leaders in health promotion evaluation, the RCT remains the bulwark for many public health practitioners who are either highly sympathetic to health promotion or would even classify themselves as health promoters. When control of the setting and population under study can be achieved for the time of the trial, and where there is a focus on a single intervention with an expected dichotomous outcome of success or failure, the RCT is indeed a powerful methodology, and there are those who argue fiercely that the RCT or a modified version thereof can be developed for health promotion. Thus the postmodern separation implied by the rejection of a model like the RCT has not impacted on these researchers and practitioners.

Nevertheless, the strength of the RCT is directly related to rigidly meeting the restrictive assumptions of experimental design. When the severe restrictions of experimental design are not met, the utility, validity and power of the RCT diminish rapidly. The misapplication of the RCT in health promotion research is now legend (Rootman et al., 2000). Even if one rejects the strictest classical RCT model, the notions of experimental and control groups remain in studies and projects which use quasi-experimental designs, controls, and all the trappings of the RCT. Unfortunately, for many at the so-called hard end of the hard to soft science spectrum, a 'softer' health promotion methodology seems implausible. In health promotion interventions, control and experimental populations are often unlikely, if not impossible. It is part of the very nature of health promotion interventions that they operate in everyday life situations, in a particular context, involving changing aspects of the intervention; outcomes are often decidedly different from expectations; unanticipated consequences of interventions are common and sometimes better than expected outcomes.

The growth of tradition and ideology

Over the years different orientations towards health promotion have developed in the research and practice community, stemming from perspectives of public health. Roughly speaking, a dichotomy exists between two traditions which could be termed 'medical public health' and 'social public health'. These two traditions are not necessarily in conflict, but they often give rise to differing interpretations of the underlying mission of public health which in turn affects the evidence debate. Essentially, medical public health regards epidemiology as the basic science of public health with a view of causation that is linear. This perspective relies heavily on 'evidence' gathered by methodological approaches which feature experimental designs. In addition there is usually a stress on the individual as the focus of public health programmes with the goal to influence changes in behaviour. In contrast, a 'social public health' considers many disciplines to be relevant and places emphasis on the human sciences, such as sociology, politics and economics. Causation is not regarded as necessarily linear, with patterns of change and complexity as expected outcomes of interventions.

Health promotion fits historically with both of these public health traditions. However, health promotion has in addition an underlying ideology that drives its distinctiveness. Elsewhere I have argued for an ethos of health promotion which helps define the nature of the field (McQueen, 1996). This ethos is manifested through a debate primarily on methodology, but seldom on theory. This ethos also helps to shape the evidence debate. This 'ethos' in health promotion has research consequences: there is less emphasis on sophistication in quantitative analyses, and more on qualitative approaches. Further, the ethos was increasingly framed in postmodern terminology, for example one position is that sophistication in data analysis may have the effect of providing detail too elaborate or inscrutable for the general needs and use of community health workers and policy makers, introducing the paradox that some of the key notions, such as dynamism, multidisciplinarity, complexity and context, might demand rather innovative and complex data collection procedures and analyses, whether quantitative or qualitative. This ethos helped reform the evidence debate.

Evidence of health promotion effectiveness: issues

Few topics in the field of health promotion have engendered as much heated debate as that of evidence. The importance of evidence as a topic for health promotion practice should be seen in a larger context of discussions on evidence-based medicine taking place in much of the world, a debate which cannot be dismissed as pertinent only to medicine. Health promotion is also challenged by the debate (Adrian et al., 1994; Allison and Rootman, 1996; MacDonald et al., 1996; Nutbeam, 1998, Sackett et al., 1996). Today, health promotion practitioners and researchers are urged to base their work on evidence. In May 1998, the 51st World Health Assembly urged all Member States to 'adopt an evidence-based approach to health promotion policy and practice, using the full range of quantitative and qualitative methodologies' (WHO, 1998).

Notions such as 'evidence', 'effectiveness', 'investment' are rightly viewed as Western-derived, European-American, and in many ways European language concepts. Most of those who have written and write about evidence have Western approaches and Western training. These concepts and the biases inherent in them developed largely out of philosophical conjectures of the past two centuries, notably from debates around logical positivism (Bhaskar, 1997; Suppe, 1977). Logical positivism operates on the tenet that meaning is only verifiable through rigorous observation and experiment. In this context, the word 'evidence' has a very strict analytic meaning. Similarly, the randomized controlled clinical trial (RCT) and the quasi-experimental approach are largely creations of a Western literature and reflect a reification of the positivist notion. Many social sciences, particularly anthropology and sociology, have alternative, but none the less Western-derived approaches to assessing evidence and the effectiveness of interventions.

If there are alternative approaches to the issues of evidence from developing countries, they are less readily accessible even on the global Internet. Yet, the Internet is a hope for the future once access to it becomes more readily available globally. Nevertheless there is another consideration; that is the urgency of emerging public health problems outside the West. We may not have the luxury or time to develop alternative approaches before the problems being faced significantly develop.

Should health promotion programmes in the developing world simply proceed with the assumption that they will use approaches that have been shown to meet evidence criteria drawn up in the West? Should there be caution in accepting a Western-based evidence criterion for health promotion? Can developing countries in their search for best practice offer better guidance on how best to evaluate programmes with minimal resources? Would other approaches be useful and/or transportable to those many Western countries with great inequities in population health? Addressing these questions is not easy, but they need to be recognized as legitimate concerns.

While the evidence debate in the West has been prolific, voices from developing countries are still missing from the debate. This lack of developing country participation is exacerbated by a debate that has been mainly conducted in the English language by those educated in a European-American context. Furthermore, the debate has been largely dominated by a privileged academic elite. The debate must find a way to uncover approaches used by developing nations that are meaningful and these must be incorporated into the existing body of the 'evidence debate'. However, the mechanism for this remains very unclear and one can even question the legitimacy of such an elite positing an appropriate mechanism for inclusion in the debate.

References

Adrian, M., Layner, N. and Moreau, J. (1994) Can life expectancies be used to determine if health promotion works? *American Journal of Health Promotion*, 8 (6): 449–61.

Allison, K. and Rootman, I. (1996) Scientific rigor and community participation in health promotion research: are they compatible? *Health Promotion International*, 11 (4): 333–40.

Bhaskar, R. (1997) *A Realist Theory of Science*. 2nd edn. New York: Verso.

Doyle, J., Waters, E., Yach, D., McQueen, D., De Francisco, A., Stewart, T., Reddy, P., Gulmezoglu, A.M., Galea, G. and Portela, A. (2005) Global priority setting for Cochrane systematic reviews of health promotion and public health research, *Journal of Epidemiology and Community Health*, 59: 193–7.

IUHPE (1999) The evidence of health promotion effectiveness: a report for the European Commission by the International Union for Health Promotion and Education. Brussels–Luxembourg: ECSC–EC–EAEC.

Jones, C. and McQueen, D. (2005) The European region's contribution to the global programme on health promotion effectiveness (GPHPE). *Promotion and Education*, Supplement 1: 9–10.

MacDonald, G. et al. (1996) Evidence for success in health promotion: suggestions for improvement. In Leathar, D. (ed.), *Health Education Research: Theory and Practice*, 11 (3): 367–76.

McQueen, D.V. (1996) The search for theory in health behaviour and health promotion, *Health Promotion International*, 11: 27–32.

McQueen, D.V. (2002) The evidence debate, invited editorial in *Journal of Epidemiology and Community Health*, 56: 83–4.

Nutbeam, D. (1998) Evaluating health promotion – progress, problems, and solutions, *Health Promotion International*, 13 (1): 27–44.

Rootman, I., Goodstadt, M., McQueen, D., Potvin, L., Springett, J. and Ziglio, E. (eds) (2000). *Evaluation in Health Promotion: Principles and Perspectives*. Copenhagen: World Health Organization Regional Office for Europe.

Sackett, D.L., Rosenberg, W.M.C., Muir Gray, J.A., Haynes, R.B. and Richardson, W.S. (1996) Evidence-based medicine: what it is and what it isn't, *British Medical Journal*, 312: 71–2.

SAJPM (Supplement to American Journal of Preventive Medicine) (January 2000) Introducing the *Guide to Community Preventive Services*: methods, first recommendations and expert commentary, *American Journal of Preventive Medicine*, 18 (1).

Suppe, F. (ed.) (1977) *The Structure of Scientific Theories*. 2nd edn. Urbana, IL: University of Illinois Press.

World Health Assembly (1998) *Resolution WHA 51.12 on Health Promotion*. Agenda Item 20, 16 May 1998. Geneva: WHO.

World Health Organization (1984) Health Promotion: concepts and principles. Report of a working group, available online at http://whqlibdoc.who.int/euro/-1993/ICP_HSR_602_m01.pdf

World Health Organisation (1998) *WHO Health Promotion Glossary*. Geneva: WHO.

Zaza, S., Briss, P. and Harris, K. (2005). *The Guide to Community Preventive Services*. Oxford: Oxford University Press.

Chapter 16

The Anthropometry of Barbie: Unsettling Ideals of the Feminine Body in Popular Culture

Jacqueline Urla and Alan C. Swedlund

It is no secret that thousands of healthy women in the United States perceive their bodies as defective. The signs are everywhere: from potentially lethal cosmetic surgery and drugs to the more familiar routines of dieting, curling, crimping, and aerobicizing, women seek to take control over their unruly physical selves. [...]

It is this conundrum of somatic femininity, that female bodies are never feminine enough, that they must be deliberately and oftentimes painfully remade to be what 'nature' intended – a condition dramatically accentuated under consumer capitalism – that motivates us to focus our inquiry into deviant bodies on images of the feminine ideal. Neither universal nor changeless, idealized notions of both masculine and feminine bodies have a long history that shifts considerably across time, racial or ethnic group, class, and culture. Body ideals in twentieth-century North America are influenced and shaped by images from classical or 'high' art, the discourses of science and medicine, and increasingly via a multitude of commercial interests, ranging from mundane life insurance standards to the more high-profile fashion, fitness, and entertainment industries. Each have played contributing, and sometimes conflicting, roles in determining what will count as a desirable body in the late-twentieth-century United States. In this chapter, we focus our attention on the domain of popular culture and the ideal feminine body as it is conveyed by one of pop culture's longest lasting and most illustrious icons: the Barbie doll. [...]

We begin by tracing Barbie's origins and some of the image makeovers she has undergone since her creation. From there we turn to an experiment in the anthropometry of

---

Edited from: Urla, J. and Swedland, A.C. (1998) The anthropometry of Barbie: unsettling ideals of the feminine body in popular culture, in J. Terry and J. Urla (eds), *Deviant Bodies: Critical Perspectives and Popular Culture*. Bloomington, IN: Indiana University Press, pp. 277–313. Reproduced with permission from the authors.

Barbie to understand how she compares to standards for the 'average American woman' that were emerging in the postwar period. Not surprisingly, our measurements show Barbie's body to be thin – very thin – far from anything approaching the norm. Inundated as our society is with conflicting and exaggerated images of the feminine body, statistical measures can help us to see that exaggeration more clearly. But we cannot stop there. As our brief foray into the history of anthropometry shows, the measurement and creation of body averages have their own politically inflected and culturally biased histories. Standards for the 'average' American body, male or female, have always been imbricated in histories of nationalism and race purity. [...]

A doll is born

[...] Marketed as the first 'teenage' fashion doll, Barbie's rise in popularity also coincided with, and no doubt contributed to, the postwar creation of a distinctive teenage lifestyle. Teens, their tastes, and their behaviors were becoming the object of both sociologists and criminologists as well as market survey researchers intent on capturing their discretionary dollars. [...]

Every former Barbie owner knows that to buy a Barbie is to lust after Barbie accessories – that pair of sandals and matching handbag, canopy bedroom set, or country camper. Both conspicuous consumer and a consumable item herself, Barbie surely was as much the fantasy of US retailers as she was the panacea of middle-class parents. For every 'need' Barbie had, there was a deliciously miniature product to fulfil it. [...]

Perhaps what makes Barbie such a perfect icon of late capitalist constructions of femininity is the way in which her persona pairs endless consumption with the achievement of femininity and the appearance of an appropriately gendered body. [...] Little girls learn, among other things, about the crucial importance of their appearance to their personal happiness and to their ability to gain favor with their friends. Barbie's social calendar is constantly full, and the stories in her fan magazines show her frequently engaged in preparation for the rituals of heterosexual teenage life: dates, proms, and weddings. A perusal of Barbie magazines, and the product advertisements and pictorials within them, shows an overwhelming preoccupation with grooming for those events. Magazines abound with tips on the proper ways of washing hair, putting on makeup, and assembling stunning wardrobes. Through these play scenarios, little girls learn about [...] the importance of hygiene, occasion-specific clothing, knowledgeable buying, and artful display as key elements to popularity and a successful career in femininity.

Barbie exemplifies the way in which gender in the late twentieth century has become a commodity itself, 'something we can buy into ... the same way we buy into a style' (Willis, 1991: 23). In her insightful analysis of the logics of consumer capitalism, cultural critic Susan Willis pays particular attention to the way in which children's toys like Barbie and the popular muscle-bound 'He-Man' for boys link highly conservative and narrowed images of masculinity and femininity with commodity consumption (1991: 27). In the imaginary world of Barbie and teen advertising, observes Willis, being or becoming a teenager, having a 'grown-up' body, is inextricably bound up with the acquisition of certain commodities, signalled by styles of clothing, cars, music, etc. [...]

Barbie is a survivor

[...] As the women's movement gained strength in the seventies, the media and popular culture felt the impact of a growing self-consciousness about sexist imagery of women. The toy industry was no exception. Barbie, the ever-beautiful bride-to-be, became a target of some criticism and concern for parents who worried about the effects such a toy would have on their daughters. Barbie buffs like BillyBoy describe the seventies as the doll's dark decade, a time when sales dipped, quality worsened as production was transferred from Japan to Taiwan, and Barbie was lampooned in the press (BillyBoy, 1987). Mattel responded by trying to give Barbie a more diversified wardrobe and a more 'now' image. A glance at Barbie's résumé, published in *Harper's* magazine in August 1990, while incomplete, shows Mattel's attempt to expand Barbie's career options beyond the original fashion model:

	Positions Held
1959–present	Fashion model
1961–present	Ballerina
1961–64	Stewardess (American Airlines)
1964	Candy striper
1965	Teacher
1965	Fashion editor
1966	Stewardess (Pan Am)
1973–75	Flight attendant (American Airlines)
1973–present	Medical doctor
1976	Olympic athlete
1984	Aerobics instructor
1985	TV news reporter
1985	Fashion designer
1985	Corporate executive
1988	Perfume designer
1989–present	Animal rights volunteer

It is only fitting, given her origin, to note that Barbie has also had a career in the military and aeronautics space industry: she has been an astronaut, a marine, and, during the Gulf War, a Desert Storm trooper. Going from pink to green, Barbie has also acquired a social conscience, taking up the causes of UNICEF, animal rights, and environmental protection. [...] Despite their efforts to dodge criticism and present Barbie as a liberated woman, it is clear that glitz and glamour are at the heart of the Barbie doll fantasy. Motz reports, for example, that in 1963 only one out of sixty-four outfits on the market was job-related. There is no doubt that Barbie has had her day as astronaut, doctor, rock star, and even presidential candidate. She can be anything she wishes to be. [...]

For anyone tracking Barbiana, it is abundantly clear that Mattel's marketing strategies are sensitive to a changing social climate. Just as Mattel has sought to present Barbie as a career woman with more than air in her vinyl head, they have also tried to diversify her otherwise lily-white suburban world. About the same time that Martin Luther King was assassinated and Detroit and Watts were burning in some of the worst race riots of the century, Barbie acquired her first black friend. 'Colored Francie' appeared in 1967, failed, and was replaced the following year with Christie, who also did not do terribly well on the market. In 1980, Mattel went on to introduce Black Barbie, the first doll with Afro style hair. She, too, appears to have suffered from a low advertising profile and low sales (Jones, 1991). Nevertheless, the eighties saw a concerted effort on Mattel's part to 'go multicultural', coinciding with a parallel preference in the pages of high-fashion magazines, such as *Elle* and *Vogue*, for racially diverse models. With the expansion of sales worldwide, Barbie has acquired multiple national guises (Spanish Barbie, Jamaican Barbie, Malaysian Barbie, etc.). In addition, her cohort of 'friends' has become increasingly ethnically diversified, as has Barbie advertising, which now regularly features Asian, Hispanic, and African American little girls playing with Barbie. Today, Barbie pals include a smattering of brown and yellow plastic friends, like Teresa, Kira, and Miko, who appear in her adventures and, very importantly, can share her clothes. This diversification has not spelled an end to reigning Anglo beauty norms and body image. Quite the reverse. When we line the dolls up together, they look virtually identical. Cultural difference is reduced to surface variations in skin tone and costumes that can be exchanged at will. Like the concomitant move toward racially diverse fashion models, 'difference' is remarkably made over into sameness, as ethnicity is tamed to conform to a restricted range of feminine beauty.

Perhaps Mattel's most glamorous concession to multiculturalism is their creation, Shani. Billed as tomorrow's African American woman, Shani, whose name, according to Mattel, means 'marvellous' in Swahili, premiered at the 1991 Toy Fair with great fanfare and media attention. Unlike her predecessors, who were essentially 'brown plastic poured into blond Barbie's mold', Shani, together with her two friends, Asha and Nichelle (each a slightly different shade of brown), and boyfriend, Jamal, created in 1992, were decidedly Afro-centric, with outfits in 'ethnic' fabrics rather than the traditional Barbie pink (Jones, 1991). The packaging also announced that these dolls' bodies and facial features were meant to be more like those of real African American women, although they too can interchange clothes with Barbie. [...]

What is striking, then, is that, while Barbie's identity may be mutable – one day she might be an astronaut, another a cheerleader – *her hyper-slender, big-chested body has remained fundamentally unchanged over the years* – a remarkable fact in a society that fetishes the new and improved. [...]

The measured body: norms and ideals

[...] As the science of measuring human bodies, anthropometry belongs to a long line of techniques of the eighteenth and nineteenth centuries concerned with measuring, comparing, and interpreting variability in different zones of the human body. [...]

It is striking that, aside from those studies specifically focused on the comparison of the sexes, women did not figure prominently in physical anthropology's attempt to quantify and typologize human bodies. [...] With males as the unspoken prototype, women's bodies were frequently described (subtly or not) as deviations from the norm: as subjects, the measurement of their bodies was occasionally risky to the male scientists, and as bodies they were variations from the generic or ideal type (their body fat 'excessive', their pelvises maladaptive to a bipedal [i.e., more evolved] posture, their musculature weak). Understood primarily in terms of their reproductive capacity, women's bodies, particularly their reproductive organs, genitalia, and secondary sex characteristics, were instead more carefully scrutinized and measured within 'marital adjustment' studies and in the emerging science of gynaecology, whose practitioners borrowed liberally from the techniques used by physical anthropologists.

In the United States, an attempt to elaborate a scientifically sanctioned notion of a normative 'American' female body, however, was taking place in the college studies of the late nineteenth and early twentieth centuries. By the 1860s, Harvard and other universities had begun to regularly collect anthropometric data on their male student populations, and in the 1890s comparable data began to be collected from the East Coast women's colleges as well. Conducted by departments of hygiene, physical education, and home economics, as well as physical anthropology, these large-scale studies gathered data on the elite, primarily WASP (White Anglo Saxon Protestant) youth, in order to determine the dimensions of the 'normal' American male and female. [...]

Standards for the average American male and female were also being elaborated in a variety of domains outside of academia. By the early part of the twentieth century, industry began to make widespread commercial use of practical anthropometry: the demand for standardized measures of the 'average' body manifested in everything from Taylorist designs for labor-efficient workstations and kitchens to standardized sizes in the ready-to-wear clothing industry (cf. Schwartz, 1986). Certainly, one of the most common ways in which individuals encountered body norms was in the medical examination required for life insurance. It was not long before such companies as Metropolitan Life would rival the army, colleges, and prisons as the most reliable source of anthropometric statistics. Between 1900 and 1920, the first medicoactuarial standards of weight and height began to appear in conjunction with new theories linking weight and health. [...] However, what began as a table of statistical averages soon became a means of setting ideal norms. Within a few years of its creation, the Dublin table shifted from providing a record of statistically 'average' weights to becoming a guide to 'desirable' weights that, interestingly enough, were notably below the average weight for most adult women. In her history of anorexia in the United States, Joan Brumberg points to the Dublin table, widely disseminated to doctors and published in popular magazines, and the invention of the personal, or bathroom, scale as the two devices most responsible for popularizing the notion that the human figure could be standardized and that abstract and often unrealistic norms could be uniformly applied (1988: 232–5).

By the 1940s the search to describe the normal American male and female bodies in anthropometric terms was being conducted on many fronts. Data on the average measurements of men and women were now available from a number of different sources, including surveys of army recruits from World War I, the longitudinal college studies, sample measurements from the Chicago World's Fair, actuarial data, and extensive data from the Bureau of Home Economics, which had amassed measurements to assist in developing standardized sizing for the garment industry. Between the two wars, nationalist interests had fueled eugenic interests and provoked a deepening concern about the physical fitness of the American people [...] and in 1945, led to the creation of one of the most celebrated and widely publicized anthropometric models of the century: Norm and Norma, the average American male and female. Based on the composite measurements of thousands of young people, described only as 'native white Americans', across the United States, the statues of Norm and Norma were the product of a collaboration between obstetrician-gynecologist Robert Latou Dickinson, well known for his studies of human reproductive anatomy, and Abram Belskie, the prize student of Malvina Hoffman, who had sculpted the Races of Mankind series. Of the two, Norma received the greatest media attention when the Cleveland Health Museum, which had purchased the pair, decided to sponsor, with the help of a local newspaper, the YWCA, and several other health and educational organizations, a contest to find the woman in Ohio whose body most closely matched the dimensions of Norma. Under the catchy headline, 'Are You Norma, Typical Woman?' the publicity surrounding this contest instructed women in how to measure themselves at the same time that it extolled the virtues of Norma's body compared to those of her 'grandmother', Dudley Sargent's composite of the 1890s woman. Within ten days, 3,863 women had sent in their measurements to compete for the $100 prize in US War Bonds that would go to the woman who most resembled the average American girl.

Although anthropometric studies such as these were ostensibly descriptive rather than prescriptive, the normal or average and the ideal were routinely conflated. Nowhere is this more evident than in the discussions surrounding the Norma contest. Described in the press as the 'ideal' young woman, Norma was said to be everything an American woman should be in a time of war: she was fit, strong-bodied, and at the peak of her reproductive potential. Commentators waxed eloquent about the model character traits – maturity, modesty, and virtuosity – that this perfectly average body suggested. Curiously, although Norma was based on the measurements of living women, only about one percent of the contestants came close to her proportions. Harry Shapiro, curator of physical anthropology at the American Museum of Natural History, explained in the pages of *Natural History* why it was so rare to find a living, breathing Norma. Both Norma and Norman, he pointed out:

> … exhibit a harmony of proportion that seems far indeed from the usual or the average. One might well look at a multitude of young men and women before finding an approximation to these normal standards. We have to do here then with apparent paradoxes. Let us state it this way: the average American figure approaches a kind of perfection of bodily form and proportion; the average is excessively rare. (Shapiro, 1945: 51)

[...] Norma and Norman were thus more than statistical composites, they were ideals. It is striking how thoroughly racial and ethnic differences were erased from those scientific representations of the American male and female. Based on the measurements of white Americans, eighteen to twenty-five years old, Norm and Norma emerged carved out of white alabaster, with the facial features and appearance of Anglo-Saxon gods. Here, as in the college studies that preceded them, the 'average American' of the postwar period was to be visualized only as a youthful white body.

However, they were not the only ideal. The health reformers, educators, and doctors who approved and promoted Norma as an ideal for American women were well aware that her sensible, strong, thick-waisted body differed significantly from the tall, slim-hipped bodies of fashion models in vogue at the time. Gebhard and others tried through a variety of means to encourage women to ignore the temptations of 'vanity' and fashion, but they were ill equipped to compete with the persuasive powers of a rapidly expanding mass media that marketed a very different kind of female body. As the postwar period advanced, Norma would continue to be trotted out in home economics and health education classes. But in the iconography of desirable female bodies, she would be overshadowed by the array of images of fashion models and pinup girls put out by advertisers, the entertainment industry, and a burgeoning consumer culture. These idealized images were becoming, as we will see below, increasingly thin in the sixties and seventies while the 'average' woman's body was in fact getting heavier. With the thinning of the American feminine ideal, Norma and subsequent representations of the statistically average woman would become increasingly aberrant, as slenderness and sex appeal – not physical fitness – became the premier concern of postwar femininity.

The anthropometry of Barbie: turning the tables

As the preceding discussion makes abundantly clear, the anthropometrically measured 'normal' body has been anything but value-free. Formulated in the context of a race-, class-, and gender-stratified society, there is no doubt that quantitatively defined ideal types or standards have been both biased and oppressive. Incorporated into weight tables, put on display in museums and world's fairs, and reprinted in popular magazines, these scientif-ically endorsed standards produce what Foucault calls 'normalizing effects', shaping, in not altogether healthy ways, how individuals understand themselves and their bodies. Nevertheless, in the contemporary cultural context, where an impossibly thin image of women's bodies has become the most popular children's toy ever sold, it strikes us that recourse to the 'normal' body might just be the power tool we need for destabiliz-ing a fashion fantasy spun out of control. It was with this in mind that we asked students in one of our social biology classes to measure Barbie to see how her body compared to the average measurements of young American women of the same period. Besides esti-mating Barbie's dimensions if she were life-sized, we see the experiment as an occasion to turn the anthropometric tables from disciplining the bodies of living women to measur-ing the ideals by which we have come to judge ourselves and others. [...]

Since one objective of the course was to learn about human variation, our first task in understanding more about Barbie was to consider the fact that Barbie's friends and family do represent some variation, limited though it may be. Through colleagues and donations from students or (in one case) their children we assembled seventeen dolls for analysis. [...] To this sample we subsequently added the most current versions of Barbie and Ken (from the 'Glitter Beach' collection) and also Jamal, Nichelle, and Shani, Barbie's more recent African American friends. [...]

Barbie and Shani's measurements reveal interesting similarities and subtle differences. First, considering that they are six inches taller than 'Army Norma', their measurements tend to be considerably less *at all points*. 'Army Norma' is a composite of the fit woman soldier; Barbie and Shani, as high-fashion ideals, reflect the extreme thinness expected of the runway model. To dramatize this, had we scaled Barbie to 5' 4", her chest, waist and hip measurements would have been 32" – 17" – 28", clinically anorectic to say the least. There are only subtle differences in size, which we presume intend to facilitate the exchange of costumes among the different dolls. We were curious to see the degree to which Mattel has physically changed the Barbie mold in making Shani. Most of the dif-ferences we could find appeared to be in the face. The nose of Shani is broader and her lips are ever so slightly larger. However, our measurements also showed that Barbie's hip circumference is actually larger than Shani's, and so is her hip breadth. If anything, Shani might have thinner legs than Barbie, but her back is arched in such a way that it tilts her buttocks up. This makes them appear to protrude more posteriorly, even though the hip depth measurements of both dolls are virtually the same (7.1"). Hence, the tilting of the lumbar dorsal region and the extension of the sacral pelvic area produce the visual illusion of a higher, rounder butt. This is, we presume, what Mattel was referring to in claiming that Shani has a realistic, or ethnically correct, body (Jones, 1991).

One of our interests in the male dolls was to ascertain whether they represent a form closer to average male values than Barbie does to average female values. Ken and Jamal provide interesting contrasts to 'Army Norm', but certainly not to each other. Their post-cranial bodies are identical in all respects. They, in turn, represent a somewhat slimmer, trimmer male than the so-called fit soldier of today. Visually, the newer Ken and Jamal appear very tight and muscular and 'bulked out' in impressive ways. The US Army males tend to carry slightly more fat, judging from the photographs and data presented in the 1988 study.

Indeed, it would appear that Barbie and virtually all her friends characterize a somewhat extreme ideal of the human figure, but in Barbie and Shani, the female cases, the degree to which they vary from 'normal' is much greater than in the male cases, bordering on the impossible. Barbie truly is the unobtainable representation of an imaginary femaleness. But she is certainly not unique in the realm of female ideals. Studies tracking the body measurements of *Playboy* magazine centerfolds and Miss America contestants show that between 1959 and 1978 the average weight and hip sizes for women in both of these groups have decreased steadily (Wiseman et al., 1992). Comparing their data to actuarial data for the same time period, researchers found that the thinning of feminine body ideals was occurring at the same time that the average weight of American women was actually increasing. A follow-up study for the years 1979–88 found this trend continuing into the eighties: approximately sixty-nine percent of *Playboy* centerfolds and sixty percent of Miss America contestants were weighing in at fifteen percent or more below their expected age and height category. In short, the majority of women presented to us in the media as having desirable feminine bodies were, like Barbie, well on their way to qualifying for anorexia nervosa.

Our Barbies, our selves

[…] The imperative to manage the body and 'be all that you can be' – in fact, the idea that you can *choose* the body that you want to have – is a pervasive feature of consumer culture. Keeping control of one's body, not getting too fat or flabby – in other words, conforming to gendered norms of fitness and weight – are signs of an individual's social and moral worth. But, as feminists Susan Bordo, Sandra Bartky, and others have been quick to point out, not all bodies are subject to the same degree of scrutiny or the same repercussions if they fail. It is women's bodies and desires in particular where the structural contradictions – the simultaneous incitement to consume and social condemnation for overindulgence – appear to be most acutely manifested in bodily regimes of intense self-monitoring and discipline. 'The woman who checks her make-up half a dozen times a day to see if her foundation has caked or her mascara run, who worries that the wind or rain may spoil her hairdo has become just as surely as the inmate of the Panopticon, a self-policing subject, a self committed to a relentless self surveillance' (Bartky, 1990: 80). Just as it is women's appearance that is subject to greater scrutiny, so it is that women's desires, hungers, and appetites are seen as most threatening and in need of control in a patriarchal society.

This cultural context is relevant to making sense of Barbie and the meaning her body holds in late consumer capitalism. In dressing and undressing Barbie, combing her hair, bathing her, turning and twisting her limbs in imaginary scenarios, children acquire a very tactile and intimate sense of Barbie's body. Barbie is presented in packaging and advertising as a role model, a best friend or older sister to little girls. Television jingles use the refrain, 'I want to be just like you', while look-alike clothes and look-alike contests make it possible for girls to live out the fantasy of being Barbie. [...] In short, there is no reason to believe that girls (or adult women) separate Barbie's body shape from her popularity and glamour.

This is exactly what worries many feminists. As our measurements show, Barbie's body differs wildly from anything approximating 'average' female body weight and proportions. Over the years her wasp-waisted body has evoked a steady stream of critique for having a negative impact on little girls' sense of self-esteem. While her large breasts have always been a focus of commentary, it is interesting to note that, as eating disorders are on the rise, her weight has increasingly become the target of criticism. [...]

There is no doubt that Barbie's body contributes to what Kim Chernin (1981) has called 'the tyranny of slenderness'. But is repression all her hyper-thin body conveys? Looking once again to Susan Bordo's work on anorexia, we find an alternative reading of the slender body – one that emerges from taking seriously the way anorectic women see themselves and make sense of their experience:

> For them, anorectics, [the slender ideal] may have very different meaning; it may symbolize not so much the containment of female desire, as its liberation from a domestic, reproductive destiny. The fact that the slender female body can carry both these (seemingly contradictory) meanings is one reason, I would suggest, for its compelling attraction in periods of gender change. (Bordo, 1990: 103)

Similar observations have been made about cosmetic surgery: women often explain their experience as one of empowerment, taking charge of their bodies and lives (Balsamo, 1993 [sic]; Davis, 1991). What does this mean for making sense of Barbie? We would suggest that a subtext of agency and independence, even transgression, accompanies this pencil-thin icon of femininity. One could argue that, like the anorectic body she resembles, Barbie's body displays conformity to dominant cultural imperatives for a disciplined body and contained feminine desires. As a woman, however, her excessive slenderness also signifies a rebellious manifestation of willpower, a visual denial of the maternal ideal symbolized by pendulous breasts, rounded stomach and hips. Hers is a body of hard edges, distinct borders, self-control. It is literally impenetrable. Unlike the anorectic, whose self-denial renders her gradually more androgynous in appearance, in the realm of plastic fantasy Barbie is able to remain powerfully sexualized, with her large, gravity-defying breasts, even while she is distinctly non-reproductive. Like the 'hard bodies' in fitness advertising, Barbie's body may signify for women the pleasure of control and mastery, both of which are highly valued traits in American society and predominantly associated with masculinity (Bordo, 1990: 105). Putting these elements together with her apparent independent wealth can make for a very different reading of Barbie than the one we often find in the popular press. To paraphrase one Barbie-doll owner: she owns a Ferrari and doesn't have a husband – she must be doing something right! [...]

References

Balsamo, Anne (1992) 'On the Cutting Edge: Cosmetic Surgery and the Technological Production of the Gendered Body'. *Camera Obscura,* 28: 207–38.

Bartky, Sandra Lee (1990) 'Foucault, Femininity, and the Modernisation of Patriarchal Power'. In *Femininity and Domination: Studies in the Phenomenology of Oppression*, pp. 63–82. New York: Routledge.

Billy Boy (1987) *Barbie Her Life and Times, and the New Theater of Fashion.* New York: Crown.

Bordo, Susan R. (1990) 'Reading the Slender Body'. In *Body/Politics: Women and the Discourses of Science.* Ed. Mary Jaconus, Evelyn Fox Keller, and Sally Shuttleworth, pp. 83–112. New York: Routledge.

Brumberg, Joan Jacobs (1988) *Fasting Girls: the History of Anorexia Nervosa.* Cambridge, MA: Harvard University Press. Reprint, New York: New American Library.

Chernin, Kim (1981) *The Obsession: Reflections on the Tyranny of Slenderness.* New York: Harper & Row.

Davis, Kathy (1991) 'Remaking the She-Devil: a Critical Look at Feminist Approches to Beauty'. *Hypatia,* 6 (2): 21–43.

Jones, Lisa (1991) 'Skin Trade: a Doll is Born'. *Village Voice,* 26 March, p. 36.

Schwartz, Hill (1986) *Never Satisfied: a Cultural History of Diets, Fantasies and Fat.* New York: Free Press.

Shapiro, Harry L. (1945) *Americans Yesterday, Today, Tomorrow.* Man and Nature Publications. (Science Guide No. 126). New York: The American Museum of Natural History.

Willis, Susan (1991) *A Primer for Daily Life.* London and New York: Routledge.

Wiseman, C., J. Gray, J. Mosimann, and A. Ahrens (1992) 'Cultural Expectations of Thinness in Woman: an Update'. *International Journal of Eating Disorders,* 11 (1): 85–9.

Chapter 17

Feminist Research and Health

Gayle Letherby

Introduction

In this chapter, I focus on the politics and practice of feminist research in relation to health, drawing on a range of empirical examples. I begin, in 'Politics and praxis', with a consideration of the philosophies behind, and approaches to, research from a feminist perspective and follow this, in 'Methods and methodologies', by arguing that it is not the methods themselves that characterise research as feminist but the way in which methods are used. In 'Subjectivity and involvement in research', I reflect on emotional involvement in research as well as involvement and detachment, and in 'Men and "other" "others"', I consider just who should be the focus of feminist research. Finally, in 'The importance of feminist health research', I reassert the value of feminist research on health.

Politics and praxis

As I have argued elsewhere, I believe that the main concern of feminist researchers has been and continues to be the knowing/doing relationship: that is, how what we do affects what we get (Letherby, 2003, 2004). Feminist researchers have been critical of male-dominated knowledge production and the methodological claims made by researchers who argue that their work is objective and value-free. They argue that all research involves some element of the researcher's personhood – in terms of values, opinions, interests and approaches, and that the researched are themselves people who influence the research process as well as providing data for the final research product (e.g., Cotterill and Letherby, 1994; Stanley and Wise, 1993; Wilkinson and Kitzinger, 1996). Thus, in all research the product cannot be separated from the conditions of its production (Olsen, 1980). What is distinctive about feminist research is that it admits this. Renate Duelli Klein (cited by Wilkinson, 1986: 14) argues that within feminist research 'conscious subjectivity' replaces the 'value-free objective' of traditional research. She argues that this is an approach that is not only more honest, but helps to break down the power relationship between researcher and researched. Feminists insist that not only is the 'personal political', but 'the personal is also theoretical'.

So, for many, feminist research is feminist theory in action, the aim being to understand the world and change it. Feminism, then, is openly political in that it celebrates and is grounded in the daily experiences of women, and by focusing on experience it is able to challenge mainstream ('malestream') knowledge. However, more recently there has been a concern to move beyond a consideration of the differences between women and men and consider differences between and among women as well as consider when, and how, women's and men's lives intersect (e.g. Doyal, 1995; Maynard, 1994 and see below).

The relationship between gender and health began to be taken seriously as a research topic in the 1970s. It was then that gender began to be considered alongside other variables, such as 'race' and ethnicity, socio-economic status, and geographical area when explaining patterns and experience of health and illness. It is no coincidence that at the same time there was also a growth in feminist research and in the activity of the women's movement, which both contributed directly to the growth of the women's health movement. However, at this time researchers equated studies of gender, health and illness almost exclusively with women. It was not until the growth of interest in men's studies in the 1980s that the relationship between concepts of health, masculinity, men's lives and their experience of illness began to be seriously considered.

Methods and methodologies

Historically, feminists have been particularly critical of the survey method, and it was/is its epistemological appropriation by those who argue for 'objective value-freedom' and the tendency of researchers to concentrate on male concerns that was/is the issue here (Graham, 1984; Oakley, 1981; Stanley and Wise, 1993). In response to this, feminists argued that the in-depth interview that takes a life-history approach is a good way of achieving an 'equal' relationship between interviewer and interviewee. By letting individuals tell 'their story', this method allows the researched an active part in the research process and project as well as making the researcher more vulnerable (Graham, 1984; Oakley, 1981; Stanley and Wise, 1993). So, the argument goes, this enables the production of research for women rather than research about or of women (Bowles and Klein, 1983; Oakley, 1981). Ann Oakley (2000) gives an example of a research project that could be described as 'research of women' rather than 'research for women'. She cites a large research project on the social origins of depression and notes that the study resulted in a convincing explanation of the relationship between women's depression and their oppression. But there was no concern with whether or how women defined themselves as depressed, only with how the state of women's mental health could be exposed and fitted into a system of classification developed by a profession of 'experts' on mental health (psychiatrists). Also, the researchers did not begin with a desire to study the situation of women or set out to give women a chance to understand their experience as determined by the social structure of the society in which they lived. The primary aim of the data was to study depression and women were selected as respondents because they are easier (and therefore cheaper) to interview, being more likely than men to be at home and therefore available during the day.

However, there are potential problems with claiming the in-depth interview as an equalising method of research, not least because, as Caroline Ramazanoglu (1989) points out, women are divided by other variables (e.g., race, class, and sexuality), and this is likely to affect the research process and the research relationship. This is reflected in that researchers who are committed to incorporating respondents from different 'races' and classes in their work may need to be prepared to allow more time and money for respondent recruitment and data collection. In these instances, access to respondents, the building of trusting relationships and coping with language differences are just some of the things that might take more time and effort than expected. Recruitment of respondents was an issue in a research project concerned with the relationship between race, class and gender inequality and well-being and mental health among full-time employed professional, managerial and administrative women in the USA. The researchers spoke at meetings and wrote for newspapers as well as using 'snowballing' techniques (word of mouth among respondents) in order to encourage respondents to come forward (Cannon et al., 1991). Other researchers have found that working-class women are less likely to respond to requests for research in written form, especially on 'official' stationery. This happened to Kay Standing (1998) in her research on lone mothers and she suggests that a mistrust of authority and the style and language that requests are written in are relevant here.

Even when women are willing to be involved in research it is important to consider that the very fact that women are 'happy to talk' may be an indication of their powerlessness and respondents may later regret what they reveal in research (Finch, 1984). This may be particularly true when the research focuses on sensitive and/or taboo topics, examples of which include dying and death, reproductive identity and reproductive experiences, long-term illness, caring responsibilities and other health-related issues. When researching people less powerful than themselves – which include the large amount of women who either self-select or are approached to be involved in health research – researchers have a responsibility to be aware of the power imbalance in the research relationship (see below). However, it is important not to over-pacify respondents and to remember that within a research relationship power can shift and change. In addition, respondents may have their own 'political' reasons for research involvement. As one of my respondents said to me in my research on 'infertility' and 'involuntary childlessness',[1] 'I can't say this publicly but you can, you can be my soapbox' (see Letherby, 2003, for further discussion on power in research relationships).

Despite these qualifications, the in-depth interview is still advocated by many feminists as a method that encourages a participatory/equalising research relationship and a good way to 'find out about people's lives'. However, several researchers and writers have emphasised that it is important not to dismiss the quantitative and that to establish a new orthodoxy of qualitative research is just as restrictive as the utilisation of traditional research methods (Jayaratne and Stewart, 1991; Kelly et al., 1994; Letherby, 2004; Letherby and Zdrodowski, 1995; Oakley, 1998). So, appropriate methods should be chosen to suit research programmes rather than research programmes being chosen to 'fit' favourite techniques. It is not the methods 'but the framework within which they are located, and the particular ways in which they are deployed' that makes research feminist (Kelly et al., 1994: 46). Liz Kelly et al. argue that by using only small-scale studies the researcher can be misled into believing that s/he has some knowledge that has not actually been collected. They use the example of work on sexual abuse and domestic violence, arguing that most work on these areas has drawn on the experiences, interviews and discussion with women who have, somehow, made their lives public. For example, most research on domestic violence is focused on women in refuges and this does not tell us if what is found here applies to those women suffering abuse who have not voiced their experiences. Kelly et al. (1994) argue that if feminist research is to be about women's experiences, we must use our power as researchers to ensure that we have accessed all these experiences and use whatever method it takes.

Subjectivity and involvement in research

As noted above, traditional research processes argued for the objective and value-free production of knowledge: a 'scientific' social science. From this perspective the research process is value-free, coherent and orderly – in fact 'hygenic' (Kelly et al., 1994; Stanley and Wise, 1993). Among other criticisms of this approach is the point that power is a fundamental aspect of all research relationships. The researcher usually has control over, for example, the construction of the questionnaire, the order in which the questions are asked in a qualitative interview, the frequency and timing of visits to a research site and the associated status that this brings. Furthermore, it is the researcher who is more often than not responsible for the final analysis and presentation of the data. Thus, researchers 'take away the words' of respondents and have the power of editorship. So, it is important to acknowledge that researchers often have the objective balance of power throughout the research project and have control of both the material and authoritative resources. With all of this in mind, Judith Stacey (1991: 144) argues that 'elements of inequality, exploitation, and even betrayal are endemic to [research]'.

In recognition of research as a subjective experience, Barbara Katz-Rothman (1996: 50) goes so far as to suggest that there has been a fundamental shift in methodological thinking, where an 'ethic of involvement has replaced an ethic of objectivity'. From this perspective, writing from personal experience rather than from a position of 'detached objectivity' is likely to give the writer 'credentials'. The suggestion here, though, is that we can only speak about (and therefore research) issues of which we have personal experience, which could lead to more research on already privileged groups, and implies that women who come from minority groups have a 'duty' to represent 'others' like them. Manjit Bola (1996), an Asian woman who has vitiligo (white patches of skin), experienced this when researching the pregnancy experience of white, middle-class women as people assumed that her work was about the pregnancy experiences of Asian women or about vitiligo.

Whatever the researchers' connection to the research topic prior to the beginning of a research project, emotional connections and involvement are inevitable, whether it be the distress experienced when researching the experience of women living and dying of breast cancer or the anger felt when uncovering bigoted medical professional practice. Feminist researchers acknowledge that emotion is not only a significant part of the research process but often a source of insight into the relationship between the process of research and the ultimate research product (e.g. Lee-Treweek and Linkogle, 2000; Letherby, 2003).

Men and 'other' 'others'

In her book on men's attitudes to menstruation, Sophie Laws (1990: 13) writes that 'feminist research must go beyond the study of women to work out ways of studying for women if it is not to remain essentially a liberal rather than a radical liberatory force'. While writing specifically about reproduction, Ellen Annandale and Judith Clark (1996: 33) note: we should remain 'cognizant of the possibility that "patriarchal discourse need not be seen as homogeneous and uniformly oppressive" ... for women or uniformly liberating and unproblematic for men, and that women do not need to be portrayed as inevitable victims and men as victors'. Thus, men can be victims, women can be powerful, men and women often share experiences of powerlessness. We also need to know what men think about women and about female oppression. This suggests that feminists need to study men's as well as women's experiences and that pro-feminist men need also to work towards a critical analysis of gender. Thus, as David Morgan (1981, 1992) argues, 'taking gender seriously' means bringing men back in. He stresses that if we accept that man is not the norm and woman the deviation, we need to consider the social construction of both femininity and masculinity. However, 'taking gender into account' is (arguably) particularly hard for male researchers as 'the massive weight of the taken-for-granted ... conspires with the researchers' own gender to render silent what should be spoken' (Morgan, 1981: 96).

In addition, as noted above, an understanding of the differences between women in terms of power and privilege is a vital part of the feminist project. For example, as Jenny Douglas (1998) notes, the health status of black and minority ethnic women in the UK reflects the interaction between their experiences of race, gender, class and culture. So, health and well-being are determined in these groups of women by a complex mixture of social and psychological influences and biological and genetic factors. Further, individuals do not have to be black to experience racism as attention to the historical and contemporary experience of Jewish and Irish people demonstrates (Maynard, 1994).

The importance of feminist health research

We know that the material conditions of women's lives worldwide are worse than those of men. For example, and particularly relevant here, violence against women is often sanctioned by culture and/or religion, as in foot-binding and female genital mutilation; male-defined female 'ideals' are arguably internalised by women themselves, manifested, not least, in anorexia and cosmetic surgery. In addition, economic, social and cultural factors prevent many women from meeting their physical and psychological health needs. Thus: 'Gender differences are not only biologically determined, culturally constructed, or politically imposed, but also ways of living in a body and thus of being in the world' (Blake, 1994: 678).

Men and women are exposed to different health risks and have access to different amounts and types of resource for maintaining or promoting their own health, plus they have different levels of responsibility for the care of others (Doyal, 1998). When ill they may define their symptoms in different ways and have very different strategies for coping, seeking help from different sources. They may also respond very differently to treatment. Despite the plethora of pro-feminist research on health, these gender differences, which clearly have profound implications for the planning of health care, have so far received little attention from those in the biomedical tradition (Doyal, 1998). Yet, we also know that men are more at risk of some illnesses and at times the similarities between female and male experience are more important than the differences between them, and that there are differences other than gender that are also necessary to consider.

Feminist-informed research on health, which interrogates its own practice as well as the issues under scrutiny, recognises the complexity of the relationship between gender and health and is therefore crucial to a better understanding of the gendered aspects of health experience and health needs.

Note

1 I write 'infertility' and 'involuntary childlessness' in singe quotation marks to highlight the problems of definition.

References

Annandale, Ellen and Clark, Judith (1996) 'What is gender? Feminist theory and the sociology of human reproduction', *Sociology of Health and Illness,* 18 (1): 17–44.

Blake, C. Fred (1994) 'Foot-binding in neo-Confucian China and the appropriation of female labor', *Signs: Journal of Women in Culture and Society,* 19(31): 676–711.

Bola, Manjit (1996) 'Questions of legitimacy? The fit between researcher and researched', in Wilkinson, S. and Kitzinger, C. (eds), *Representing the Other: a Feminism and Psychology Reader.* London: Sage.

Bowles, Gloria and Klein, Renate Duelli (eds) (1983) *Theories of Women's Studies.* London: Routledge and Kegan Paul.

Cannon, L.W., Higgenbotham, E. and Leung, M.L.A. (1991) 'Race and class bias in qualitative research on women', in Fonow, M.M. and Cook, J.A. (eds), *Beyond Methodology: Feminist Scholarship as Lived Experience.* Bloomington, IN: Indiana University Press.

Cotterill, Pamela and Letherby, Gayle (1994) 'The person in the researcher', in Burgess, R. (ed.), *Studies in Qualitative Methodology* (Vol. vi). London: Jai Press.

Douglas, Jenny (1998) 'Meeting the health needs of women from black and minority ethnic communities', in Doyal, L. (ed.), *Women and Health Care Services.* Buckingham: Open University Press.

Doyal, Lesley (1995) *What Makes Women Sick?: Gender and the Political Economy of Health.* Basingstoke: Macmillan.

Doyal, Lesley (ed.) (1998) *Women and Health Care Services.* Buckingham: Open University Press.

Finch, Janet (1984) '"It's great to have someone to talk to": the ethics and politics of interviewing women', in Bell, C. and Roberts, H. (eds), *Social Researching: Politics, Problems, Practice.* London: Routledge and Kegan Paul.

Graham, Hilary (1984) *Women, Health and the Family.* Brighton: Wheatsheaf.

Jayaratne, Toby Epstein and Stewart, Abigail J. (1991) 'Quantitative and qualitative methods in the social sciences: current feminist issues and practical strategies', in Fonow, M.M. and Cook, J.A.

(eds), *Beyond Methodology: Feminist Scholarship as Lived Experience*. Bloomington, IN: Indiana University Press.

Katz-Rothman, Barbara (1996) 'Bearing witness: representing women's experiences of prenatal diagnosis', in Wilkinson S. and Kitzinger C. (eds), *Representing the Other: a Feminism and Psychology Reader*. London: Sage.

Kelly, Liz, Burton, Sheila and Regan, Linda (1994) 'Researching women's lives or studying women's oppression? Reflections on what constitutes feminist research', in Maynard, M. and Purvis, J. (eds), *Researching Women's Lives from a Feminist Perspective*. London: Taylor and Francis.

Laws, Sophie (1990) *Issues of Blood: the Politics of Menstruation*. Basingstoke: Macmillan.

Lee-Treweek, Geraldine and Linkogle, Stephanie (eds) (2000) *Danger in the Field: Risk and Ethics in Social Research*. London: Routledge.

Letherby, Gayle (2003) *Feminist Research in Theory and Practice*. Buckingham: Open University Press.

Letherby, Gayle (2004) 'Quoting and counting: an autobiographical response to Oakley' *Sociology*, 38 (1): 175–90.

Letherby, Gayle and Zdrodowski, Dawn (1995) 'Dear researcher: the use of correspondence as a method within feminist qualitative research', *Gender and Society,* 9: 5.

Maynard, Mary (1994) '"Race", gender and the concept of "difference" in feminist thought', in Afshar, A. and Maynard, M. (eds), *The Dynamics of 'Race' and Gender: Some Feminist Interventions*. London: Taylor and Francis.

Morgan, David (1981) 'Men, masculinity and the process of sociological inquiry', in Roberts, H. (ed.), *Doing Feminist Research*. London: Routledge and Kegan Paul.

Morgan, David (1992) *Discovering Men*. London: Routledge.

Oakley, Ann (1981) 'Interviewing women: a contradiction in terms?', in Roberts, H. (ed.), *Doing Feminist Research*. London: Routledge.

Oakley, Ann (1998) 'Gender, methodology and people's ways of knowing: some problems with feminism and the paradigm debate in social science', *Sociology*, 32 (4): 707–32.

Oakley, Ann (2000) *Experiments in Knowing: Gender and Method in the Social Sciences*. Cambridge: Polity Press.

Olsen, Tillie (1980) *Silences*. London: Virago.

Ramazanoglu, Caroline (1989) 'On feminist methodology: male reason versus female empowerment', *Sociology*, 26 (2): 201–12.

Stacey, Judith (1991) 'Can there be a feminist ethnography?', in Gluck, B. and Patai, D. (eds), *Women's Words, Women's Words, Women's Words: the Feminist Practice of Oral History*. New York: Routledge.

Standing, Kay (1998) 'Writing the voices for the less powerful: research on lone mothers', in Ribbens, J. and Edwards, R. (eds), *Feminist Dilemmas in Qualitative Research*. London: Sage.

Stanley, Liz and Wise, Sue (1993) *Breaking Out Again: Feminist Ontology and Epistemology* London: Routledge.

Wilkinson, Sue (ed.) (1986) *Feminist Social Psychology: Developing Theory and Practice*. Buckingham: Open University.

Wilkinson, Sue and Kitzinger, Celia (eds) (1996) *Representing the Other: a Feminism and Psychology Reader*. London: Sage.

Chapter 18

Researching the Views of Diabetes Service Users from South Asian Backgrounds: a Reflection on Some of the Issues

Cathy E. Lloyd

Diabetes is a major health concern of the 21st century, with the incidence and prevalence of this condition increasing rapidly (Department of Health, 2002). The diagnosis of diabetes has both immediate and longer-term consequences for individuals, with alterations in lifestyle, diet and medication regimes among the short-term and the development of complications such as diabetic retinopathy, renal failure and coronary artery disease among the most serious long-term effects. Ideally, the care of diabetes requires a dual approach, with people with the condition carrying out self-care activities for themselves in partnership with a number of different health-care professionals. Indeed self-care has been identified as the cornerstone of diabetes care and the National Service Framework for diabetes has recommended the promotion of skills for diabetes self-management in order to optimise health outcomes (Department of Health, 2002). Given the centrality of diabetes self-management to policy and practice, it follows that research in this area, in particular with regard to identifying optimal ways of supporting those with diabetes, is required. This chapter discusses the difficulties of researching the views and life experiences of people with diabetes, with particular reference to issues around diabetes self-management, in those whose main language is not English.

Although there has been a relatively short history of research in diabetes self-care, the number of publications in this field has increased in recent years. Large epidemiological studies in the USA and the UK have measured the long-term outcomes of diabetes and its complications according to different modes of self-care (The DCCT Research Group, 1993; Matthews, 1999). Smaller-scale studies of varying types have also been carried out investigating levels of self-care and the factors that impact on health behaviours, the impact of the external environment on self-care and, more recently, a growing body of literature has appeared on empowerment and diabetes self-care (e.g. Anderson and

Funnell, 2000; Davies et al., 2005). At the present time, there remains controversy with regard to the optimal ways of delivering support for diabetes self-care or a 'one-size-fits-all' strategy that can be recommended to people with diabetes, given the myriad differences in circumstances, motivations and context. For example, the two main types of diabetes affect people at different ages, require differing self-care regimens, and although both carry the risk of complications, such as eye disease and renal failure, this differs according to duration of disease as well as other factors such as long-term levels of glucose in the blood. There are a range of psychosocial implications too, for instance employment (some jobs are closed to those with Type 1 diabetes), sexual health (including impotence) and the effects of stress on diabetes (Lloyd et al., 2005).

Most of the published literature in this area is centred on Caucasian populations in the west, with a dearth of studies carried out and reported in non-English-speaking populations. The experiences of, for example, minority ethnic groups in the UK or the USA, are rarely researched, even in a field (such as diabetes) where they comprise a large section of the patient population. Studies have, in the main, utilised self-complete questionnaires, or biomedical data which is collected on large groups of individuals which is then statistically analysed and reported in peer-reviewed journals with a biomedical focus. Most funding for research in diabetes supports a similar type of research – biomedical and/or laboratory based. Every week there are articles in both the professional journals and the lay media proclaiming yet another breakthrough in science, the discovery of another gene linked to diabetes or its complications. The views and real-life experiences of those who live with diabetes on a daily basis are rarely researched and even less likely to be published. A random selection of two 2005 issues of *Diabetic Medicine*, the professional journal of Diabetes UK, revealed that out of 41 original articles published, only two were related to psychosocial issues in diabetes, the vast majority being either epidemiological or clinical studies usually around genetic susceptibility or risk of developing diabetes complications.

The reasons for this lack of psychosocial research in those with diabetes are varied and remain open to speculation. Research into new drugs to medicate the effects of diabetes is big business. Sometimes drug research includes a sub-study of psychosocial aspects of the new treatment (e.g. O'Hare et al., 2004), however funding for psychosocial research in its own right remains rare. The perceived validity of the 'scientific method', large databases containing 'hard' data on hundreds of 'subjects' and the centrality of the gold standard randomised controlled trial remain obstacles to researchers wishing to understand more about the personal implications of diabetes, including the factors that influence diabetes self-care. Alongside this, while some psychosocial research utilises quantitative methods (e.g. research into diabetes and depression, Anderson et al., 2001), researchers wishing to use qualitative methods face a further barrier. In diabetes, 'hard' data is typified by blood glucose levels – the HbA1c value (often dreaded by patients and revered by medics) is the gold standard. 'Soft' data, captured through observation or interviewing, may not be considered sufficiently 'scientific' and may be too much open to interpretation. Importantly, however, those studies that have been carried out show that self-care is strongly associated with blood glucose levels. The research has huge implications at both a personal level as well as in terms of health-care costs, given the well-established causal relationship between poor glucose control and the development of diabetes complications (The DCCT Research Group, 1993; Matthews, 1999). Although the correlation between blood glucose levels and various aspects of diabetes self-care can be statistically demonstrated, the reasons why self-care is often poor are difficult to elucidate via quantitative methods.

All is not lost, however. The traditional biomedical approach to researching diabetes and its care is shifting and includes not only HbA1c as an outcome measure, but satisfaction with treatment, depression and anxiety research, and other studies evaluating specific interventions in diabetes. Yet, as this shift occurs, we are presented with a new set of problems. It is not difficult to collect blood from any person, with consent, and the results (blood sugar levels, cholesterol, etc.) are easy for health-care professionals to interpret against standard values or 'normal ranges'. Research into discovering the experiences of patients, their emotional state, or their difficulties with self-care strategies are a whole different ball game. A range of influences are at play, not just gender or ethnicity, or social class, but the entire range and cultural context in which people live their everyday lives. Inequalities in access to services, acknowledged to be a key factor in determining health status, have rarely been researched in terms of the experiences of people from minority ethnic communities (Rhodes et al., 2003).

My own research recently brought these issues sharply into focus when I was asked to identify two suitable questionnaires for use in a sub-study of a risk factor intervention trial in South Asian patients with diabetes. The sub-study was aimed at identifying deficits in knowledge and poor self-efficacy in diabetes self-management, in order to better tailor diabetes education services. I identified two appropriate questionnaires and arranged for these to be translated and back-translated according to accepted methods. My job was to explain to the research assistants (three link workers) how these questionnaires were to be implemented and then analyse the data once it had been collected. However, there were particular difficulties encountered during the administration of these questionnaires, as outlined below.

The two (self-complete) questionnaires had been translated into Urdu and Bengali, as these were the two main languages spoken and written by the South Asian population under investigation. However, during the translation process it became clear that some English words had a completely different meaning (or even none at all) in Bengali or Urdu. Consulting with the link workers during the research process was vital and led to the (albeit limited) success of carrying out the study, as they were able to point out that, while the questionnaires had been entirely accurately translated, they were frequently unusable in this particular study population. The majority of the study participants were unable to read or write either Urdu or Bengali and used a spoken-only language (Mirpuri or Sylheti). The link workers subsequently agreed a version of Mirpuri that could be used during data collection, with the responses to the questions recorded on the Urdu translation of the questionnaires. As none of the link workers spoke Sylheti, only the Bengali written questionnaire could be used in the study. This meant that those potential study participants who spoke only Sylheti and did not read/write Bengali were effectively excluded from this study.

A total of 1700 adults with Type 2 diabetes from South Asian backgrounds were recruited to the intervention study. The first 175 were asked to complete a knowledge and a self-care questionnaire and 107 (61 per cent) agreed to do so. Although this was a fairly high response rate, only 14 questionnaires were completed by the person with diabetes, the rest being completed by the link workers or (on six occasions) by a relative. Out of the nine people who spoke Bengali or Sylheti, only one of them completed a questionnaire and this was with the help of a relative. All those approached who spoke Pashto (a dialect of a region in Pakistan) declined to participate. In subsequent interviews with the link workers, designed to elucidate some of the problems they faced in carrying out this research, several key issues came to light.

The most common problem experienced by the link workers was the time required to complete the two questionnaires. Each study participant was allocated 30 minutes in which to have all his/her medical history, personal details and various clinical measures collected as well as to complete several questionnaires. Even explaining the rationale behind the questionnaires took up valuable time. A further common problem reported by the link workers was the frequent negative reactions they received from the participants, who were often uncomfortable about their perceived lack of knowledge and were concerned about giving incorrect answers to the questions. Previous research has also demonstrated that poor knowledge of diabetes, fear of the condition and its complications, and the stigma attached to diabetes, are common in South Asian people with diabetes (Curtis et al., 2003; Greenhalgh et al., 1998). Rankin and Bhopal (2001) have reported in their research in South Asian populations that there is often a misunderstanding of the term 'diabetes', with many individuals being unable to provide a description of diabetes or suggest any risk factors for developing this condition. Difficulties related to understanding terminology were also common and were compounded by the fact that the link workers were trying to determine how much the patient knew about their diabetes. If they explained the words contained in the questions, this would have meant they had given the answers to the questions.

It is important to note that for a small minority of participants the completion of these questionnaires was a positive experience. This was evident for those individuals who wanted to know more about their diabetes, and was influenced by their understanding that identifying the gaps in their knowledge could lead to more diabetes education in that area and thus improve their knowledge and could lead to changes in self-care. However, for most of them, being asked questions about their knowledge of diabetes and their self-care practices was an uncomfortable experience that they would not wish to repeat. Vyas et al. (2003) have suggested that, even when interpreters are used to collect data, the way information is collected is still a crucial issue. So what are the implications for collecting information and seeking out the views of those people from South Asian backgrounds who currently utilise health-care services in the UK?

The South Asian population in the UK is one of the fastest growing populations with Type 2 diabetes. It is over four times more common and age of onset is earlier (Chowdhury and Lasker, 2002; Department of Health, 2002). In Birmingham, where the risk factor intervention study was carried out, approximately 25% of the population of Birmingham are of South Asian origin, and people of Mirpuri (Pakistani) and Bangladeshi-Sylheti origin are well represented in this. A number of particular problems with regard to the management of the condition in this group have been observed, in particular the cultural and communication difficulties which often make appropriate support of self-management of diabetes more difficult (Baradaran and Knill-Jones, 2004; Greenhalgh et al., 1998; Vyas et al., 2003). However, a small study recently demonstrated that the use of Asian support workers, or Asian link workers, markedly improves patient outcomes, in terms of increased knowledge and understanding of their diabetes, improved attendance rates at clinics and at education sessions (Curtis et al., 2003). In our sub-study it was clear that the link workers' role was of pivotal importance, although not without limitations. They did not, between them, speak all the languages that were required in order to encourage participation and, when assisting those who required help in completing the questionnaires, they had to rely on their memories of the agreed words to be used in Mirpuri. Maximising the chance of meeting standardised data collection procedures meant reliance was also placed on the link workers' skills in accurately recording responses, avoiding the use of leading questions or answering for the respondent.

While the translations were seen to have been accurate, and also culturally sensitive, the content of the questionnaires and the actual mode of data collection were often seen as inappropriate by both those collecting the data and those providing the data (i.e. the study participants). A recent systematic review of the process of translation and adaptation of health-related quality of life measures (Bowden, 2003) suggested that there is currently a misguided preoccupation with the scales being used rather than a focus on the actual concepts being scaled, with too much reliance on unsubstantiated claims of conceptual equivalence. When questionnaires are translated, it is frequently the case that any cultural differences are not accounted for (Froman and Schmitt, 2003; Greenhalgh et al., 1998; Hunt, 1994; Hunt and Bhopal, 2004). One might argue that both the content and the design of the scale are equally important, although success in either aspect cannot be fully achieved if the specific needs of the target population are not addressed. In this case the need for assisted completion or finding other ways of collecting data which does not involve having to complete questionnaires in a written form appears to be crucial.

Not only must the needs of the potential study participants be considered, however. The needs of those who are charged with the task of collecting the data must also be taken into account if success is to be achieved. The link workers who attempted to collect this data were all highly trained in working with people with diabetes and using standard forms for the collection of personal and medical information. However, none of them had used translated questionnaires before and this could have impacted on how they worked in this regard. If the link workers were unsure of how to use these questionnaires, this may well have influenced patients' willingness to take part and so may have impacted on response rates. Training and experience in the administration of translated questionnaires are thus critical for studies such as these. This, alongside greater involvement in all other aspects of the research process may well influence the success (or otherwise) or the research, not just the response rate. Health-care professionals' communication with patients has been seen as crucial in previous research in this area (Curtis et al., 2003; Rhodes et al., 2003). The use of interpreters can be difficult, lead to role conflict and relies heavily on communication skills (Hsieh, 2006). In this research, the link workers agreed that the time taken to work with them to develop an agreed form of Mirpuri to be used when required was invaluable and gave them a chance to voice their concerns with regard to the data collection methods. This positive perception of increased involvement in the research process was reflected in the higher response rate in Mirpuri speakers. The high refusal rate in those participants who spoke Bengali/Sylheti was simply because none of the link workers spoke either of these languages, thus making communication difficult. This is not an issue confined to research but one that confronts all health services staff (i.e. that of attempting to meet the needs of all sections of the patient population in an equitable manner). At the same time, the dangers of assuming similarities in the experiences of all persons identified as belonging to a particular ethnic group must also be acknowledged.

Conclusion

This chapter has highlighted some of the difficulties in collecting data in groups whose main or only written/spoken language is not English, and questions some of the strategies currently used in research to collect information. It is clear from our experiences that the role of the link worker (or indeed other data collector) is of primary importance, as is the need to involve those out in the field in the research process. Equally valid, I would argue, are the experiences of the 'researched' or service users, whose input into the research process is increasingly being considered as vital to the success of any project. Success in research is not just about using an appropriate methodological approach, but also involving both the researchers and the researched at each step along the way. Consultation with both health service workers and service users in the development of alternative, valid, coherent modes of data collection seems to be the only appropriate way forward.

References

Anderson, R.M. and Funnell, M. (2000) *The Art of Empowerment: Stories and Strategies for Diabetes Educators.* American Diabetes Association, Alexandria, VA.

Anderson, R.J., Freedland, K.E., Clouse, R.E. and Lustmann, P.J. (2001) The prevalence of comorbid depression in adults with diabetes: a meta-analysis, *Diabetes Care*, 24: 1069–78.

Baradaran, H. and Knill-Jones, R. (2004) Assessing knowledge, attitudes and understanding of type 2 diabetes amongst ethnic groups in Glasgow, Scotland, *Practical Diabetes International*, 21 (4): 143–8.

Bowden, A. and Fox-Rushby, J.A. (2003) A systematic and critical review of the process of translation and adaptation of generic health-related quality of life measures in Africa, Asia, Eastern Europe, the Middle East, South America, *Social Science and Medicine*, 57: 1289–1306.

Chowdhury, T.A. and Lasker, S.A. (2002) Complications and cardiovascular risk factors in South Asians and Europeans with early onset type 2 diabetes, *Quarterly Journal of Medicine*, 95 (4): 241–6.

Curtis, S., Beirne, J. and Jude, E. (2003) Advantages of training Asian diabetes support workers for Asian families and diabetes health care professionals, *Practical Diabetes International*, 20 (6): 215–18.

Davies, M.J., Heller, S., Khunti, K. and Skinner, T.C. (2005) The DESMOND (Diabetes Education and Self Managment for Ongoing and Newly Diagnosed) programme: from pilot phase to randomised control trial in a study of structured group education for people newly diagnosed with Type 2 diabetes mellitus, *Diabetic Medicine*, 22 (2): 108.

Department of Health, (2002) *National Service Framework for Diabetes: Standards of Core Document. 2002*, http://www.doh.gov.uk/nsf/diabetes/.

Froman, R.D. and Schmitt, M.H. (2003) Thinking both inside and outside the box on measurement articles, *Research in Nursing & Health*, 26: 335–6.

Greenhalgh, T., Helman, C. and Chowdhury, A.M. (1998) Health beliefs and folk models of diabetes in British Bangladeshis: a qualitative study, *British Medical Journal*, 316: 978–83.

Hsieh, E. (2006) Conflicts in how interpreters manage their roles in provider–patient interactions, *Social Science & Medicine*, 62: 721–30.

Hunt, S.M. (1994) Cross-cultural comparability of quality of life measures, in *International Symposium on Quality of Life and Health* (pp. 25–7). Blackwell Verlag, Berlin.

Hunt, S.M., and Bhopal, R. (2004) Self report in clinical and epidemiological studies with non-English speakers: the challenge of language and culture, *Journal of Epidemiology and Community Health*, 58: 618–22.

Lloyd, C.E., Mith, J. and Winger, K. (2005) Stress and diabetes: a review of the links, *Diabetes Spectrum*, 18: 121–7.

Matthews, D.R. (1999) The natural history of diabetes-related complications: the UKPDS experience, *Diabetes, Obesity and Metabolism*, 1: 7–13.

O'Hare, P., Raymond, N.T., Mughal, S., Dodd, L., Hanif, W., Ahmed, Y. et al. (2004) Evaluation of enhanced diabetes care to patients of South Asian ethnicity: the United Kingdom Asian Diabetes Study (UKADS), *Diabetic Medicine*, 21: 1357–65.

Rankin, J. and Bhopal, R. (2001) Understanding of heart disease and diabetes in a South Asian community: cross-sectional study testing the 'snowball' sample method, *Public Health*, 115: 253–60.

Rhodes, P., Nocon, A. and Wright, J. (2003) Access to diabetes services: the experiences of Bangladeshi people in Bradford, UK, *Ethnicity & Health*, 8: 171–88.

The DCCT Research Group (1993) The effect of intensive treatment of diabetes on the development and progression of long-term complications in insulin-dependent diabetes, *New England Journal of Medicine*, 329: 977-86.

Vyas, A., Haidery, A.Z., Wiles, P.G., Gill, S., Roberts, C. and Cruickshank, J.K. (2003) A pilot randomized trial in primary care to investigate and improve knowledge, awareness and self-management among South Asians with diabetes in Manchester, *Diabetic Medicine*, 20: 1022–6.

Chapter 19

Complexity and Complicity in Researching Ethnicity and Health

Yasmin Gunaratnam

Over the past two decades I have been involved in research in academia and in the voluntary sector on questions of 'race' and ethnicity in health and social care. During this time I have seen an increasing research interest in ethnicity. Although such interest feels important in that it has provided insights into the long marginalised health experiences of those categorised as being 'minority ethnic' (see Aspinall and Jacobson, 2004), I remain uncertain and ambivalent about its value. What has further contributed to my ambivalence has been my growing awareness of levels of complicity in research, where tensions in the meanings of the word between 'complex or involved' and 'partnership in an evil action' (Marcus, 1998) raise uncomfortable questions about the non-innocence of research on ethnicity in relation to wider processes and structures of racism and oppression.

In what follows, I examine methodological and ethical dilemmas in research on ethnicity. This exploration is not so much about providing technical fixes that can solve our research dilemmas and 'problems'. Rather, I want to provoke discussion and thought about how we might develop responsible research practices within a policy context that is marked by a voracious appetite for approaches that simplify, objectify and tame the meanings and effects of ethnicity and difference. Drawing upon the work of feminist and postcolonial writers, I elaborate upon Kum-Kum Bhavnani's (1993) three criteria of reinscription, micropolitics and difference as elements which we can use to enhance our thinking and doing of research.

Kum-Kum Bhavnani: 'reinscription, micropolitics and difference'

In an article in the *Women's Studies International Forum* in 1993, Kum-Kum Bhavnani used an engagement with the feminist writer Donna Haraway's (1988) concept of 'feminist objectivity' to develop her thinking about ethical research on difference. Haraway's concept of feminist objectivity is deliberately subversive of positivist claims that research can be a-historical, value-free and objective. Instead, Haraway has contended that:

> Feminist objectivity is about limited location and situated knowledge,not about transcendence and splitting of subject and object. It allows us to become answerable for what we learn to see. (Haraway, 1988: 583)

The ethical and political issue of accountability in research – becoming 'answerable for what we learn to see' – has been central to the development of feminist, black feminist and postcolonial methodological writing (Bhavnani and Phoenix, 1994; Gunaratnam, 2003; Visweswaran, 1994). This concern recognises the entangled relationships between research and wider social contexts marked by racisms and other forms of oppression in which the very categories that we think with, and the research methods that we use, can never be 'objective'. The impetus behind much feminist and postcolonial methodological writing has thus been concerned with how 'to produce different knowledge and to produce knowledge differently' (Lather, 2001: 200).

In developing Haraway's ideas and emphasis on research as involving partial insights, social and historical positions and accountability between researchers, research participants and communities, Bhavnani offers the three criteria of reinscription, micropolitics and difference as providing a framework that can be used to guide and judge research that is concerned with social difference. For Bhavnani, research should not be complicit with dominant representations of different social groups, so that it reproduces social inequalities.

Through the idea of reinscription, Bhavnani suggests that researchers need to ask themselves two main questions: 'Does this work/analysis define the researched as either passive victims or as deviant?' 'Does it reinscribe the researched into prevailing representations?' (1993: 98). The second concept of 'micropolitics' refers to whether research findings discuss the micropolitical processes involved in the research: 'What are the relationships of domination and subordination which the researcher has negotiated and what are the means through which they are discussed in the research report?' (1993: 98). In the third criterion of 'difference' Bhavnani suggests that researchers ask: 'In what ways are questions of difference dealt with in the research study – in its design, conduct, write-up, and dissemination?' (1993 98).

Drawing upon my own qualitative research experiences and wider research on ethnicity and health, I will look at and elaborate upon the three criteria of reinscription, micropolitics and difference. Due to restrictions of space, I will concentrate upon the former two criteria, including a discussion of difference throughout.

Reinscription

While the questions Bhavnani suggests that researchers ask themselves when addressing reinscription are important and relevant – and more than a decade after Bhavnani's paper was written – I want to look at a related aspect of reinscription which marks my current experience of research on ethnicity and health. For me, a significant challenge in relation to reinscription relates to how our research can reaffirm racialised power relations by essentialising difference. By essentialising, I am referring to a process of thought and knowledge production that implies an 'internal sameness and external difference or otherness' (Werbner, 1997: 228) and which can lead to lazy generalisations and a lack of critical engagement with relationships of power.

In my experience, the aim of not wanting research to essentialise the identities and experiences of research participants must begin with a radical examination of the terminology and categories that we use to research ethnicity and the levels at which these are used. In general, I try to avoid using the term 'minority ethnic', because it homogenises the experiences and social positions of very different groups. In addition, as Brah (1996) has pointed out, the use of the term 'minority' has a history based in pathological representations of women, colonial 'subjects' and working classes, while also serving to discourage a critical analysis of power relations. For Brah, the simplistic numerical 'minority'/'majority' dichotomy and its repeated circulation has the effect of 'naturalising rather challenging the power differential' (Brah, 1996: 187). That is to say, the term 'minority' can obscure relationships to power, in which individuals who are in a 'minority' position because of their ethnicity can be in a 'majority' position in relation to another aspect of their identity. This is why our acceptance and unproblematic use of current terminology can reiterate rather than disrupt and challenge existing social power relations.

However, while all social categories involve an erasing of heterogeneity within the category (Sayyid, 2000), there are times, such as when we are interpreting large quantitative data sets, when it is relatively easy, as Sheldon and Parker (1992) have pointed out, to suspend our epistemological concerns about the status and meaning of broad ethnic categorisations. Yet, our relationships to research on ethnicity are also more complicated than the naivety that Sheldon and Parker suggest, because despite the limitations of the broad categories that are used in research, such categories can still serve a purpose in identifying health inequalities (see Aspinall and Jacobson, 2004; and Smaje, 1996).

For instance, the third of the national surveys of NHS patients (Airey et al., 2002) used the broad categories of 'Black', 'South Asian' and 'White'. Nevertheless, the finding that among cancer patients, 32 per cent of South Asian patients did not completely understand their diagnosis, compared to 25 per cent of black patients and 19 per cent of all patients can be a valuable starting point in exploring inequalities of care within services. What is important when we work with such categorisations of ethnicity in research is that we remain aware of what is gained and what is lost in the process and the levels of categorisation and generalisation. In the face-to-face interactions of qualitative research, for example, we might use such categories as 'White', 'Black' or 'South Asian' in the initial stages of research, but these categories can also be opened to more rigorous questioning and deconstruction in the process of analysing and representing research.

My own ways of negotiating what I have called the 'treacherous bind' (Gunaratnam, 2003) of terminology to describe something of the collective experience of those in socially marginalised ethnic groups are both evolving and imperfect. What underlies my continuing struggle with terminology is the belief that language to describe the complex positions and experiences of ethnicity should be difficult, contested and troubling. This is why I abhor the use of the term 'BME' (Black and minority ethnic). Constructed as a convenient short-hand to roll off the tongue with ease, I feel that it inhibits critical thought and dialogue. When writing and speaking in academic fora, I have used the jarring term 'minoritised' ethnic groups to draw attention to the active processes of social categorisation that are involved in terminology. More than this, the harshness of the term 'minoritised' helps to foreground relations of power. This discursive strategy has not been so sustainable in the voluntary sector where time for critical debate is often undermined by scarce resources and funding criteria. My compromise has been to attempt to highlight the problematic nature of terminology by talking about groups 'categorised as being minority ethnic' or 'racialised as being minority ethnic' and then using the term in scare quotation marks so that it is not normalised. However, in order to forge partnership working, to write collaboratively, campaign and to do research, I have noticed the term 'minority ethnic' creeping into my vocabulary. 'Complex or involved' or 'partnership in an evil action?'

Reinscription and qualitative research

One strategy of avoiding 'reinscription' that I have used in my qualitative research in the palliative care field is to not take the accounts of research participants at face value. This psychosocial approach has been influenced by poststructuralist and psychoanalytic theories of knowledge (Hollway and Jefferson, 2000), which suggest that the accounts of research participants are constructions rather than transparent representations of 'reality'. In my qualitative interviews, I look for the points of tension and contradiction within inter-view accounts and I use these points of tension to 'disassemble' (Knowles, 1999) broad ethnic categories and to understand something of the lived experience of ethnicity and its changing relationships to other social differences (Gunaratnam, 2003).

For example, James, a Kenyan patient with AIDS whom I interviewed in my hospice research (see also Gunaratnam, 2004), talked about the tribe that he came from as being a 'proud people', telling me that 'the ethnicity has got some proudness. They're a proud people ... I still carry that pride within ... you really have pride.' Yet, when I asked James whether he had any contact with the Kenyan community where he lived, he told me:

> No. No. And I don't want to have anything to do with the Kenyan community ... with this disease, they tend to actually prey on you ... they spread out rumours to the rest of the community, which is quite damaging.

By recognising the painful tensions in James's account between being a 'proud Kenyan' and 'living with AIDS', it was possible to grasp something of the ways in which AIDS, as an illness that carries social and moral meanings (Lather and Smithies, 1997), can rupture the 'we-ness' of ethnic identifications. In this context, the very failure of ethnic identifica-tions to represent experience 'fully' can be a grounds through which we can sometimes glimpse the contradictory and emotional dimensions of identity in everyday lived lives.

To draw upon arguments made by Stuart Hall (1993) in a different context, the more we are able to use our research practices to recognise ethnic identifications as being multiple and contested, the more we are able to ask the significant questions of 'which identity?', 'whose identity?' and 'which version?'. By questioning and breaking down the meanings of ethnic categories in this way, it is also possible to challenge processes of reinscription in research *and* in the accounts of research participants, by recognising how other social identities, such as those relating to gender, class or health, interact with and inflect lived experiences of ethnicity (Knowles, 1999).

Micropolitics

In relation to the micropolitical interactions in research, Bhavnani highlights the complicated power relationships between herself as a South Asian, middle-class woman researcher and her young male and female working-class research participants from a range of different South Asian, African Caribbean and White British backgrounds (see also Phoenix, 2001). Bhavnani discusses how her research relationships were unpredictable, both inverting *and* reproducing disparities of power, having 'structural domination and structural subordination in play on both sides' (1993: 101).

Of particular interest is Bhavnani's suggestion that research which is based upon 'matching' between the identities of researchers and research participants, or which assumes commonalities of identity and experience, often fails to address power relationships in research and how these relationships are connected to the knowledge that is produced about difference. In relation to the broader discussion, what I want to draw attention to is how, if we are concerned with ethical relationships in research, we must question both what appear to be purely technical research practices and the institutional contexts in which research takes place. I will use the example of ethnic matching in research to examine these issues further.

Practices of ethnic matching, between practitioners and service users and/or local communities, occupy a central position in discussions about cross-cultural research and 'culturally competent' service provision and practice in health care (see Alexander, 1999; Chambers and Obrey, 2004; Kai and Hedges, 1999; Papadopoulos and Lees, 2002; Papadopoulos et al., 1998 for examples). In a discussion of 'culturally competent' nurse research, Papadopoulos and Lees (2002) advocate ethnic matching as an example of 'ethnic sensitivity'. They suggest that matching should be practised 'whenever possible' because it:

> [...] encourages a more equal context for interviewing which allows more sensitive and accurate information to be collected. A researcher with the same ethnic background as the participant will possess 'a rich fore understanding' (Ashworth, 1986) and an insider/emic view (Leininger, 1991; Kauffman, 1994), will have more favourable access conditions and the co-operation of a large number of people (Hanson, 1994) and a genuine interest in the health and welfare of their community (Hillier and Rachman, 1996). (Papadopoulos and Lees, 2002: 261)

This statement by Papadopoulos and Lees, encapsulates many of the assumptions that are made about commonality and difference in research on ethnicity, in which ethnic correspondence is constructed as the best all-round solution to the complexities of communicating across difference. What is noteworthy in this example is that ethnic commonalities are not just seen as a way of overcoming cultural and linguistic differences in research interactions, they are also promoted as reducing emotional distances between the interviewer and the research participant (see also Bhopal, 2001; Dunbar et al., 2002). That is, ethnicity is seen as a form of interactional and emotional capital that can be exploited to build rapport and co-operation, and to gain access to the subjectivity (processes of self and sense making) of minoritised research participants, enabling researchers to move from 'outsiders' to 'insiders' (see Ryen, 2002 for further discussion).

It is this assumption that is ethically and politically dangerous in research because it can essentialise 'race' and ethnicity as fixed, singular categories of difference, producing and obscuring the micropolitics of research. There are three specific 'dangers' that I wish to highlight. First, such strategies can serve to define the experiences of individuals and groups primarily in relation to their ethnicity. Second, experiences of ethnicity, but also language and its meanings, are treated as uncontested, rather than as multiple and changing. And third, as Gail Lewis (2000: 127) has pointed out in relation to matching practices in social work, 'no room is allowed for the possibility of shared understandings, correspondences of experiences or fluidity across group boundaries, nor indeed of heterogeneity within groups.

In questioning the assumptions, and the rationale behind ethnic matching in research, my aim is not to deny the possibility or the value of points of connection across ethnicity, culture and language. Rather, I want to move away from essentialist ideas of 'commonality' that suggest a naturalised affinity in communication, interpretation and understanding between members of the same ethnic/cultural/linguistic group (see Gunaratnam 2003: Chapter 4, for further examples). The challenging of such essentialism can be especially important in negotiating the micopolitics of research on ethnicity in health, where essentialism can be encouraged not only by funding agencies, but also by some of the community 'representatives' with whom we work.

A qualitative study by Elam and Chinouya (2000) on extending national health surveys to include black African populations living in the UK, is one of the few Department of Health funded studies that I have come across that discusses critically some of the micropolitics of expectations and demands for ethnic matching strategies in research:

> There was an expectation that research conducted by community members would be genuine, non-judgemental and tailored to community needs. However, benefits of matching need to be balanced against generational differences; regional animosity; and a reluctance to talk openly for fear of personal circumstances reaching community members in the UK and those in home towns of Africa. The latter concern arises from the strong links many Africans have with relatives in Africa; the desire to protect dependants living in Africa from problems people have in the UK; the stigma attached to poor health in general and to poor mental health, TB, and HIV in particular; and concerns that poor health may impede Asylum applications. (Elam and Chinouya, 2000: 9)

The realities of challenging essentialism throughout the research process (for example, in applying for funding, recruiting researchers and research participants, in fieldwork and analysis) are complicated and difficult. For instance, while in academic research, discussion of micropolitical issues in research is acceptable and often encouraged and valued, it is much more difficult for these discussions to be a legitimate part of the research reports of research funded by government agencies. It is also the case that even though I remain critical of strategies such as ethnic matching at a conceptual and political level, I recognise that essentialist ideas about commonality and difference have served to provide research jobs (though often marginalised, insecure and badly paid) for those researchers and interviewers racialised as being 'minority ethnic' (Twine, 2000).

Ann Phoenix (2001) has further suggested that matching practices in research can be exploitative of some minoritised research participants. This is because research participants can believe that the minoritised interviewer has some control over the research, when frequently 'the black interviewer has little control over the trajectory of the research or the analysis of data' (Phoenix, 2001: 214). The paradox in much contemporary research on ethnicity and health is that apparent concern with enabling the participation of 'ethnic minorities' in research as participants is frequently achieved through the very compounding, manipulation and exploitation of racialised, gendered and class-related inequalities in research structures and practices. A critical task in challenging complicity in research on ethnicity thus relates to how, as researchers and readers, we can find, connect, and do something about the collision of 'micro' and 'macro' inequalities throughout the research process.

Conclusion

Through a discussion of Bhavnani's criteria of reinscription, micropolitics and difference, I hope to have shown some of the challenges of researching ethnicity. The development of ethical and accountable research that runs counter to the essentialist threads that weave so casually through many current approaches to ethnicity and health is a difficult, risky and uncertain business. In 'real-world' research it can mean questioning inadequate and homongenising conceptual categories and then having little choice but to work with these same categories in order to secure research funding, communicate with stakeholders, publish, and engage with policy debates. It can also mean facing up to the complicities of research that may be concerned with alleviating inequalities in health, but which concretise inequalities at the micropolitical levels of research. Caught between the inviting simplicity and neatness of essentialist approaches to ethnicity and the need to 'do something' about health and social inequalities, our recognition and attention to the complexities and complicities of research have much to offer.

References

Airey, C., Becher, H., Erens, B. and Fuller, E. (2002) *National Surveys of NHS Patients. Cancer: National Overview 1999/2000*. London: Department of Health.

Alexander, Z. (1999) *Study of Black, Asian and Ethnic Minority Issues*. London: Department of Health.

Ashworth, P. (1986) *Qualitative Research in Psychology*. Pittsburgn, PA: Duquesne University Press.

Aspinall, P. and Jacobson, B. (2004). *Ethnic Disparities in Health and Health Care: a Focused Review of the Evidence and Selected Examples of Good Practice*. London: London Health Observatory.

Bhavnani, K.-K. (1993) Tracing the contours of feminist research and feminist objectivity, *Women's Studies International Forum*, 6 (2): 95–104.

Bhavnani, K. and Phoenix, A. (eds) (1994) *Shifting Identities, Shifting Racisms: a Feminism and Psychology Reader*. London: Sage.

Bhopal, K. (2001) Researching South Asian women: issues of sameness and difference in the research process, *Journal of Gender Studies*, 10 (3): 279–86.

Brah, A. (1996) *Cartographies of Diaspora: Contesting Identities*. London: Routledge.

Chambers, C. and Obrey, A. (2004) Creating an inclusive environment for black and minority ethnic nurses, *British Journal of Nursing*, 13 (22): 1355–7.

Dunbar, C. Jr, Rodriguez, D. and Parker, L. (2002) Race, subjectivity and the interview process, in J. Gubrium and J. Holstein (eds), *Handbook of Interview Research: Context and Method*. Thousand Oaks, CA: Sage, pp. 279–98.

Elam, G. and Chinouya, M. (2000) *Feasibility Study for Health Surveys among Black African Populations Living in the UK: Stage 2 – Diversity among Black African Communities*. London: National Centre for Social Research.

Gunaratnam, Y. (2003) *Researching 'Race' and Ethnicity: Methods, Knowledge and Power*. London: Sage.

Gunaratnam, Y. (2004) Skin matters: 'race' and care in the health services, in J. Fink (ed.), *Care: Personal Lives, Social Policy*. Bristol: Policy Press, pp. 112–44.

Hall, S. (1993) Culture, community, nation, *Cultural Studies*, 7 (3): 349–63.

Hanson, E. (1994) Issues concerning the familiarity of researchers with the research setting, *Journal of Advanced Nursing*, 20 (3): 940–2.

Haraway, D. (1988) Situated knowledges: the science question in feminism and the privilege of partial perspective, *Feminist Studies*, 14 (3): 575–99.

Hillier, S. and Rachman, S. (1996) Childhood development and behavioural and emotional problems as perceived by Bangladeshi parents in East London, in D. Kelleher and S. Hillier (eds), *Researching Cultural Differences in Health*. London: Routledge, pp. 38–68.

Hollway, W. and Jefferson, T. (2000) *Doing Qualitative Research Differently: Free Association, Narrative and the Interview Method*. London: Sage.

Kai, J. and Hedges, C. (1999) Minority ethnic community participation in needs assessment and service development in primary care: perceptions of Pakistani and Bnagladeshi people about psychological distress, *Health Expectations*, 2: 7–20.

Kauffman, K. (1994) The insider/outsider dilemma: field experience of a white researcher 'getting in' a poor black community, *Nursing Research*, 43: 179–83.

Knowles, C. (1999) Race, identities and lives, *Sociological Review*, 47 (1): 110–35.

Lather, P. (2001) Postbook: working the ruins of feminist ethnography, *Signs*, 27 (1): 199–227.

Lather, P. and Smithies, C. (1997) *Troubling the Angels: Women Living with HIV/AIDS*. Boulder, CO: Westview Press.

Leininger, M. (ed.) (1991) *Culture Care, Diversity and Universality: A Theory of Nursing*. New York: NLN Press.

Lewis, G. (2000) *'Race', Gender, Social Welfare: Encounters in a Postcolonial Society*. Cambridge: Polity Press.

Marcus, G. (1998) *Ethnography Through Thick and Thin*. Princeton, NJ: Princeton University Press.

Papadopoulos, I. and Lees, S. (2002) Developing culturally competent researchers, *Journal of Advanced Nursing*, 37 (3): 258–64.

Papadopoulos, I., Tilki, M. and Taylor, G. (1998) *Transcultural Care: a Guide for Health Care Professionals*. Dinton: Quay Books.

Phoenix, A. (2001) Practising feminist research: the intersection of gender and 'race' in the research process, in K.-K. Bhavnani (ed.), *Feminism and Race*. Oxford: Oxford University Press, pp. 203–19; originally published in M. Maynard and J. Purvis (eds) (1994) *Researching Women's Lives*. London: Taylor Francis, pp. 49–71.

Ryen, A. (2002) Cross-cultural interviewing, in J. Gubrium and J. Holstein (eds), *Handbook of Interview Research: Context and Method*. Thousand Oaks, CA: Sage, pp. 335–54.

Sayyid, S. (2000) Beyond Westphalia: nations and diasporas – the case of the Muslim umma, in B. Hesse (ed.), *Un/settled Multiculturalisms: Diasporas, Entanglements, Transruptions*. London: Zed Books, pp. 33–50.

Sheldon, T. and Parker, H. (1992) The use of 'ethnicity' and 'race' in health research: a cautionary note, in W.I.U. Ahmad (ed.), *The Politics of 'Race' and Health*. Bradford: Race Relations Unit, University of Bradford and Ilkey Community College, pp. 53–78.

Smaje, C. (1996) The ethnic patterning of health: new directions for theory and research, *Sociology of Health and Illness*, 18: 139–71.

Twine, F.W. (2000) Racial ideologies and racial methodologies, in F.W. Twine and J. Warren (eds), *Racing Research, Researching Race*. New York: New York University Press, pp. 1–34.

Visweswaran, K. (1994) *Fictions of Feminist Ethnography*. Minneapolis: University of Minnesota Press.

Werbner, P. (1997) Essentialising essentialism, essentialising silence: ambivalence and multiplicity in the constructions of racism and ethnicity, in P. Werbner and T. Modood (eds), *Debating Cultural Hybridity: Multi-Cultural Identities and the Politics of Anti-Racism*. London: Zed Books, pp. 226–54.

Part IV
Promoting Public Health through Public Policy

Introduction

Jenny Douglas

The *Ottawa Charter for Health Promotion* of 1986 has been highly influential in focusing public health action on developing healthy public policy and putting health on the agendas of organisations and sectors which have not focused previously on health. In 2005, the *Bangkok Charter*, building upon the values and principles of the *Ottawa Charter* and subsequent global health promotion conferences, identified action required to address the determinants of health in a globalised world. The contributions in Part IV are concerned with developing healthy public policy in the context of increasing globalisation and exploring the links between public health, politics and economics.

Ilona Kickbusch and Birahim Seck set the scene in Chapter 20. Outlining global health issues which transcend national boundaries, they argue that in order to understand the present state of global health there needs to be greater awareness of the governance issues which impede global health action. They suggest a new conceptual map for global public health, concluding that in order for all global actors to become more responsive and accountable for their contribution to the health of the world's populations, legal and regulatory frameworks must be put in place and that there needs to be a focus on political mechanisms to ensure that the poorest people of the world have access to health.

In Chapter 21, Hilary Graham provides an overview of the links between poverty and health over time and compares national and global trends. She argues that social and economic policies hold the key to improving the life chances of poor groups and concludes by raising questions about the ethics of current public policy, proposing that human development and not economic development should be shaping national and global policies for the 21st century.

The importance of recognising that actions at a global level affect our ability to improve health at a local level is explored by Ronald Labonte in Chapter 22. He examines the effects of global economic policies on health. Although addressing issues of global trade can seem a huge task to individuals involved in promoting public health, Ronald Labonte sets out action that individual health promoters can take based upon skills developed through health promotion practice. He argues that health promoters cannot afford to ignore issues such as globalisation.

In the 21st century, events such as 11 September 2001 have focused attention on the impact of terrorism on the health of individuals. In Chapter 23, John Middleton and Victor Sidel argue that the principal responsibility for the public health community is to understand the nature of terrorism in order to tackle its root causes – gross inequalities in the world's access to resources, poverty and inequality in health. They conclude that support of human rights and pursuit of social justice are essential for improved public health.

In Chapter 24, Mike Rowson evaluates some of the evidence used in debates about the complex relationship of income and health in developing countries and the impact of globalisation on health, arguing that there is no straightforward relationship between globalisation, income and health. He suggests that the effects of income on health are dependent upon patterns of social organisation and that governments can do a lot to protect the health of the vulnerable.

Often the poorest people in a society are the people who have been forced to migrate there for a whole host of reasons, including war, natural disasters, political persecution or persistent poverty and famine. In the final contribution in Part IV, Natalie Grove, Anthony Zwi and Pascale Allotey explore how forced migrants are constructed and portrayed as 'not belonging' and as the 'other'. They argue that an understanding of 'othering' is important to public health and outline how othering, whether based on disability, gender, health status, sexuality or ethnicity, can lead to social marginalisation of groups and limit their access to health and other services. The authors conclude that respect for human rights at an individual level is key to effective public health at a population level.

Chapter 20

Global Public Health

Ilona Kickbusch and Birahim Seck

Great achievements have been made in global disease control in recent decades: small pox has been eradicated, polio has nearly been defeated, many parts of the world are now free of measles and other childhood diseases. However, while some diseases have been controlled successfully, others such as malaria and tuberculosis are fighting back with renewed ferocity. Global restructuring, combined with the continued spread of HIV/AIDS, the advent of new diseases such as SARS, the rise of natural disasters, and the threat of an influenza pandemic, have created a global health crisis which threatens to undermine the gains made so far. Global health, as a new dimension of public health action, 'addresses those health problems, issues and concerns that transcend national boundaries, may be influenced by circumstances or experiences in other countries, and are best addressed by co-operative actions and solutions' (Institute of Medicine, 1997). But despite the acknowledgement of the global health challenge what we find is a lack of long-term commitment at both national and international levels.

In consequence, the disease crisis is the result of a governance crisis. Despite long years of development aid and many activities by an increasing number of players, the responsiveness, efficacy and performance of the global health system have been weakened through a neglect of public health systems within countries and a lack of political will to engage in collective action at the global level. Increased mortality and morbidity are the outcome of unfit governance structures and the combined challenge of poverty and disease – not a lack of proven interventions. Despite new global commitments (United Nations, 2000), we are presently in a situation that all progress achieved so far towards health and well-being could be wasted unless effective global health policies are formulated, and commitments are made to implement them nationally and internationally.

This chapter argues that in order to understand the present state of global health we need to understand some of the governance issues which seriously impede the global health action. It is structured as follows. Part I presents the extent of the disease crisis, part II maps out the central systemic weaknesses of the present global health governance system and part III discusses some strategic directions for change.

Part I: The extent of the disease crisis

The extent of the disease crisis can be illustrated by seven critical developments.

AIDS

The AIDS epidemic continues to outstrip global and national efforts to contain it. A new report shows that despite the huge global campaign, the new Global Fund on AIDS, Tuberculosis and Malaria, and a substantial amount of funds and resources, the total number of people living with the human immunodeficiency virus (HIV) has reached its highest level: an estimated 40.3 million (36.7–45.3 million) people are now living with HIV. Close to 5 million people were newly infected with the virus in 2005 (UNAIDS/WHO, 2005). Africa remains the most affected, but the pandemic is growing in Central and Eastern Europe and the countries of the former Soviet Union, as well as Russia, India and especially China (Zhu et al., 2005).

Malaria

The fight against Malaria is also being lost despite the considerable efforts and resources being mobilized to confront the disease. New estimates show the rising trends of the pandemic. The World Health Organization (WHO) estimates that approximately 300 million people worldwide are affected by malaria and between 1 and 1.5 million people die from it every year. Previously extremely widespread, malaria is now mainly confined to Africa, Asia and Latin America. The problems of controlling malaria in these countries are aggravated by inadequate health structures and poor socioeconomic conditions. The situation has become even more complex over the last few years with the increase in drug resistance.

Tuberculosis

In 1993 the WHO declared tuberculosis 'a global health emergency'. It is estimated that there are 8.3 million new cases of tuberculosis (TB) and almost 2 million deaths worldwide annually, making it the second leading cause of death globally from an infectious disease (Corbett et al., 2003: 1009). There is growing concern about the emergence of multidrug-resistant strains, which now affect up to 50 million people. According to the WHO, one-third of deaths of those who are HIV-positive are tuberculosis related. Tuberculosis kills more young people and adults than any other infectious disease. The WHO predicts that by 2020 nearly one billion people will be newly infected with TB, and of them 70 millions will die.

The epidemics of tobacco and obesity

The non-communicable diseases epidemic that began in industrialized countries is spreading to low and middle-income nations (WHO, 2001). Approximately 177 million people are currently living with diabetes, and the number of people with the disease is projected to more than double by 2030, especially in developing nations (WHO, 2004). Tobacco is responsible for about 5 million deaths each year, particularly among poor populations and poor countries. The total number of people who smoke is increasing (WHO, 2003).

Maternal and child mortality

The 2005 *World Health Report* (WHO, 2005) shows that pregnancy, childbirth and their consequences are still the leading cause of death, disease and disability among women of reproductive age in developing countries. In Africa, the lifetime risk of maternal death is one in 16, compared to one in 28,000 in rich countries. About 10.6 million children still die before reaching their fifth birthday and most deaths are attributable to a handful of avoidable conditions.

Rise of natural disasters

Earthquakes and hurricanes have become deadlier and more regular. The 2004 'Christmas tsunami in the Indian Ocean, Hurricane Katrina on the US Gulf Coast, and the Pakistan earthquake together have left nearly 300,000 dead and millions homeless' (Bohannon, 2005: 1883). The aftermath of disasters is associated with public health consequences, including mortality, injury, infectious disease, psychosocial effects, displacement and homelessness, damage to the health-care infrastructure, disruption of public health services, transformation of ecosystems, social dislocation, and loss of jobs (Shultz et al., 2005: 21–35).

SARS, the Avian influenza and a potential human influenza pandemic

There are now growing concerns regarding a possible outbreak of a human influenza pandemic. The Avian influenza, known as H5N1, is now spreading through bird populations across Asia and has recently reached Europe. The global community is on alert as it fears that the virus will mutate and spread from human to human. The Asian Development Bank predicts that such an outbreak could kill 3 million people in Asia, trigger economic carnage in the region worth almost US $300 billion and push the world into a recession. As a result, donor countries have pledged US $1.9 billion to confront the threat of a global pandemic. Urgent priorities have focused on health and veterinarian services, aiming to prevent the virus mutating and spreading from human to human.

Part II: The governance crisis

The global diseases and emerging threats outlined above indicate the weakening of public health systems throughout the world. Paradoxically, these diseases occur where public health solutions do exist. This raises not only the issue of why there has been such a significant failure in health and development in the past, but also the point that present-day public health structures and processes are no longer sufficient to deal with major seminal trends occurring in relation to health and society. We argue that the present global health crisis is not primarily one of disease, but of governance. In this section we highlight four major concerns, which are an expression of this governance crisis.

Concern 1: The lack of sustainable health systems

Progress in global health is first and foremost dependent on the performance of health systems at the national and local levels. International health development investments have been mainly based on implementing specific programmes rather than sustaining health systems infrastructure and capacity building for frontline health workers. Indeed, during the last two decades many countries have been forced, as a part of international agreements such as the Washington Consensus (Kuczynski and Williamson, 2003), to reduce public spending on health. According to WHO, nearly 20 per cent of member states spend less that US$ 15 per capita on health (WHO, 2003). Shortages of human resources plague the health systems of the developing world. The lack of health workers is impeding progress, particularly in sub-Saharan Africa and the 'brain drain' of health workers is weakening already fragile health systems. In most countries there is insufficient investment in national capacities for public health and other basic infrastructures such as water and sanitation. Failures of health systems disproportionately impact the poor. They suffer from a lack of health-care coverage and are forced to pay for their treatment. In India, for example, families pay 80 per cent of their health costs out of their own pockets.

The SARS and the Avian influenza outbreaks have been another warning sign that global health security is challenged by two key systemic components:

1   The weakest link: a functioning primary health-care system in the poorest countries.
2   The accountability, transparency and cooperation between all the players at the global governance level.

Concern 2: The consequences of global restructuring

The restructuring of the global economy has led to a very different socioeconomic–political context of health. Public health is not yet prepared – both in its mind set and its organizational structure – to face the major changes that have occurred as a consequence of globalization. Some of these changes, as outlined by Kelley Lee (2003), include the erosion of the ability of a country to set a national health policy in the face of global pressures, the changing balance of power among public and private sector actors in health, and the weak protection of public health in other global policy arenas, such as multilateral trade agreements of the World Trade Organization (WTO).

Globalization impacts on the determinants of health and, as a result, the poorest countries are feeling the devastating effects of global health disparities. While there is an increasing recognition that investments in health are of prime importance (WHO Commission on Macroeconomics and Health, 2001) to ensure the participation of the poorest in economic and social development, the redirection of policies has been slow to follow. In many cases health agendas and economic growth and investment agendas compete rather than complement one another, and innovation is focused on the needs of the rich rather than the poor countries – as in pharmaceutical development, for example.

Migration issues are also of major concerns in this new restructured world as they mostly affect the poorest. Currently, there are 175 million international migrants in the world (International Organization for Migration, 2003) and according to UNHCR, the number of displaced people in the world has increased more than fourfold from 5.4 million in 1980 to 22.3 million in 2000 (UNHCR, 1998, 2000).

Concern 3: The 'unstructured plurality' of the global health system

Global health has no defined centre of action and creates a new political space (Kickbusch, 2003). It is characterized by a growing and complex assemblage of actors, which interacts on a wide variety of converging and conflicting interests, mainly at policy level. This governance characteristic has been termed as 'unstructured plurality' (Beck and Lau, 2004). The key new players are:

- *Business actors* in health have become central. Health is now one of the largest private markets in the world. Industries that endanger health, such as the tobacco and alcohol industries, are among the most influential global industries, as are industries with a high relevance to health, such as the food industry. Medical and pharmaceutical research is a key area of research and technology development, and a major factor in innovation and competition between companies, regions and nations (World Economic Forum, 2006).
- *Other international agencies and groupings* Health has become a central component in the agendas of non-health organizations such as the World Trade Organization and the World Bank, as well as in deliberations of groupings such as the G8 and the World Economic Forum (Labonte et al., 2004; Ollila, 2005).
- A growing number of *highly diverse new organizations, networks and alliances* focusing on discrete and measurable areas of action have superseded the traditional division of delivery mechanisms between bilateral and multilateral health agencies (Richter, 2004). For example, new organizations such as the Global Fund on AIDS, Tuberculosis and Malaria and UNAIDS have been established to address priority problems and an increasing number of public–private partnerships, such as the Global Alliance on Vaccines and Immunization (GAVI), are engaged in reducing the infectious disease burden in the poorest countries.
- A *set of strong new non-state players* is defining priorities and approaches. Non-governmental organizations (NGOs) have become much more prominent both in setting agendas and in delivering services. Private foundations have gained high influence through their resource-based power in global health, in particular the Bill and Melinda Gates Foundation, which spends about US$ 1 billion on global health annually. The pharmaceutical industry and other parts of the private sector are increasingly involved in not-for-profit activities and alliances to improve health in rich and poor countries (Stansfield, 2002; Hilts, 2005).
- *Regional organizations* such as the European Union, ASEAN, OAS (Organization of American States) and the OECD have significantly strengthened their health portfolios. In parallel, a spectrum of municipal actors are engaging in worldwide cooperation to address local problems.

This new set of players – in particular the public–private partnerships, global funds and alliances – aims to provide better results (in particular more efficiency and effectiveness) than the international state-based system (i.e. the United Nations organizations), to provide a greater focus on technical agendas rather than politics, and to be more inclusive by involving a wide range of stakeholders. But concerns are growing that the redirection of global health functions from interstate mechanisms to this polycentric group of actors is not fulfilling its promise.

Concern: 4 The lack of global accountability

The unstructured plurality of players has brought new concerns, raising the issue to what extent they are efficiently advancing the global health agenda. Indeed, with the fragmentation of activities and competition, the lack of transparency and accountability and the growing disparities in power between rich and poor as well as strong and weak players, it has become difficult to discern whom to hold responsible for success or failure and, for instance, to whom to impute the present global health crisis.

In view of the global challenges it is no longer sufficient to work – even if successfully – programme by programme, but it is critical to have a systematic effort to build health systems and human resources for health throughout the developing world. Therefore programme accountability must be linked to a more systemic accountability on the contribution of each actor to the functioning of the overall impact and contribution to the national health system and the system of global health. For example, we have witnessed that even as more initiatives, medicines and resources have become available in the global health arena, countries most in need do not have the infrastructure and the frontline health workers to get the treatments to the people. Accountability must be for the contribution to the system as a whole.

Part III: Steps towards a new conceptual map

It is clear that ethical, technical and political issues must interface in new ways to produce results. What follows are six key dimensions of a new conceptual map for global public health:

1. Health as a global public good

The present system of development aid, international agencies and voluntary actors is not organized to deliver global and transnational public goods, except in the area of trade. This must change. The critical step is to recognize health as a global public good that cuts across borders, generations, and populations (Kaul et al., 1999). The global health challenges require not just good national policies, but also strong global responses and international collective action (Smith et al., 2003). First steps are being undertaken to pool sovereignty for health and create new binding regimes such as the 2005 International Health Regulations, the International Framework Convention on Tobacco Control and new policies on intellectual property rights. New financing models are essential for a global public good (GPG) approach (Kaul and Conceição, 2006) and are increasingly being explored. Examples are the International Finance Facility, designed to frontload aid to help meet the Millennium Development Goals (Department for International Development/HM Treasury, 2003) and a tax on airline travel recently introduced by France to fund HIV/AIDS, malaria and tuberculosis programmes.

2. A rights based approach

During the past few years there has been a growing focus on health as human rights, and an increasing global attempt to develop a conceptual framework which explores the reciprocal influences of health and human rights. This is a reflection of the move from a state-based international system to one that also recognizes the rights of individuals. The present director of Human Rights Watch has highlighted the difficulty of holding governments to account for violations of social and economic rights (Roth, 2004). But there is a growing national and international jurisprudence on the right to health, and while the legal content of the right to health is not yet well established, it represents one of the biggest global public health challenges of the 21st century.

3. Health as a key component of global and human security

In an interdependent world disease outbreaks are a threat to the security of states, of individuals and of the global community as a whole. Nation states are increasingly integrating health issues into their security and foreign policy strategies. Issues of health are now part of the agenda of the Security Council of the United Nations and are of increasing concern to development and investment banks and the private sector. But we need to ensure a concept of collective human security and combine forces to address global and transnational risks through a joint system of regimes, surveillance, preparedness and response. Such a system must clearly separate all forms of military surveillance from public health. A priority must be the establishment of a global surveillance infrastructure and a rapid health response force which could be financed through new forms of global risk insurance or taxation.

4. Global health governance for interdependence

Global health governance needs to establish mechanisms that take into account the reality of interdependence, the plurality, diversification and number of actors in the global health arena. As the role of the nation state has shifted towards an intermediary position between external (global) and internal (domestic) policy demands (Kaul and Conceição, 2006), the role of international organizations will need to change to build policy consensus between a wide range of different players. An organization such as the WHO will need a new role to ensure policy coherence in global health. It should be able to ensure transparency and accountability in global health governance and play a brokering role in relation to the health impacts of policies of other agencies. The WHO must make certain that the new collaborative arrangements in global health evolve into networks and regimes of governance. This could include a new kind of accountability and reporting system that is requested of all international health actors.

5. Health as a key factor of sound business practice and social responsibility

Companies must be more accountable for global public goods, in particular those that improve health. New business models and new forms of philanthropy have now become part of the work of the World Economic Forum and many public–private partnerships. Also, companies are exploring the reach of their products and services beyond the traditional consumer base in order to include disadvantaged populations. Pharmaceutical companies have been called on to engage in differentiated pricing and in research for 'forgotten' diseases such as malaria and tuberculosis, thereby increasing the capacity of poor countries to access treatments and support the WHO. Health philanthropic activity by companies is significantly on the rise and business has started to work in partnership with development agencies. Several CEOs have taken the lead in creating foundations, for example Bill Gates, George Soros and Ted Turner.

6. The ethical principle of health as global citizenship

Social and economic inequities, including health, must rigorously be addressed at the international level through sustained action. Rich nations must not only increase their foreign aid to the minimum 0.7 per cent GNP, but also reduce poverty via trade, investment, migration, environment, security and technology. Ethical norms must apply to international relations. As inequities in health become increasingly obvious, the notion of health as a human right is gaining support. Nigel Dower (2003: 132) points out:

> If citizens are increasingly motivated by global concerns, then cosmopolitan goals enter domestic policy in that way and people can be effective global citizens by being effective global-oriented citizens of their own states.

Conclusion

At present, the unstructured plurality of the global health system is an impediment to progress. But we cannot turn back the clock to a clearly circumscribed international system. The challenge will be to move forward and create the synergies needed, but also to put into place the legal and regulatory frameworks to ensure that all global actors will become more responsible and accountable for their contribution to the health of the world's populations. We know what creates health and disease. We now need to focus on the political mechanisms to ensure that the poorest people of the world get access to health as an expression of their right as global citizens.

References

Beck, U. and Lau, C. (2004) *Entgrenzung und Entscheidung.* Edition Zweite Moderne Suhrkamp, Frankfurt.

Bohannon, J. (2005) Breakthrough of the year: Disasters – searching for lessons from a bad year, *Science*, 310 (5756): 1883.

Corbett, E.L., Watt, C.J., Walker, N., Maher, D., Williams, B.G., Raviglione, M.C. and Dye, C. (2003) The growing burden of tuberculosis: global trends and interactions with the HIV epidemic, *Archives of Internal Medicine*, 163 (9): 1009–21.

Department for International Development/HM Treasury (2003) *International Finance Facility.* HM Treasury, London.

Dower, N. (2003) *An Introduction to Global Citizenship.* Edinburgh University Press, Edinburgh.

Hilts, P. (2005) *Rx for Survival: Why We Must Rise to the Global Health Challenge.* Penguin, New York.

Institute of Medicine (1997) *America's Vital Interest in Global Health.* National Academy Press, Washington DC.

International Organization for Migration (2003) *World Migration 2003.* IOM, Geneva.

Kaul, I. and Conceição, P. (2006) *The New Public Finance: Responding to Global Challenges.* Oxford University Press, New York.

Kaul, I., Grunberg, I. and Stern, M. (eds) (1999) *Global Public Goods: International Cooperation in the 21st Century.* UNDP, New York.

Kickbusch, I. (2003) Global health governance: some theoretical considerations in a new political space, in Lee, K. (ed.), *Health Impacts of Globalization.* Palgrave Macmillian, Basingstoke.

Kuczynski, P.-P. and Williamson, J. (eds) (2003) *After the Washington Consensus.* Institute for International Economics, Washington DC.

Labonte, R., Schrecker, T., Sanfers, D. and Meeus, W. (2004) *Fatal Indifference: the G8, Africa and Global Health.* UCT Press, Ottawa, ON.

Lee, K. (2003) *Globalization and Health: an Introduction.* Palgrave Macmillian, Basingstoke.

Ollila, E. (2005) Global health priorities: priorities of the wealthy?, *Globalization and Health*, www.globalizationandhealth.com/content/1/1/6 (accessed 3 March 2006).

Richter, J. (2004) Public–private partnerships for health: a trend with no alternatives?, *Society for International Development*, 47 (2): 43–8.

Roth, K. (2004) Defending economic, social and cultural rights, *Human Rights Quarterly*, 26: 63–73.

Shultz, J.M., Russell, J. and Espinel, Z. (2005) Epidemiology of tropical cyclones: the dynamics of disaster, disease, and development, *Epidemiologic Reviews*, 27 (1): 21–35.

Smith, R., Beaglehole, R., Woodward, D. and Drager, N. (2003) Global public goods for health, in Smith, R., Beaglehole, R., Woodward, D. and Drager, N. (eds), *Global Public Goods for Health: Health Economic and Public Health Perspectives.* Oxford University Press, Oxford, pp. 271–8.

Stansfield, S. (2002) Philanthropy and alliances for global health, in Kaul, I., Conceição, P., Le Goulven, K. and Mendoza, R.U. (eds), *Providing Global Public Goods: Managing Globalization.* Oxford University Press, New York.

UNAIDS/WHO (2005) *AIDS epidemic update.*, December. UNAIDS/World Health Organisation, Geneva.

UNHCR (1998) *State of the World's Refugees.* UNHCR, Geneva.

UNHCR (2000) *State of the World's Refugees.* UNHCR, Geneva.

United Nations (2000) *United Nations Millenium Declaration.* Official document A/55/L.2 of the UN General Assembly. United Nations, Geneva.

WHO (2001) *World Health Report 2001.* World Health Organisation, Geneva.

WHO (2003) *World Health Report 2003.* World Health Organisation, Geneva.

WHO (2004) Diabetes Mellitus Fact Sheet No. 138. Available at: http://www.who.int/mediacentre/ factsheets/fs138/en/ (accessed 3 March 2006).

WHO (2005) *World Health Report 2005: Make Every Mother and Child Count*. WHO, Geneva.

WHO Commission on Macroeconomics and Health (2001) *Macroeconomics and Health: Investing in Health for Economic Development*. December. World Health Organisation, Geneva.

World Economic Forum (2006) *Global Governance Initiative Third Annual Report*. Available at: http://www.weforum.org/pdf/Initiatives/GGI_Report06.pdf (accessed 3 March 2006).

Zhu, Tuo Fu, Wang, Chun Hui, Lin, Peng and He, Na (2005) High risk populations and HIV–1 infection in China, *Cell Research*, 15: 852–7.

Chapter 21

Poverty and Health: Global and National Patterns

Hilary Graham

Introduction

Poverty is linked to poor health over time, across and within societies, and despite changes in the major causes of death. But it is not only the poor whose health is compromised by their living conditions. The link between poverty and poor health is part of a wider relationship between an individual's socioeconomic circumstances and their health. It is part of a 'social gradient' in which middle-income groups enjoy better health than those in poverty, but fail to reach the levels of health achieved by those higher up the socioeconomic ladder.

The chapter begins by briefly describing data sources before mapping the enduring association between poverty and poor health. It concludes by discussing explanatory and policy perspectives on the poverty/poor health relationship.

Measuring poverty and health

The record-keeping systems required to capture the health effects of poverty are available only for a minority of the world's population. While 80 per cent of the European population have such systems, this is true for less than 5 per cent of the poorer regions of the world (Sen and Bonita, 2000).

In rich countries, relative measures of poverty are used (i.e. relative to average living standards). An example of a relative poverty line is a household income below 60 per cent median household income (adjusted for household size and composition), the one now used by the British government. It is very similar to 50 per cent of mean household income, another widely used measure of poverty (Department of Work and Pensions,

2006). Non-income based indicators of living conditions are also used, like educational attainment and occupation (and for children, parents' occupations).

In middle and low-income countries, a large proportion of the population is engaged in subsistence agriculture and the informal economy. This makes income-based measures less useful. Indicators based on housing quality and access to amenities (e.g. a home with a solid floor and roof, access to piped water) and ownership of assets (like land, animals and farming materials) are therefore used instead (Wagstaff, 2000; Blakely et al., 2005). Nonetheless, incomplete and unreliable data mean that little is known about poverty and health in countries where over 80 per cent of the population lives.

For cross-country analyses where standardised measures are needed, gross domestic product per person (GDP) is the most widely used measure of national income. It captures the scale of global inequalities in wealth, with annual GDP in 2001 ranging from $34,000 in the USA and $24,000 in the UK, to under $600 in the poorest countries of Africa (World Bank, 2003a). The World Bank has also established an international poverty line, based on the typical poverty line in low-income countries in the mid-1980s. People living on less than US$1 a day (uprated in 1993 to $1.08) are defined as living in 'extreme poverty'; those living on less than $2 a day are defined as poor. On this measure, 23 per cent of the population of low- and middle-income countries are in extreme poverty; when less than $2 a day is taken as the poverty line, the proportion rises to 56 per cent (World Bank, 2003a).

Mortality-based measures like infant mortality (stillbirths and deaths in the first year of life) and life expectancy are important indicators of health, particularly in countries where death rates are high. Where data permit, these are supplemented by measures of the quality of people's health, like 'disability-free life expectancy' and 'healthy life expectancy', which estimate the years an individual lives in good health. In addition, child development – physical, cognitive and psychological – is increasingly recognised as a major influence on adult health, with studies highlighting how poor childhood conditions compromise healthy development, and have lifelong effects on health in adult life (Graham and Power, 2004).

The scale of poor–rich inequalities in health is sensitive to the measures used to capture them. In both high-income and lower-income countries, inequalities tend to be larger for objective measures of health, like mortality, than for subjective measures, like self-assessed health. This is because people's expectations of health rise with income, with poorer groups more likely to tolerate disease and disability than better-off groups. However, while the magnitude of poor–rich differences varies across measures, the health inequalities that they reveal are consistently to the disadvantage of the poor.

Poverty and health over time

Evidence of a link between poor conditions and poor health dates back to ancient China, Greece and Egypt (Krieger, 1997; Whitehead, 1997). But it is only over the last 100 years or so that reliable data have been routinely collected. As the first industrialising nation, Britain provides a window on historical patterns.

In mid-19th century Britain, mortality rates stood at 23 per 1000 and one in five children died before their fifth birthday (Farr, 1885; Charlton and Murphy, 1997). High mortality rates were associated with marked inequalities in the health of rich and poor. For example, in the

1860s, death rates among children aged 0–5 years stood at 460 per 1000 in poor cities like Liverpool and 175 per 1000 in prosperous districts like Hampstead (Farr, 1885). From the late 19th century, death rates fell rapidly, a decline driven primarily by improvements in the living and working conditions of the urban poor and, in particular, by investment in municipal public health: in clean water and sanitation, in improved housing and in the regulation of the food supply (McKeown, 1979; Szreter, 1988; Doran and Whitehead, 2004).

With health improving for both rich and poor, absolute difference in their death rates narrowed (when death rates fall in all groups, mortality differences between them typically become smaller). However, relative differences in health – in the risk of death in poorer groups compared with better-off groups – remained pronounced (Pamuk, 1985; Drever and Bunting, 1997). It is a pattern captured in trends for infant mortality using Britain's traditional socioeconomic classification, based on five broad social classes. In 1911, infant mortality rates stood at 153 per 1000 among children born into the poorest circumstances (social class V) and 76 per 1000 among children born into best circumstances (social class I), representing an absolute difference in death rates of 77 deaths per 1000 per year (Registrar General, 1913). By the 1930s, infant mortality rates had fallen in all social classes, to under 80 per 1000 in social class V and under 40 per 1000 in social class I (an absolute difference of less than 40 deaths per 1000 per year) (Woolf, 1947). But, while absolute differences shrank, relative differences remained pronounced. Children born into the poorest circumstances in the 1930s were still twice as likely to die before their first birthday as children in the best-off families.

In recent decades, there is evidence of a widening health gap. This is because the rate of health gain in poorer groups has failed to keep pace with that achieved by better-off groups. Women's life expectancy in England and Wales illustrates this trend (Figure 21.1), with the gap at the end of the 1990s wider in both absolute and relative terms than it was in the early 1970s. Since 2000, there has been no narrowing of inequalities in male and female life expectancy (Department of Health, 2005).

Poverty and health across countries

As in the UK, global health improved across the 20th century: by 2001, global life expectancy had reached 66.7 years, an increase of eight years in two decades (UNDP, 2003). But national histories demonstrate the fragility of health gains, as the examples of HIV/AIDS in sub-Saharan Africa and social upheaval in the former USSR illustrate (Sen and Bonita, 2000). In South Africa, HIV/AIDS has reversed the upward trend in life expectancy: at 47 years in 2001, it is ten years lower than it was in 1980 (World Bank, 2003a). In the early 1990s, political and economic disruption in former Soviet countries like Russia and Estonia brought a rapid fall in life expectancy. While evidence is patchy, key factors appear to be the sharp increase in poverty and income inequalities resulting from market liberalisation and the weakening of welfare safety nets (Leinsalu et al., 2003). Behavioural factors are also implicated, with social disruption and greater poverty associated with higher alcohol consumption and an increase in alcohol-related deaths (Leon et al., 1997; McKee, 2003).

Whether life expectancy is rising or falling, it is the poor whose health suffers most. Thus, life expectancy is typically at its lowest in low-income countries and highest in

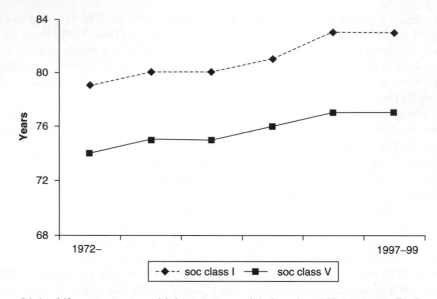

Figure 21.1   Life expectancy at birth, women social class I and V, 1972–99, England and Wales
Source: Donkin et al., 2002: constructed from data.

high-income countries. Shorter lives are often ones spent in poor health and with more disability. In sub-Saharan Africa, the region of the world with the lowest life expectancy, it is estimated that 18 per cent of total life expectancy is spent living with disability; in countries where life expectancy is high, like Japan, around 8 per cent of the average lifespan are years of disability (Mathers et al., 2000).

Figure 21.2 captures the broad relationship between national wealth and national health first charted by Samuel Preston (Preston, 1975). Among the poorest countries, increases in GDP are strongly associated with improvements in life expectancy: at this point in the income distribution, the line linking income and health is almost vertical. Among richer countries, the curve flattens out, with higher incomes bringing diminishing health benefits. Because the marginal health gains of extra income are much greater at the lower end of the income range, a redistribution of income from richer to poorer can be expected to increase the health of poorer societies more than it damages the health of the rich (Deaton, 2003).

As Figure 21.2 makes clear, there are 'outlier' countries with lower or higher life expectancies than their wealth would predict. One example, the world's richest country, the USA, with a lower life expectancy (77.0) than countries with much lower GDP, like Sweden (79.7) and Japan (80.7), and an infant mortality rate which is more than twice as high. Another is Sri Lanka, with a GDP which is half of that of Brazil but a higher life expectancy (73.1 versus 68.1) and a lower infant mortality rate (17 versus 31 per 1000) (World Bank, 2002; UNDP, 2003). The mediating factor is government investment in services which universalise access to key health resources, including clean water and sanitation, basic education, and health care (Sen, 1999). Since its independence in 1948, Sri Lanka has an equity-oriented approach to economic development, spending a relatively high proportion of GDP on poverty alleviation and population-wide sanitation, education

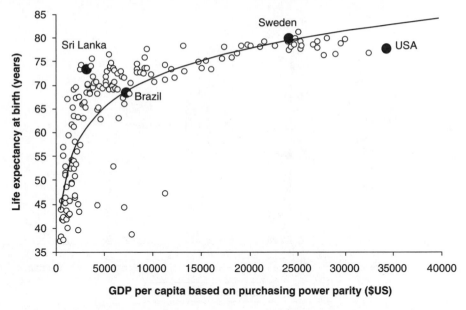

Figure 21.2   Gross domestic product per person (US$), adjusted for purchasing power parity, and life expectancy in 159 countries, 2001 (logarithmic trend line)
Source: World Bank, 2003a: constructed from data.

and health care (Drèze and Sen, 1989; Fernando, 2000; WHO Regional Office for SE Asia, 2004). As a result, over 75 per cent have access to safe drinking water, literacy rates are high (90 per cent), nearly 100 per cent of pregnant women receive antenatal care and are attended at birth by trained personnel and over 80 per cent of children receive the full complement of immunisations by their first birthday. Infectious disease rates, including HIV, are also low (World Bank, 2003b; WHO Regional Office for SE Asia, 2004).

Poverty and health within countries

Within societies, death rates are typically highest among the poorest (Kunst et al., 1998; World Bank, 2004). Figure 21.3 focuses on children aged 0–5 to illustrate the link between poverty and mortality in poorer countries. While there are marked national differences both in mortality rates and in the magnitude of the poor/rich gap, it is poor children who are at greater risk of death. Inequalities in health are matched by inequalities in access to the determinants of health, with publicly funded health care failing 'to reach the poor in almost all developing countries' (Wagstaff, 2002: 102, see also Schellenberg et al., 2003). A study using the international poverty line (living on less than US$1 a day/US$1–2 a day/and more than US$2 a day) revealed clear income gradients in health risks, with poverty associated with child malnutrition and limited access to water and sanitation (Blakely et al., 2005).

In rich societies, better socioeconomic circumstances – whether measured by income, education or occupation – are again associated with better health (Mackenbach et al., 2004).

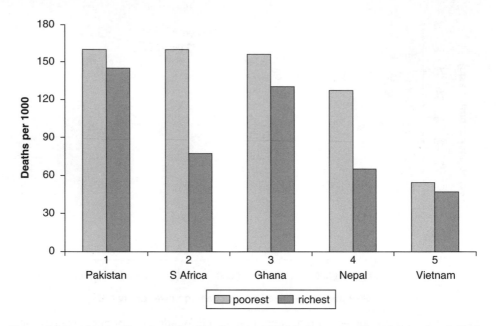

Figure 21.3   Under-five mortality (deaths per 1000) in the poorest and richest quintile in low-income and middle-income countries
Source: Wagstaff, 2000: constructed from data.

Figure 21.4 captures this association for self-assessed health. It is based on the British 2001 census, where respondents were asked to rate their health as 'good', 'fairly good' or 'not good' (Doran et al., 2004). Figure 21.4 uses the National Statistics Socioeconomic Classification (NS–SEC), which has replaced the traditional social class classification in Britain. Its major socioeconomic groups are managerial and professional, intermediate, and routine and manual occupations. The stepwise relationship between worsening socioeconomic conditions and poorer health which the figure reveals is found for major causes of death, including coronary heart disease.

While health inequalities are evident across societies, the poor endure poorer health in some countries than in others. For example, GDP is very similar in Sweden and Britain, but the poorest groups in Sweden can expect to live longer than the poorest in Britain (Kunst et al., 1998). Nepal's GDP is one-tenth of South Africa's, but its poorest children have a greater likelihood of surviving to age 5 (Figure 21.3).

... and despite changes in the major causes of death

Historically, the process of industrialisation has brought changes in patterns of disease, with infectious and nutrition-related diseases giving way to non-infectious diseases as the major cause of death. The 'epidemiological transition' is the term given to this shift in the burden of ill-health.

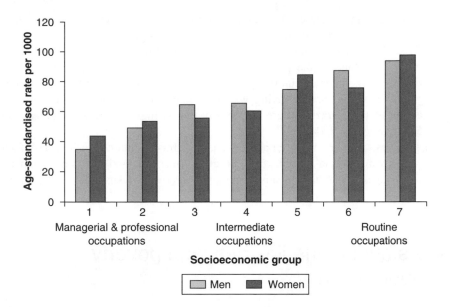

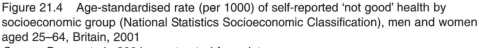

Figure 21.4   Age-standardised rate (per 1000) of self-reported 'not good' health by socioeconomic group (National Statistics Socioeconomic Classification), men and women aged 25–64, Britain, 2001
Source: Doran et al., 2004: constructed from data.

Beginning in the UK and the countries of western Europe, rapid industrialisation left the urban poor without access to clean water, sanitary housing and an adequate diet – and, in consequence, at risk of infectious and nutrition-related diseases. In mid-19th-century Britain, the average age of death for labourers in cities like Manchester was 17; for the gentry and professional classes it was 38 (Lancet, 1843). From the early 20th century, circulatory disease (heart disease and stroke) and lung cancer took an increasing toll, with mortality initially higher among affluent groups. But the socioeconomic profile of chronic disease has changed, as risk factors like smoking and obesity have increasingly became markers of poverty. Since the 1960s, socioeconomic gradients in heart disease and cancer have steepened as the death rates from these diseases have fallen more rapidly in richer than poorer groups. In consequence, socioeconomic inequalities in key measures of health have widened (Department of Health, 2005; Mackenbach, 2005). Figure 21.1 provides an example.

In poorer countries, infectious and nutrition-related diseases are still major causes of death, including malaria, measles, tuberculosis and HIV/AIDs. But the drive for economic growth has disrupted traditional food systems, diets and patterns of tobacco use, and increased consumption of processed foods and manufactured cigarettes. As a result, poor communities can simultaneously provide new markets for the tobacco and 'junk food' (energy dense, nutrient poor) industries – and lack clean water and sewage disposal (de Beyer et al., 2001; Leatherman and Goodman, 2005). For example, in Bangladesh, where more than 80 per cent of the population live on less than US$2 a day, smoking rates among men aged 35–49 stand at over 70 per cent (Efroymson et al., 2001; World Bank, 2003a).

In consequence, poorer countries face 'a double burden of disease', with high rates of acute, infectious diseases persisting alongside an increase in chronic non-infectious diseases (Monteiro et al., 2004; Yusuf et al., 2004). As in older richer societies, chronic diseases are initially diseases of affluence. But, as countries get richer, the socioeconomic profile of risk factors like smoking and obesity changes (Efroymson et al., 2001; Blakely et al., 2005). For example, the positive association between wealth and obesity found among women in low-income countries (e.g. India) flattens in low-to-middle income countries (e.g. South Africa) before giving way to a negative association in upper-middle income countries (e.g. Brazil) where the obesity risk is higher in lower socioeconomic groups (Monteiro et al., 2004).

As this suggests, the link between poverty and health is maintained, as new risk factors emerge and new diseases take hold. It is reproduced over time and across places: persisting despite changes in the mechanisms through which poverty takes a toll on health (Link and Phelan, 1995).

Understanding the link between poverty and poor health

An enduring association between poverty and poor health suggests, but does not demonstrate, that living on a low income compromises health. Poverty could instead be the outcome of poor health. Longitudinal studies confirm that poor health does indeed pull individuals into poverty. But, while important for individuals struggling with illness, such effects have been found to play only a modest role in the association between poverty and poor health across the population as a whole. Studies suggest, too, that long-term income is more strongly related to health than current income, with the result that the strength of the association between social conditions and health may be underestimated when only measured at one point in time (Davey Smith et al., 1997; Benzeval and Judge, 2001).

Such evidence supports a 'lifecourse perspective' on poverty and health. This is one which recognises that, from before birth and across life, the social and physical environment leaves imprints on body systems (Kuh and Ben-Shlomo, 2003). Thus, poverty before and during pregnancy can deprive the mother of key nutrients, compromising foetal development and leaving the child vulnerable to chronic disease in later life (Barker, 1998). After birth, poor children continue to be at greater risk of exposure to health-damaging environments and behaviours both in childhood and in adulthood (Figure 21.5). As a result, death rates among middle-aged men and women born into poorer families are double those of men and women growing up in better-off circumstances, with the increased risk of death remaining after adjustment for adult socioeconomic position (Kuh et al., 2002). Circumstances in adulthood have an additional health effect, with disadvantage further increasing the risk of poor health and premature death (Blane, 1999). As this suggests, children who escape from poverty have better health in adulthood than those who endure persisting disadvantage across their lives.

While circumstances at all life stages influence health, childhood is especially important. This is in part because, as a period of rapid development, there is heightened sensitivity to environmental influences. In addition, childhood and adolescence is the formative period

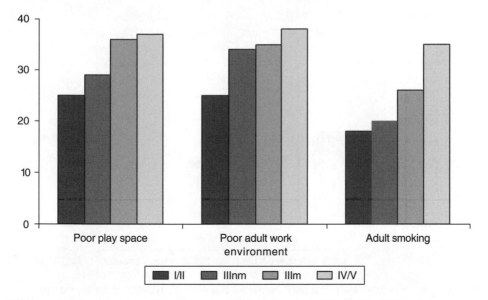

Figure 21.5   Exposure to risk factors in childhood and adulthood by childhood social class (father's occupation at birth) in the 1958 British birth cohort study
Social class: I/II = professional & managerial; IIInm = skilled non-manual; IIIm = skilled manual; IV/V = semi- & unskilled manual.
Source: Power and Mathews, 1997: constructed from data.

for adult health behaviours like smoking, which take a heavy toll on health in adulthood. These life stages are also important for adult socioeconomic position, with educational trajectories influencing career opportunities and lifetime earnings (Graham and Power, 2004).

Conclusion

Three broad conclusions can be drawn from this brief review.

First, poor children and poor adults are disproportionately exposed to the risk factors and diseases driving death rates in the societies of which they are part. Risk factors and diseases change during the course of economic development, but their health costs are borne by the poor.

Secondly, the poorer health of poorer groups captures, in stark relief, the broader relationship between social and health inequalities. Inequalities in living standards become, in a literal sense, embodied in health: in inequalities in birth weight, child development and body shape and size as well as in disease, disability and death.

Thirdly, social and economic policies hold the key to improving the life chances and the health chances of poor groups. The evidence reviewed in this chapter underlies how policies can secure, and equalise access to, basic health resources like sanitation,

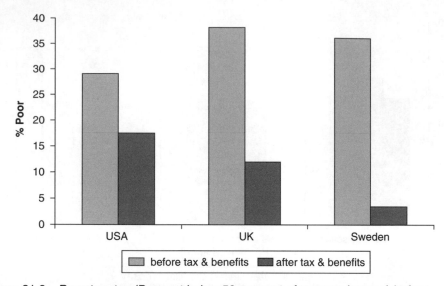

Figure 21.6   Poverty rates (Per cent below 50 per cent of average income) before
and after income transfers (tax and welfare benefits), 1995.
Source: Ritakallio, 2002: constructed from data.

nutrition, income and education. Poverty-alleviating policies in high-income countries
provide an example. Figure 21.6 maps poverty rates before and after payment of tax and
receipt of welfare benefits in Sweden, the UK and the USA. While taxes and benefits
reduce poverty rates in all three countries, the effectiveness of their welfare systems
varies. The Nordic system, with inclusive provision of benefits pegged to average
incomes, is more efficient than systems which rely on low-income and means-tested benefits (USA and UK): the poverty rate in Sweden falls from 36 per cent to 3 per cent.
Investment in welfare services, including education, housing and health care, is also
redistributive, with a greater proportionate impact on the living standards of poorer than
richer households (Graham, 2002).

   Investment in public services also reaps dividends in poorer countries. A review of countries
with low GDP but high life expectancy concluded that 'the quality of life can be vastly raised,
despite low incomes, through an adequate program of social services', including basic education and health care (Sen, 1999: 49; see also UNDP, 1990 and 2003). In line with Amartya
Sen's view, the United Nations Human Development Index measures not economic performance and industrial output, but access to health (life expectancy), knowledge (literacy levels)
and a decent standard of living (GDP) to assess the quality of people's lives (UNDP, 1990).

   The link between poverty and poor health, enduring despite economic growth and in the
richest societies, is opening up a wider debate about the ethics of public policy. Should
increasing wealth or improving health be the first and fundamental priority? Evidence that
the public health infrastructure and welfare policies matter most for poor groups lends support to the view that human development, not economic development, should be shaping
national and global policies for the 21st century.

References

Barker, D.J.P. (1998) *Mothers, Babies and Health in Later Life*, Churchill Livingstone, Edinburgh.

Benzeval, M. and Judge, K. (2001) Income and health: the time dimension, *Social Science and Medicine*, 52: 1371–90.

Blakely, T., Hales, S., Kieft, C., Wilson, N. and Woodward, A. (2005) The global distribution of risk factors by poverty level, *Bulletin of the World Health Organisation*, 83, 2: 118–26.

Blane, D. (1999) The life course, the social gradient and health. In *Social Determinants of Health* (Eds M. Marmot and R.G. Wilkinson), Oxford University Press, Oxford.

Charlton, J. and Murphy, M. (1997) Trends in causes of mortality: 1841–1994 – an overview. In *The Health of Adult Britain 1841–1994* (Ed. Office for National Statistics), The Stationery Office, London.

Davey Smith, G., Hart, C., Blane, D., Gillis, C. and Hawthorne, V. (1997) Lifetime socioeconomic position and mortality: prospective observational study, *British Medical Journal*, 314: 547–52.

Deaton, A. (2003) Health, inequality and economic development, *Journal of Economic Literature*, XLI: 113–58.

De Beyer, J., Lovelace, C. and Yürekli, A. (2001) Poverty and tobacco, *Tobacco Control*, 10: 210–11.

Department of Health (2005) *Tackling Health Inequalities: a Programme for Action Status Report*, Department of Health, London.

Department of Work and Pensions (2006) *Households Below Average Income (HBAI) Statistics 1994/5–2004/5*. Department of Work and Pensions, London.

Donkin, A., Goldblatt, P. and Lynch, K. (2002) Inequalities in life expectancy by social class, 1972–1999, *Health Statistics Quarterly*, 15: 5–15.

Doran, T., Drever, F. and Whitehead, M. (2004) Is there a north–south divide in social class inequalities in health? Cross-sectional study using data from the 2001 census, *British Medical Journal*, 328: 1043–5.

Doran, T. and Whitehead, M. (2004) Do social policies and political context matter for health in the United Kingdom? In *The Political and Social Contexts of Health* (Ed. V. Navarro), Baywood Publishing, New York.

Drever, F. and Bunting, J. (1997) Patterns and trends in male mortality. In *Health Inequalities* (Eds F. Drever and M. Whitehead), Office for National Statistics, London.

Drèze, J. and Sen, A. (1989) *Hunger and Public Action*, Clarendon Press, Oxford.

Efroymson, D., Ahmed, S., Townsend, J., Alam, S.M., Dey, A.R., Saha, R., Sujon, A.I., Ahmed, K.U. and Rahman, O. (2001) Hungry for tobacco: an analysis of the economic impact of tobacco consumption on the poor in Bangladesh, *Tobacco Control*, 10, 3: 212–17.

Farr, W. (1885) Life and death in England. In *Vital Statistics: Memorial Volume of Selections from the Reports and Writings of William Farr* (Ed. N.A. Humphreys), The Sanitary Institute of Great Britain, London. Reprinted in *Bulletin of the World Health Organisation*, 2000, 78, 1: 88–96.

Fernando, D. (2000) Health care systems in transition III. Sri Lanka, Part 1: an overview of Sri Lanka's health care system, *Journal of Public Health Medicine*, 22, 1: 14–20.

Graham, H. (2002) Building an interdisciplinary science of health inequalities: the example of life-course research, *Social Science and Medicine*, 55, 11: 2007–18.

Graham, H. and Power, C. (2004) *Childhood Disadvantage and Adult Health: a Lifecourse Framework*, Health Development Agency, London (www.hda.nhs.uk/evidence).

Krieger, N. (1997) Measuring social class in US public health research, *American Review of Public Health*, 18: 341–78.

Kuh, D.L. and Ben-Shlomo, Y. (eds) (2003) *A Life Course Approach to Chronic Disease Epidemiology: Tracing the Origins of Ill Health from Early to Adult Life*, 2nd edition, Oxford University Press, Oxford.

Kuh, D., Hardy, R., Langenberg, C., Richards, R. and Wadsworth, N.E.J. (2002) Mortality in adults aged 26–54 related to socioeconomic conditions in childhood and adulthood: post war birth cohort study, *British Medical Journal*, 325: 1076–80.

Kunst, A.E., Groenhof, F., Mackenbach, J.P. and EU Working Group on Socioeconomic Inequalities in Health (1998) Mortality by occupational class among men 30–64 years in 11 European countries, *Social Science and Medicine*, 46, 11: 1459–76.

Lancet (1843) Editorial, *The Lancet*, no. 1040, 5 August: 657–61.

Leatherman, T.L. and Goodman, A. (2005) Coca-colonization of diets in the Yucatan, *Social Science and Medicine*, 61: 833–46.

Leinsalu, M., Vägero, D. and Kunst, A.E. (2003) Estonia 1989–2000: enormous increase in mortality differences by education, *International Journal of Epidemiology*, 32: 1081–7.

Leon, D.A., Chenet, L., Shkolnikov, V.M., Zakharov, S, Shapiro, J., Rakhmanova, G., Vassin, S. and McKee, M. (1997) Huge variation in Russian mortality rates 1984–94: artefact, alcohol or what?, *The Lancet*, 350: 383–8.

Link, B.G. and Phelan, J. (1995) Social conditions as fundamental causes of disease, *Journal of Health and Social Behaviour*, Extra Issue: 80–94.

Mackenbach, J.P. (2005) *Health Inequalities: Europe in Profile*, An independent expert report commissioned by and published under the auspices of the UK Presidency of the European Union, Erasmus MC University Medical Center, Rotterdam.

Mackenbach, J.P., Martikainen, P., Looman, C.W.N., Dalstra, J.A.A., Kunst, A.E., Lahelma, E. and members of the SEdHA working group (2004) The shape of the relationship between income and self-assessed health: an international study, *International Journal of Epidemiology*, 34: 286–93.

McKee, M. (2003) Commentary: winners and losers, *International Journal of Epidemiology*, 32: 1087–8.

McKeown, T. (1979) *The Role of Medicine: Dream, Mirage or Nemesis?* Basil Blackwell, Oxford.

Mathers, C.D., Sadana, R., Salomon, J.A., Murray, C.J.L. and Lopez, A.D. (2000) Healthy life expectancy in 191 countries 1999, *The Lancet*, 357: 1686–90.

Monteiro, C.A., Moura, E.C., Conde, W.L. and Popkin, B.M. (2004) Socoieconomic status and obesity in adult populations of developing countries: a review, *Bulletin of the World Health Organisation*, 82, 12: 940–6.

Pamuk, E.R. (1985) Social class inequality in mortality from 1921 to 1972 in England and Wales, *Population Studies*, 39: 17–31.

Power, C. and Matthews, S. (1997) Origins of health inequalities in a national population sample, *Lancet*, 350: 1584–9.

Preston, S.H. (1975) The changing relationship between mortality and economic development, *Population Studies*, 29: 231–48.

Registrar General (1913) *Registrar General's 74th Annual Report, 1911*, Registrar General Office, London.

Ritakallio, V.-M. (2002) Trends in poverty and income inequality in cross-national comparison, *European Journal of Social Security*, 4, 2: 151–77.

Schellenberg, J.A., Victora, C.G., Mushi, A., de Savigny, D., Schellenberg, D. et al. (2003) Inequities among the very poor: health care for children in rural southern Tanzania, *The Lancet*, 361: 561–6.

Sen, A. (1999) *Development as Freedom*, Oxford University Press, Oxford.

Sen, K. and Bonita, R. (2000) Global health status: two steps forward, one step back, *The Lancet*, 356: 577–82.

Szreter, S. (1988) The importance of social intervention in Britain's mortality decline *c.* 1850–1914, *Social History of Medicine*, 1: 1–37.

UNDP (1990) *Human Development Report 1990: Concept and Measurement of human development*, United Nations Development Programme, New York.

UNDP (2003) *Human Development Report 2003*, United Nations Development Programme, New York.

Wagstaff, A. (2000) Socioeconomic inequalities in child mortality: comparisons across nine developing countries, *Bulletin of the World Health Organisation*, 78, 1: 19–29.

Wagstaff, A. (2002) Poverty and health sector inequalities, *Bulletin of the World Health Organisation*, 80, 2: 97–105.

Whitehead, M. (1997) Life and death over the millennium. In *Health Inequalities* (Eds F. Drever and M. Whitehead), Office for National Statistics, London.

WHO Regional Office for SE Asia (2004) *Country Health Profiles: Sri Lanka*, World Health Organisation Regional Office for SE Asia, New Delhi, http://w3.whosea.org/cntryhealth/srilanka (accessed 27.11.05).

Woolf, B. (1947) Studies on infant mortality, part II: social aetiology of stillbirths and infant deaths in county boroughs of England and Wales, *British Journal of Medicine*, 2: 73–125.

World Bank (2002) *World Development Indicators CD-ROM*, World Bank, Washington DC.

World Bank (2003a) *World Development Indicators CD-ROM*, World Bank, Washington DC.

World Bank (2003b) *Issue Brief HIV/AIDS: Sri Lanka*, World Bank, Washington DC, http://Inweb18.worldbank.org/sar/sa.nsf/Countries/Sri+Lanka (accessed 27.11.05).

World Bank (2004) *Round II Country Reports on Health, Nutrition, Population Conditions among Poor and Better-Off in 56 Countries*, World Bank, Washington DC: http//web.worldbank.org/poverty/health/data (accessed 27.11.05).

Yusuf, S., Ounpuu, S., and Hawken, S. (2004) Effect of potentially modifiable risk factors associated with myocardial infarction in 52 countries (the INTETHEART study): case-control study, *The Lancet*, 364: 937–52.

Chapter 22

Health Promotion, Globalisation and Health

Ronald Labonte

Introduction

When health promoters gather to talk shop, much of their exchange is on their local work. What's new in substance abuse prevention programmes? Are we rising to the new challenges of obesity and diabetes? What have we learned about improving the health of migrant communities? How effective have we become in overcoming social exclusion? These are all important questions. But we are also increasingly aware that actions at a global level are affecting our abilities to improve health at a local level. From the threat of new plagues (and their challenge to public health systems that have been allowed to languish in many countries) to deadly bush fires and storms (exacerbated by global climate change) to the failure of the world's nations to act effectively against the greatest pandemic (HIV) since Europe's Black Death, 'globalisation' is no longer a fact of our lives that we can ignore. Contemporary globalisation is characterised by a constellation of processes by which nations, businesses and people are becoming more connected through communication exchange, cultural diffusion, travel and, most importantly, economic integration.

Contemporary globalisation is really about the global reorganisation of production

Those born in wealthier countries only began to confront globalisation when free trade agreements threatened their manufacturing, textile and agricultural sectors. Transnational

---

This chapter is an expanded and updated version of the article: Labonte, R. (2004) An unabashedly opinionated (but evidence-based) overview of globalisation's challenge to health, *VicHealth Letter,* Summer: 14–18; reproduced with permission.

companies reorganised themselves into global production chains to take maximum advantage of lower labour costs and tax regimes, and less costly environmental regulations and social programmes in different countries of the world. The North American Free Trade Agreement opening borders between Canada, the USA and Mexico, for example, spurred the rapid growth of Mexican *maquiladoras* – special 'export-processing zones' that often denied human rights (such as the right to organise unions), lacked adequate living and workplace health and safety standards, and violated already lax environmental standards (Frey, 2003). While providing employment to some otherwise poor Mexicans – often young women who were considered more docile – at the cost of job-losses in Canada and the USA, the *maquiladoras* nonetheless failed to contribute to Mexico's overall economic development because they existed outside its domestic economy (ILO, 1998).

Box 22.1   Free trade is not fair trade

A key plank in contemporary globalisation is 'free trade' – the unimpeded flow of goods, services, capital and (to a much lesser degree) skilled labour across national borders. With the birth of the World Trade Organisation (WTO) in 1995, trade agreements became more than simply lowering border barriers. They began to limit the 'policy flexibilities' of national governments in ways that could imperil public health. The most well known are:

- TRIPS Agreement (Agreement on Trade-Related Intellectual Property Rights), which, by extending patent protection, can limit access to essential medicines, particularly in poorer countries, and reduce public funding available for other health investments.
- GATS Agreement (General Agreement on Trade in Services), which, by 'locking in' existing levels of privatisation and requiring countries to continue to liberalise their service sectors, could prevent the extension of public health care funding and provision.

Other agreements can affect broader health determinants by requiring governments to adopt domestic health and environment regulations that are 'least trade restrictive', and that are justified by costly and sometimes controversial scientific risk assessments. Current trade rules, largely influenced by wealthier countries' interests, still allow rich nations to continue to subsidise and protect areas of their economy (such as agriculture) where poorer countries have some advantage, while requiring poorer nations to open their economies to rich countries' products. Most importantly, free trade is not fair trade. As the World Commission on the Social Dimensions of Globalisation recently concluded, equal rules for unequal players only produce unequal results (World Commission, 2004). There are some exemptions to WTO agreements for developing countries, referred to as 'special and differential treatment'. Despite repeated promises and commitments, wealthier WTO member nations have not supported actions to do so. And, as free trade talks stall at the WTO, where developing countries have organised in greater strength, the European Union and the USA are using the promise of more aid or better market access to pressurise individual nations to enter into bilateral or regional trade agreements that give greater advantage to themselves (Labonte, 2004; Labonte and Sanger, 2006a and b).

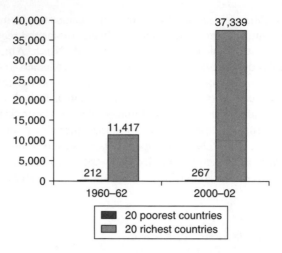

Figure 22.1   The result ... unequal growth of wealth (GDP/capita US$, 20 poorest/ richest countries)
Source: World Development indicators 2003, online verson available from http://publications.worldbank.org/ecommerce/catalog/product?item_id = 631625: constructed from data.

These developments of the 1990s were a wake-up call for many of the wealthy world's middle and working class to a new and harsher global order from which their privileged national geography no longer guaranteed protection. Given the importance to health of such determinants as secure work, adequate income and welfare safety nets, it would be hard to argue against extending the 'enabling, mediating and advocating' strategies of the Ottawa Charter to local mobilisations against globalisation's economic or environmental threats – even if it does make health promotion's mandate bigger, messier and more political.

Which started with poorer countries first

At least a decade before free trade agreements began to complete capitalism's project of global market integration, much of the developing world was already suffering from the damaging impacts of two of its earlier strategies:

1. Structural adjustment loan conditions imposed by the World Bank and International Monetary Fund (IMF) on indebted poor countries. These conditions followed a standard neo-liberal economic prescription:

   - Liberalisation: reduce tariffs – border taxes – on imported goods.
   - Privatisation: sell-off profitable state-owned assets.
   - Deregulation: reduce state controls over foreign investors and the private sector.
   - State minimalism: reduce public spending to the most basic of services, target the poor only and implement cost-recovery (user charge) programmes (Milward, 2000).

These structural adjustment policies did help some countries improve their economic indicators by reducing runaway inflation and increasing growth and foreign investment. But these policies did not lower overall global poverty (the single biggest risk factor for disease), were singularly negative for health in Africa (Breman and Shelton, 2001) and often increased gender inequities in access to jobs, goods and services (Elson and Cagatay, 2000). They also helped to concentrate even more global assets into the hands of transnational corporations and to quadruple global inequalities in wealth from their already inequitable 1960 level (Figure 22.1).

2. Currency speculation, made possible by computers and capital market liberalisation. Country after country (from Mexico, Brazil and Russia to most of Southeast Asia) saw their currencies first rise as 'hot money' (so-called portfolio investments) entered, and then plunge as investors cashed out their winnings. Every affected country experienced increased poverty, decreased health, social and environmental spending, and lowered economic growth (O'Brien, 2002). The 'casino capitalism' addiction of the rich was paid for by the health of the poor, particularly women and children (Strange, 1986; Gyebi et al., 2002).

These claims, while supported by evidence, are not without contention. The pro-globalisation 'story' (as economists describe their theories) is that liberalisation increases trade, which increases growth and wealth, which decreases poverty. Less poverty means better health, better health means more economic growth, and there is a 'win/win' virtuous circle (Dollar, 2001; Dollar and Kraay, 2000). But the facts have been less generous. Those countries where liberalisation did lead to growth (primarily Southeast Asia and China) did so by *not* following many of the World Bank/IMF conditions and free trade rules. Their growth did lift many people out of poverty, at the abject less than US$1/day level (an imperfect measure used by the World Bank). But it did not lift them very far. Poverty at the less than $2/day level increased over the same period (Milanovic, 2003; Wade, 2004). In every other region of the world, poverty rates increased. Economic growth has also given rise to escalating income inequalities within most nations, especially those that have grown the fastest.

The argument that economic growth is essential to sustaining better health for the world's poor may be true in the long run. But how long should we expect people to wait? Much of the convergence in life expectancies between rich and poor countries over the past 50 years can be traced to low-cost health care innovations, primary health care and education access, and improvements in sanitation and water (World Bank, 1993). It is these simple measures that have been most compromised by contemporary globalisation.

And underpins the biggest health problem of our generation

Nowhere has this been starker than in the case of the HIV/AIDS pandemic in sub-Saharan Africa. The global convergence in life expectancy diverged sharply in the early 1990s as HIV/AIDS began its grim reaping. The virus is the cause. Its denial by some leaders, poor gender equity in many countries, corrupt politicians, the sexual predations of different militaries using both rape and HIV as weapons, all contribute to the pandemic. But contemporary globalisation also has a huge debt owing. The top individual risk factor for HIV infection around the world is poverty (Basu, 2003). And global market integration – declaring much of the African continent ripe for resources, poor for consumer markets and marginal in economic returns – has helped push it deeper into poverty.

Consider Zambia, a poor southern African country that, to qualify for World Bank and IMF loans to pay its debts, was obliged to open its borders to textiles, many of them second-hand cast-offs that began life as charity donations in wealthier countries. Its 'inefficient' domestic manufacturing could not compete. Thirty thousand jobs disappeared and 132 of 140 textile mills closed operations, which the World Bank now acknowledges as 'unintended and regrettable consequences'of the adjustment process (Jeter, 2002). Previously employed workers were forced to eke out a living as insecure street vendors in the underground, and untaxed, 'informal' economy. In the early 1990s, user charges for schools, imposed partly because of the loss of public revenues following collapse of the textile sector, led to increased dropout and illiteracy rates – just at a time when the HIV pandemic began to surge (Commission for Africa, 2005). Zambia today has one of the continent's highest rates of HIV/AIDS.

Then there is the collapse of public health systems in many African countries, partly the result of structural adjustment conditionalities that capped public spending and health sector reforms that emphasised cost-recovery. The subsequent 'brain drain' of health professionals from Africa to wealthier nations (primarily the UK, USA, Canada, Australia and Aotearoa/New Zealand) is costing the continent hundreds of millions of dollars each year in lost training costs (IRIN, 2002). The brain drain is partly 'pull' (active recruitment) and partly 'push' (who can blame a health worker whose job is insecure or sometimes unpaid, in a system lacking many of the essential basics, for wanting a better place to practise her skills?). But it has been described as the most serious crisis affecting the future of African health care and its ability to turn around the pandemics of HIV/AIDS, tuberculosis and malaria.

But rich countries seem more concerned with national security than with human development

It would be simplistic to blame contemporary globalisation for the HIV/AIDS or other disease pandemics in Africa. But it would be naïve to ignore its role. As the new millennium dawned, the global community of countries imperfectly constituted as the United Nations consolidated a list of Millennium Development Goals (MDGs) that it thought must be, and could be, achieved by the year 2015 to begin to turn things around. Most of these goals concern health or health determinants. All of these goals were endorsed by all nations, with the wealthiest declaring that the poorest should not lack for the resources necessary to attain them.

The rhetoric of the rich world, however, has not been matched by action. For over 20 years, most of the world's wealthier nations – the 'donor' countries – have pledged to contribute at least 0.7 per cent of their gross national income (a measure that replaces the older measure of the gross domestic product, or GDP) to official development assistance (ODA).

Very few have and ODA rates actually fell dramatically in most donor countries during the 1990s. There have been some recent promises to increase ODA; the European Union countries have pledged to reach the 0.7% target by 2015, though the USA and Japan – both important donor countries – have not. Even with promised increases, the sums still represent less than half of the estimated amounts of money many poorer nations need to meet the MDGs, or improve their people's health. Moreover, much of this development assistance is 'phantom aid', so-called because the poor nations receiving it must use it to purchase expensive goods or services from the donor country rather than from within their own country.

This problem is worsened by the fact that, with the recent exception of sub-Saharan Africa, poor countries actually send to wealthy nations far more money in debt servicing costs than they receive in ODA. The debt crises of the 1980s arose first with the sudden high costs of oil imports (causing developing countries to borrow heavily), but were compounded by high interest rates and other fiscal policies of the lending nations that multiplied the debt burden many times over. Most indebted countries have already paid back more than the principal of their loans, but remain almost as heavily in debt as they began (Martin, 2004; UNCTAD, 2004).

Wealthy countries began a programme of debt relief in 1998 for the poorest and most indebted countries (the HIPC or Heavily Indebted Poor Country programme), run by the World Bank and IMF. But the programme has been inadequate and, even with more generous debt cancellation announced at the G8 summit in the UK in 2005, will find most developing countries trapped in a downwards spiral of debt. Countries receiving partial debt cancellation must also follow the structural adjustment rules laid down by the IMF and World Bank, despite these having been largely destructive and unhealthy in the past (Labonte and Schrecker, 2006).

The costs of creating greater global health equity are not cheap. But the rich world does not lack in the ability to pay. Indeed, more money is being spent annually on increased border security, militarisation and tax cuts than on ODA and debt cancellation combined (Labonte et al., 2004). The issue is one of where the public and private sectors of the world's elite nations choose to invest their money, and how the world's publics can influence those choices.

Yet there are solutions, if we can create the political will

To influence those choices, health promoters need to know what global 'healthy public policy' options can, and should, be advocated. Some examples already exist: the Kyoto Protocol on Greenhouse Gas Emissions, the Framework Convention on Tobacco Control (the world's first public health international covenant), and new funding programmes such as the Global Fund to fight AIDS, Tuberculosis and Malaria. And there is no shortage of other possible and achievable policy alternatives[1], including:

- Fair trade rules, in which rich countries open their markets to goods from poorer ones, while allowing poorer countries more flexibilities under trade rules to develop their economies using the same policies of potectionism and subsidisation as the already wealthy nations once used.

- Fulfilment by the rich world of development assistance commitments, and untying such assistance from the purchase of donor country goods or services.
- Cancellation of poor countries' debts, including a recognition that under international law much of this debt – poorly loaned and allowed to be 'stolen' by corrupt leaders often with the knowledge of the lending country or institution – should be considered 'odious' and uncollectible.
- New forms of global taxation to fund wealth redistribution and human development on a global scale. These could include taxes on currency exchange (which would also quell health-damaging speculation), arms trade (which may reduce the deadly trafficking of small arms that are the real weapons of mass destruction in many poor nations), carbon emissions (which could lower the pace of climate change) and international travel/jet fuel (which is already being introduced by France and will fund its overseas aid for HIV/AIDS programmes).
- Closure of tax haven countries, many of which operate under UK or US protectorate status. These countries are used by transnational companies and their highly paid executives to hold their wealth exempt from taxation. Between 8 and 13 trillion dollars sit in such tax havens (the low estimate comes from the IMF, the high estimate from the international Tax Justice Network). Using the low estimate and assuming a 5 per cent return, taxed at 40 per cent, this would raise US \$160 billion a year (UNRISD, 2000) – about the estimated amount required in extra financing to reach the Millennium Development Goals.
- Radical reform of the World Bank and IMF, including replacing the neo-liberal economic conditionalities of present loans and grants with health/human development conditionalities, such as increased public spending on education, health care, water/ sanitation, gender equity and other interventions known to improve health equity; and giving the debtor nations equal voice in decision-making in these institutions.[2]

Ultimately, we need a new global governance system that is explicitly rights-based and ethical. It must be democratic in both representation and participation, and strong enough to begin the task of re-regulating a capitalism that has been freed from national oversight, and of imposing upon global corporations, entrepreneurs and transnational elites some reciprocal obligations for equity, health and environmental sustainability. How we might achieve this is the greatest and most important health promotion task of our lives.

And there are strategies and tools already in our health promotion practice kit

There is no blueprint for how we might achieve this goal. But there are some steps health promoters can take. First, we can align with the local chapters/organisations of the larger global social movement for health and justice. One such group is The People's Health Movement, a global network of health activists founded in 2000 that has participated in many global justice actions and in 2005 launched its own international 'right to health' campaign. With 'circles' in many different countries, it has become a powerful voice in the international arena for the principles that have underpinned health promotion practice first encapsulated in the 1986 *Ottawa Charter for Health Promotion*.[3]

Secondly, we can build empowering health promotion partnerships that link poorer nations with wealthier ones. Many of these already exist, partly through the funding mechanism of ODA, or through the new proliferation of international public–private partnerships for health, such as the Global Fund to Fight AIDS, Tuberculosis and Malaria. Many of these new initiatives suffer the same 'top-down' problem of early health promotion, with a focus on specific diseases, treatments or behaviour change without sufficient attention to the social and economic determinants of these diseases. Many health promoters are skilled in good 'bottom up' and more empowering development approaches that can be diffused through these global partnerships. Look for opportunities, and seize them.

Thirdly, we can enter the growing debates over how globalisation enhances or imperils global health equity. We might do this as individuals, or by joining global social movements, or by ensuring our professional associations take strong, evidence-based positions on how globalisation should change to improve health outcomes. Health promotion has developed some useful tools over the past years that can be harnessed to issues central to contemporary globalisation, such as applying the techniques of health impact assessment to trade or ODA policies, using capacity-building forms of evaluation to health projects funded through ODA or the new global health partnerships, or working with our national health ministries to promote more international health 'laws' like the Framework Convention on Tobacco Control (the obesity pandemic that arises, in part, from increased global trade in unhealthy but profitable 'foods' is a good next target).

Finally, at a personal level, as we confront the hugeness of these tasks, there is a fourth essential step. We need to practise optimism, not as a personality trait or a sunny-sided disposition, but as a disciplined act of political resistance. We have reached a point in human history where we measure our actions less by our estimates of success, and more by our awareness that, failing to act, we are only guaranteeing their failure.

Notes

1 One of the largest mobilisations on these issues was the global 2005 Make Poverty History campaign, which focused on Africa and the need for increased aid, decreased debt and fairer trade. While not without its criticisms (the prominence of celebrities, the lack of African voices and the moderation of demands), the ongoing campaign did popularise many of the basic options (see http://www.makepovertyhistory.org/).

2 For a more detailed discussion of these options, see Labonte, R., Schrecker, T. and Gupta, A.S. (2005) *Health for Some: Death, Disease and Disparity in a Globalizing Era*. Toronto: Centre for Social Justice, downloadable free at: http://www.socialjustice.org/publications.php? filter = subject), and People's Health Movement et al. (2005) *Global Health Watch 2005–2006*. London: Zed Books, (downloadable free at: http://www. ghwatch.org/), as well the companion publication *Global Health Action*.

3 For more information on the People's Health Movement, see http://www.phmovement.org/index.html.

References

Basu, S. (2003) AIDS, empire, and public health behaviourism. *Equinet Newsletter*, 28, http://www.equinetafrica.org/newsletter/index.php?issue=28 (accessed 1 February 2005).

Breman A. and Shelton, C. (2001) *Structural Adjustment and Health: a Literature Review of the Debate, Its Role-players and Presented Empirical evidence*. Paper No. WG6: 6. Cambridge, MA: Commission on Macroeconomics and Health http://www.cmhealth.org/docs/ wg6_paper6.pdf (accessed 27 May 2003).

Commission for Africa (2005) *Our Common Interest: Report of the Commission for Africa*. London: Commission for Africa.

Dollar D. (2001) *Globalization, Inequality, and Poverty since 1980*. Washington, DC: World Bank, http://econ.worldbank.org/files/2944_globalization-inequality-and-poverty.pdf (accessed 1 February 2005).

Dollar, D. and Kraay, A. (2000) *Growth is Good for the Poor*. Working Paper No. 2587. Washington, DC: World Bank, http://www.worldbank.org/research/growth/pdfiles/growthgoodforpoor.pdf (accessed 1 February 2005).

Elson, D. and Cagatay, N. (2000) The social content of macroeconomic policies. *World Development*, 28 (7): 1347–64.

Frey, R.S. (2003) The transfer of core-based hazardous production processes to the export processing zones of the periphery: the maquiladora centers of northern Mexico. *Journal of World-Systems Research*, 9 (2): 317–54.

Gyebi, J., Brykczynska, G. and Lister, G. (2002) *Globalisation: Economics and Women's Health*. London: UK Partnership for Global Health, http://www.ukglobalhealth.org/content/Text/ Globalisation_New_version.doc (accessed 1 February 2005).

ILO (1998) *Labor and Social Issues Related to Export Processing Zones*. Geneva: International Labour Organisation, http://www.ilo.org/public/english/dialogue/govlab/legrel/tc/epz/reports/ epzrepor_w61/index.htm (accessed 1 February 2005).

IRIN (2002) *Africa: Brain Drain Reportedly Costing US$ 4 billion a Year*. Nairobi: United Nations Office for the Coordination of Humanitarian Affairs, http://www.irinnews.org/report.asp?Report ID=27536&SelectRegion=Africa&SelectCountry=AFRICA (accessed 27 May 2003).

Jeter, J. (2002) The dumping ground: as Zambia courts western markets, used goods arrive at a heavy price. *Washington Post*, 22 April: A1.

Labonte, R. (2004) Globalization, health and the free trade regime: assessing the links. In Harris, R. and Seid, M. (eds), *Globalization and Health*. Boston: Brill, pp. 47–72.

Labonte, R. and Sanger, M. (2006a) A glossary of the World Trade Organization and public health: Part 1. *Journal of Epidemiology and Community Health* (in press).

Labonte, R. and Sanger, M. (2006b) A glossary of the World Trade Organization and public health: Part 2. *Journal of Epidemiology and Community Health* (in press).

Labonte, R. and Schrecker, T. (2006) The G8 and global health: what now? What next? *Canadian Journal of Public Health* (in press).

Labonte, R., Schrecker, T., Sanders, D. and Meeus, W. (2004) *Fatal Indifference: the G8, Africa and Global Health*. Cape Town: University of Cape Town Press.

Martin, M. (2004) Assessing the HIPC initiative: the key policy debates. In Teunissen, J. and Akkerman, A. (eds), *HIPC Debt Relief: Myths and Realities*. The Hague: Forum on Debt and Development (FONDAD), pp. 11–47.

Milanovic, B. (2003) The two faces of globalization: against globalization as we know it. *World Development*, 31 (4): 667–83.

Milward, B. (2000) What is structural adjustment? In Mohan, G. et al. (eds), *Structural Adjustment: Theory, Practice and Impacts*. London: Routledge, pp. 24–38.

O'Brien, R. (2002) Organizational politics, multilateral economic organizations and social policy. *Global Social Policy*, 2: 141–62.

Strange, S. (1986) *Casino Capitalism.* Oxford: Blackwell.

UNCTAD (United Nations Conference on Trade And Development) (2004) *Economic Development in Africa – Debt Sustainability: Oasis or Mirage?* New York and Geneva: United Nations.

UNRISD (2000) *Visible Hands: Taking Responsibility for Social Development*. Geneva: United Nations Research Institute for Social Development.

Wade, R H. (2004) Is globalization reducing poverty and inequality? *World Development*, 32 (4): 567–89.

World Bank (1993) *World Development Report 1993: Investing in Health*. New York: Oxford University Press.

World Commision on the Social Dimension of Globalization (2004) *A Fair Globalization: Creating Opportunities for All.* Geneva: International Labour Organization. http://www.ilo.org/public/english/wcsdg/docs/report.pdf (accessed 1 February 2005).

Chapter 23

Terrorism and Public Health

John Middleton and Victor W. Sidel

Introduction

The public health and health services communities around the globe have a long tradition of working for health improvement, transcending narrow economic concerns and the self-interest of individuals, ethnic groups, religions or countries. The need to reaffirm this global and collective ethic has never been stronger. Public health has brought together humankind in a spirit of co-operation and mutual support. The eradication of small pox and the near eradication of polio are perhaps the best examples of this spirit. The all-embracing world health strategies of 'Health for all by the year 2000' and now 'Health 21'[1] have expressed wider aspirations, including solidarity between nations and reducing inequalities in economic status, health experience and life chances. 'Health promotion is peace promotion';[2] the activity of improving population health inherently strives to reduce inequalities, to achieve fairness, and tackle environmental, economic and social causes of ill health.[3-6] The need to strengthen national and international public health networks is also apparent.[7-9]

The principal responsibility for the public health community in tackling terrorism *is to prevent it*.[10] To seek to understand the nature and motivation of terrorism is not to condone it.

Terrorism is *politically motivated violence or the threat of violence, especially against civilians, with the intent to instill fear*. Terrorism is intended to have psychological effects that reach beyond the immediate victims to intimidate a wider population, such as rival ethnic or religious groups, a national government or political party, or an entire country.[10] The term *terrorist* is applied to enemies and opponents. What is called terrorism depends

---

The authors are grateful for important contributions to the discussion of these issues to H. Jack Geiger, Barry S. Levy, Hillel Cohen, Robert Gould and Mark Sidel.

on one's point of view; terrorists become guerrillas, freedom fighters, national war heroes.[11] Groups which have been relatively powerless often use terrorist tactics, believing these represent their only effective weapon against superior force. In this context, fabricating a 'war on terrorism' is to create an endless conflict. As the terrorist becomes more disenfranchised and disempowered, and loses hope for the future, the easier it becomes to choose martyrdom. The more calculated, extreme and desperate terrorist actions become, the more demonised and dehumanised the terrorists become, in a downward spiral that harms us all.[11–13]

The terrorist attacks of 9–11 raised to a new level the scale and potential for atrocity against civilian populations. They demonstrated a new capacity and ingenuity for destruction, using limited resources from everyday life without the need for specialist knowledge. They require resilience planners and the public health community need 'to think the unthinkable' and plan for the previously unimagined.[12,13,14]

Public health is *'what we, as a society, do collectively to assure the conditions in which people can be healthy'*. It takes a society to practise public health.[15] Terrorism creates unique challenges for the public health system in planning, responses and prevention. Bioterrorism is a special kind of terrorism that can create unusual epidemics.[10,14,15,16] The anthrax attacks via the American postal system late in 2001 seemed to confirm the accessibility of agents of destruction and the familiarity with which they could wreak havoc. They further confirmed the levels of excessive paranoia, the scope for political manipulation of the masses and for damaging public mental health. Terrorist outrages of the future may well harness the essentials of modern civilisation; people may be damaged physically or psychologically or civil unrest created by the destructive use of the internet (cyberterrorism),[17] through manipulation of the media and misinformation and through disruption of water, food, power and transport.[10]

Some responses to terrorism, however, can be harmful. The scope for hoaxers adds further to panic. Vengeful responses to terrorist acts or threats may hurt innocent people. Attempts to locate, interrogate, and punish suspects may threaten domestic civil liberties and international justice.[18,19,20] And the diversion of resources from essential public health programmes for the 'war on terrorism' may lead to neglect of common health problems and disaster responsiveness.[21,22,23]

A balanced approach is needed to create appropriate security and to protect the rights and values of the society which make it worth securing.[19–21] Here we set out some of the features of terrorism and its effects on health and some of the responses needed to be 'tough on terrorism, and tough on the causes of terrorism'.

Prevention of terrorism and its consequences

Public health professionals distinguish between primary, secondary, and tertiary levels of prevention, and use this framework in developing and implementing policies and programmes. The 'Guiding Principles for a Public Health Response to Terrorism', adopted by the American Public Health Association in October 2001, have been adapted to this framework (see Box 23.1).[10]

Box 23.1   Guiding principles for a public health response to terrorism

Adapted from the statement adopted by the Governing Council of the American Public Health Association October 2001, statements arranged according to their place in primary, secondary and tertiary prevention, some items appear twice Reprinted with permission from the American Public Health Association.

Primary prevention

Article 1 of APHA statement	Address poverty, social injustice, and health disparities that may contribute to the development of terrorism.
Article 2	Provide humanitarian assistance to, and protect the human rights of, the civilian populations that are directly or indirectly affected by terrorism.
Article 3	Advocate the speedy end of armed conflicts and promote non-violent means of conflict resolution. [*To prevent circumstances in which terrorism may arise and be seen as the only way out, e.g. Iraq, Chechnya.*]
Article 10	Prevent hate crimes and ethnic, racial, and religious discrimination; promote cultural competence and diversity training, and dialogue among people and protect human rights and civil liberties.
Article 11	Advocate the immediate control and ultimate elimination of biological, chemical and nuclear weapons.
Authors' addition 1	Promote sustainable development to ensure the appropriate and fair use of resources and the protection of the environment, minimising conditions of injustice to which terrorism may be a response.
Authors' addition 2	Strengthen international laws and respect for international law among politicians. Strengthen the resources available to the United Nations for peacekeeping purposes and strengthen the mandate of the United Nations, to create binding and enforced international laws.

Secondary prevention

Article 2	Provide humanitarian assistance to, and protect the human rights of, the civilian populations that are directly or indirectly affected by terrorism.
Article 4	Strengthen the public health infrastructure (which includes workforce, laboratory and information systems) and other components of the public health system (including education, research, and the faith community) to increase the ability to identify, respond to, and prevent problems of public health importance, including the health aspects of terrorist attacks.

(Continued)	
Article 6	Educate and inform health professionals and the public to better identify, respond to, and prevent the health consequences of terrorism, and promote the visibility and availability of health professionals in the communities that they serve.
Article 7	Address mental health needs of populations that are directly or indirectly affected by terrorism.
Article 9	Assure clarification of the roles, relationships and responsibilities among public health agencies, law enforcement and first responders.

Tertiary prevention

Article 5	Ensure availability of, and accessibility to, health care, including medications and vaccines, for individuals exposed, infected, made ill, or injured in terrorist attacks.
Article 7	Address mental health needs of populations that are directly or indirectly affected by terrorism.
Article 8	Assure the protection of the environment, the food and water supply, and the health and safety of rescue and recovery professionals.
Article 12	Build and sustain the public health capacity to develop systems to collect data about the health and mental health consequences of terrorism and other disasters on victims, responders, and communities, and develop uniform definitions and standardised data-classification systems of death and injury resulting from terrorism and other disasters.
Authors' addition 3	Promote sustainable development in order to enhance resilience in the light of a terrorist action.

Primary prevention attempts to prevent disease or injury occurring. In this chapter, primary prevention is used to describe policies and actions which prevent terrorism arising. *Secondary prevention* attempts to identify and control disease at an early, treatable stage. Secondary prevention, here, is protection against harm from terrorist attack. *Tertiary prevention* attempts to prevent disabling consequences of disease or injury by helping individuals regain their optimal level of function after a disease or injury. With regard to terrorism, examples of tertiary prevention include effectively organised emergency responses, and the treatment and rehabilitation of individuals who have been seriously injured by a terrorist attack.

Of these three levels of prevention, primary prevention has the greatest human appeal and is the most cost-beneficial. We will first look at the specific roles for public health professionals in secondary and tertiary prevention.

Improving public health system capabilities to respond to health consequences of terrorist acts

The terrorist threat requires the strengthening of public health systems (Articles 4 and 12 of the APHA principles, see Box 23.1). Public health agencies have suffered from decades of under-funding.[21] Skilled resources are needed in epidemiology, surveillance, microbiological, occupational and environmental science. The effectiveness, safety, and availability of vaccines, antimicrobials and antitoxins for bio-terrorist agents need to be intensively researched and supply systems improved (Article 5). Mental health capabilities also need to be improved (Article 7). The better protection of food and water supplies and the ambient air is needed (Article 8). We also need better ways of communicating with the public and better ways of mobilising and co-ordinating the vast resources of voluntary organisations (Article 6).[10]

Roles of health professionals

Health professionals need to develop their own knowledge and understanding of manifestations of terrorist actions and maintain vigilance – many of the diseases and injuries caused by biological and chemical agents are non-specific and insidious. Health systems need to develop their collective capacity, intelligence and preparedness. Health professionals and emergency services need to ensure the availability of and knowledge about appropriate vaccines and antimicrobials, for the protection of high-risk frontline staff and for the prevention of secondary infection and contamination following a terrorist action. Health professionals need to be able to support the public health investigation of an immediate chemical or biological problem and population health surveys of long-term health consequences. There is a role for higher education in incorporating prevention of terrorism and emergency planning into the public health curriculum (Article 6).[10]

Preparedness planning/'resilience'

Resilience has come to mean *the overall ability of public services and communities to respond to and deal with 'all risks' of civil, environmental, communicable disease disasters and breaches of security*. Concern became extreme in the UK in the wake of the 2000 fuel strike, floods and the 2001 foot and mouth disease epidemic and led to the Civil Contingencies Bill which underwent further strengthening following the events of 9–11.[24]

Health professionals need to be able to inform their patients about the health consequences of terrorist attacks to enable appropriate levels of preparedness and resilience by the public (Articles 6 and 9). Public health services need to be an integral part of all civil contingencies planning, be vigilant, informed and test plans regularly.[24–26] There is a difficult balance between informing and preparedness and creating alarm.[27]

Community development

Community development practitioners have a key role to play in assisting local resilience. Maintaining and developing community networks can provide immediate human support to respond to the distress and fear caused by terrorist attacks (Article 2); it can also provide longer-term support in the event of major civil contingencies, for example providing community care during an influenza pandemic (Article 5). Community development also has a strong role in reducing poverty and injustice, strengthening communities, developing cultural competence, protecting rights and liberties, building respect and confidence between ethnic and religious groups, and in working for community safety and sustainable development (Articles 1, 2, and 10).[3,4,28]

Resilience and sustainable development

Sustainable development offers the potential to create greater resilience in communities in the event of terrorist actions. For example: households capable of 'grey water' recycling or with an independent water supply will be resistant to the contamination of water supplies; households using solar power or other renewable energy sources will be resistant to loss of power; communities where there are robust local money systems, local exchange trading or time banks will be less reliant on cash and credit should a cyber terror attack wipe out banking computers; accessible communities reliant on cycling and walking will be less at risk from fuel blockades; communities which can step up their local food supply will also have more local security.[29]

The epidemiology of violence

The public health community should take a key role in monitoring violence, including terrorist outrages, as major health threats.[30] A good example was the recent study showing the psychological resilience of Londoners after the 7-7 bombings.[31] It can also serve part of the documentation function for reconciliation.[32] Its major function is to determine prevention strategies.[33,34]

Taking actions to help prevent terrorism

Advocating the control, reduction and elimination of weapons of mass destruction

A serious attempt to prevent terrorism must include measures to control weapons of mass destruction and ultimately eliminate them (Article 11). The threat of nuclear war and nuclear winter demonstrated how the best civil defence could never offer protection from truly catastrophic scenarios.[33] Similarly, the best civil defence cannot protect against the worst possible terrorist outrage. Prevention is better than cure when there is no cure. Real biological security can only come from securing global control over weapons technologies. Public health professionals can advocate strengthening international treaties to control, and ultimately eliminate, chemical, biological and nuclear weapons in the same way that they have with specific disease control and eradication programmes.[3,4,10,12,13,31,33,34]

National policies for control of small arms explosives and incendiaries are also needed, particularly in the USA. Health professionals can help document the adverse health impact of these weapons and advocate control.[35,36]

Addressing factors that may breed terrorism

Poverty

Often terrorist movements are a response to gross inequality – extreme poverty juxtaposed against the extreme wealth of ruling classes or regimes. Gross inequality in access to environmental resources, food and water, and exploitation by multinational companies are leading to worsening levels of poverty, poorer health and poorer access to health care. For 80 per cent of the world's population, living standards are getting worse. The average African household consumed 20 per cent less in 2000 than it had in 1975. About 3 billion people live on less than US $2 per day and 1.3 billion people on less than $1 a day. The richest fifth of the world control 85 per cent of the world's wealth. Daily, more than 1 billion people drink unsafe water and infectious diseases kill more than 50,000 people a day.[7,8,9,10,34,37,38] The powerless feel humiliated and threatened[11] and may resort to protest, subterfuge, and then outright terrorism. In a world bombarded with media messages, only the biggest outrages will register in the popular consciousness.[10,11]

Religious extremism

Religious fundamentalists find a rich harvest of potential martyrs from conditions of abject poverty around the world. But for some, religious totalitarianism and intolerance is the driver. In the USA, religious extremists have bombed abortion clinics.[10] Al Qaeda arises in part from an Islamic movement called Salafiyya, the 'venerable forefathers', referring to the generation of the Prophet Mohammad, who were committed to *Jihad* or 'Holy War'. Extremist Salafis regard western civilisation as a source of evil that spreads idolatry throughout the world in the form of secularism.[10,11] It is difficult for any agency or value system – religious, scientific, cultural, political or economic – to combat any form of fanaticism, which by definition is not open to argument. The greatest chance to diffuse fanaticism is to work with the vast majority of moderates in all the great religions to achieve some common ground. Even in highly charged conflict situations, a willingness to understand the other side's viewpoint can prevent violence and sideline the extremists.[32] Instant resort to violence only confirms the fanatic in the righteousness of his or her cause and fuels distrust, dehumanisation and satanisation of 'the other'.

Promoting the protection of civil rights and human rights

Elsworthy and Rifkind describe a human security approach to protect human rights and civil society through local and international non-violent, practical and immediate responses.[32] The robust, non-violent mobilisation of the community, with the strong involvement of women, is possible and can be highly effective. They describe local actions which can defuse violence and begin to establish conditions for trust and confidence-building in conflict situations. These are:

- avoid where possible the use of more violence;
- show respect;
- improve physical conditions;
- include all parties in the peace process;
- encourage civil society and consult;
- set up centres of listening and documentation (CLDs);
- provide trauma counselling;
- train and employ a significant number of women in policing duties;
- train skilled negotiators and mediators;
- work with religious leaders;
- build bridges;
- introduce truth and reconciliation processes.

Specific examples of the success of women's initiatives come from Kenya, Sierra Leone and Mothers for Peace in Northern Ireland. Truth and reconciliation commissions have been successful in Sierra Leone, Rwanda and South Africa. In addition, there are five global dimensions:

- combine military and civilian peace-building;
- employ third-party intervention;
- cut the export of weapons;
- secure long-term support for peace processes;
- establish horizontal networks that combine legitimacy and neutrality.[32]

The examples of conflict resolution and the defence of civil society often require personal risk. This is a feature of the most decisive community development and public health practice.[3,4,32,34]

Respect for international law

The United Nations has 'become essential before it has become effective'.[10,39,40] Now more than ever, there is a need for respect and support for the United Nations and for financial and moral backing from world authorities. Under international law, national dictators are not immune from prosecution for crimes against humanity. A key tenet of international law is that the right to use armed force is limited to situations of self-defence, and then only when the United Nations Security Council has taken the necessary steps to maintain international peace and security. This is further reinforced by the guidance that the right to use force should only be where 'the necessity of that self-defence is instant, overwhelming, leaves no choice of means and no moment for deliberation.'[10] These tenets have been flouted by the USA and Britain in recent conflicts. If a new just world order is to be established, our leaders will need to develop greater respect for and commitment to a more democratic and powerful United Nations.[39,40]

Promoting a balance between response to terrorism and to other public health concerns: diversion of resources

Strengthening public health systems to respond to terrorism will strengthen some capabilities – for example, in epidemiology, surveillance and planning, in dealing with other problems of public health importance. It should enhance our ability to respond to other major threats, such as climatic change.

Yet, public health professionals should be aware that responding to and developing preparedness for terrorism may

- shift attention and divert critically needed human, financial, and other resources away from other important public health needs, adversely affecting the health and well-being of individuals and communities;
- require public health professionals and their organisations to work with the military and criminal justice agencies in ways that may compromise their trust with their communities and their freedom to communicate important public health information;
- compromise the civil rights and human rights of individuals and organisations.

Public health is a critical element in reducing or preventing inappropriate or hazardous responses to threats of future terrorism, such as the diversion of resources and attention from other urgent public health needs, adverse health effects from misuse of antibiotics and ill-conceived immunisation, and abrogation of civil rights and human rights.

We must maintain and strengthen support for other public health priorities. For example, more than 100,000 people in the UK die each year of tobacco-related disease, and another 40,000 die of alcohol-related disease. Attention to these urgent problems by health professionals, policy-makers, and the general public should not be diverted.[10,18–23]

Conclusion

Terrorism is a threat to public health and to society as a whole. Health professionals can do much to mitigate the health consequences of terrorist threats or acts, and to help prevent them. Preventing terrorism and its health consequences should be in the curricula of all schools of health. At the same time, health professionals must maintain and promote a balanced perspective that gives terrorism preparedness an appropriate priority amidst the many other health problems people suffer.

Sustainable development is necessary for resilience, for robust civil society and for good public health. The pursuit of social justice and securing human rights are essential for improved public health. Visionary leadership by public health professionals will continue to be critically important in addressing terrorism. Preventing ill-health and reducing global inequalities in health are the central roles of public health, and also happen to be the most important requirements for preventing terrorism.

Note

The authors are grateful for important contributions to the discussion of these issues to H. Jack Geiger, Barry S. Levy, Hillel Cohen, Robert Gould and Mark Sidel.

References

1. World Health Organisation. (1999) *Health 21*. Copenhagen: WHO EURO.
2. Middleton, J. (1988) Health promotion is peace promotion. *Health Promotion International,* 2 (4): 341–5.
3. Middleton, J. (2003) Health, environmental and social justice. *Local Environment,* 8 (2): 155–65.
4. Middleton, J. (1997) Public health, security and sustainable development. *Health and Hygiene,* 18: 149–54.
5. Santa Barbara, J. and MacQueen, G. (2004) Peace through health: key concepts. *Lancet,* 364: 384–6.
6. Buhmann, C.B. (2005) The role of health professionals in preventing and mediating conflict. *Medicine, Conflict and Survival,* 21 (4): 299–311.
7. Global Health Watch (2005) *An Alternative World Health Report*. London: Zed Books (in association with the People's Health Movement, Bangalore, Medact, London, Global Equity Gauge Alliance, Durban).
8. Kickbusch, I. (2004) The Leavell lecture – the end of public health as we know it: constructing global public health in the 21st century. *Public Health,* 188 (7): 463–9.
9. Brundtland, G.-H. (2000) Health and population. Fourth Reith Lecture, www.bbc.co.uk/radio4/reith2000.
10. Sidel, V. and Levy, B. (2003) *Terrorism and Public Health*. Oxford: Oxford University Press.
11. De Zulueta, F. (2006) Terror breeds terrorists. *Medicine, Conflict and Survival,* 22: 13–25.
12. Rogers, P. (2005) *Endless war: the global war on terror and the new Bush administration.* Oxford: Oxford Research Group, briefing paper, www.oxfordresearchgroup.org.uk.
13. Barnaby, F. (2002) *The new terrorism*. Also: *Waiting for terror: how realistic is the biological, chemical and nuclear threat?* Oxford: Oxford Research Group, www.oxfordresearchgroup.org.uk.
14. Gofin, R. (2005) Preparedness and response to terrorism: a framework for public health action. *European Journal of Public Health,* 15: 100–4.
15. United States Institute of Medicine (1988) *The Future of Public Health*. Washington, DC: National Academy of Sciences.
16. Watts, G. (2005) Harnessing mother nature against your fellow humans. *British Medical Journal,* 331: 1228.
17. Denning, D. (2001) Activism, Hacktivism and cyberterrorism: the internet as a tool for influencing foreign policy. In: Arquilla, J. and Ronfeldt, D.F. (eds), *Networks and Netwars: the Future of Terror, Crime and Militancy*. Santa Monica, CA: Rand Corporation National Defense Research Institute.
18. Annas, G.J. (2002) Bioterrorism, public health, and civil liberties. *New England Journal of Medicine,* 346: 1337–42.
19. Pilger, J. (2006) The death of freedom. *New Statesman,* 9 January: 10–12.
20. Sidel, M. (2004) *More Secure, Less Free? Antiterrorism Policy and Civil Liberties after September 11*. Ann Arbor: University of Michigan Press.

21. Sidel, V. (2003) Bioterrorism in the United States: a balanced assessment of risk and response. *Medicine, Conflict and Survival*, 19: 318–25.

22. Frank, E. (2005) Funding the public health response to terrorism. *British Medical Journal*, 331: 526–7.

23. Atkins, D. and Moy, E. (2005) Left behind: the legacy of hurricane Katrina. *British Medical Journal*, 331: 916–17.

24. HM Government (2004) *Civil Contingencies Act 2004*. London: Office of Public Sector Information, www.opsi.gov.uk/acts/acts 2004/20040036.htm.

25. www.ukresilience.info/ccact/index.shtm and www.epcollege.gov.uk.

26. HM Government (2005) *Preparing for Emergencies*. London: Cabinet Office, www.preparing foremergencies.gov.uk/index.shtm.

27. UK Resilience (2005) *Communicating Risk: Warning and Informing the Public*. London: Cabinet Office, www.ukresilience.info/preparedness/warningandinforming/index.shtm

28. Home Office (2005) *Preventing Extremism Together: Response to Working Group Reports (on Community Cohesion)*. London: Home Office; *Tackling Religious Extremism*. www.home office.gov.uk.

29. Middleton, J. (2003) World summit on sustainable development: what does it mean for Sandwell? In Middleton, J. (ed.), *What Works for Health in Sandwell? The 14th Annual Public Health Report for Sandwell*. West Bromwich: Sandwell Primary Care Trusts.

30. World Health Organisation (2002) *The World Report on Violence and Health*. Geneva: World Health Organisation.

31. Rubin, G.J., Brewin, C.R., Greenberg, N. et al. (2005) Psychological and behavioural reactions to the bombings in London on 7 July 2005: cross-sectional survey of a representative sample of Londoners. *British Medical Journal*, 331: 606–11.

32. Elsworthy, S. and Rifkind, G. (2005) *Hearts and Minds: Human Security Approaches to Political Violence*. London: Demos.

33. British Medical Association (1983) *The Health Effects of Nuclear War*. Report of the Board of Science and Education. London: BMA.

34. Sidel, V. (1985) Destruction before detonation. *Lancet*, ii: 1287–9.

35. Matthews, D. (2005) *War Prevention Works*. Oxford: Oxford Research Group, www.oxford researchgroup.org.uk.

36. Editorial (2000) Reducing gun deaths in the USA. *Lancet*, 356, 1367.

37. Shiva, V. (2000) Poverty and globalisation. Fifth Reith lecture, www.bbc.co.uk/radio4/reith 2000/lecture5_print.shtml.

38. United Nations Development Programme (2004) *Human Development Report*. Geneva: United Nations.

39. Lee, K. (2005) Is the UN broken and can we fix it?, *British Medical Journal*, 331: 525–6.

40. Renner, M. (2005) Security redefined. In World Watch Institute report *State of the World, 2005*. New York: W.W. Norton.

Chapter 24

Economic Change, Incomes and Health

Mike Rowson

1 Introduction

This brief chapter covers rather a lot of ground, in both subject matter and evidence. It attempts to bring together two sets of discussions about economic change and health: one that is mainly confined to the developing world and which concerns the relationship between growth in per capita income and health outcomes; and another which is mainly confined to discussions in the developed world about the (economic) sources of health inequalities. I evaluate some of the evidence used in both these debates and then use that evidence to pose some questions about globalization.

Globalization can be described as 'a process of greater integration within the world economy through movements of goods and services, capital, technology and (to a lesser extent) labour which lead increasingly to economic decisions being influenced by global conditions' (Jenkins, cited in Global Health Watch, 2005: 13). The effect of this process of economic integration on the health of people around the world has been extensively debated: does globalization create increased wealth and therefore better health for all? Or does it increase income inequalities between rich and poor within countries and worsen overall health? My purpose here is not to answer these questions definitively, but rather to show how an understanding of the debate is premised on thinking about the complex relationships between income and health, and the way those relationships are themselves mediated by a broad array of factors. I end by reviewing some strong claims made about the health effects of globalization by public health advocates.

2 Income and health – the developing country story

I take as my starting point the well-described relationship between income, expressed on the graph in Figure 24.1 as average GDP per capita (at purchasing power parities, a

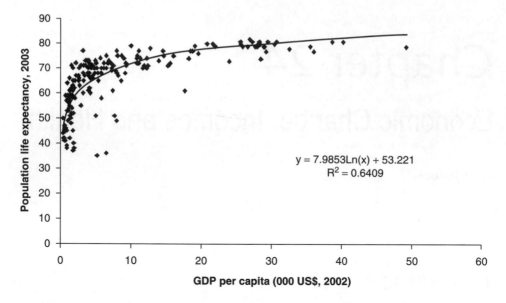

Figure 24.1   The relationship between wealth and health (GDP per captia and population life expectancy)

calculation which adjusts national income for cost of living) and life expectancy. The curvilinear relationship which the graph shows suggests two initial conclusions. First, that up to a level of around US$5,000 per capita (at PPP), life expectancy appears to be sensitive to increases in average income. A policy inference might therefore be drawn that economic policies which focus on increasing incomes will have the greatest benefit for population health in countries below this standard of living. This appears to make sense, as income has the potential to give people the capacity to exist healthily: to be able to buy nutritious food, live in a healthy environment with access to clean water and proper sanitation and to be able to purchase health care and education.

A second inference that can be made from Figure 24.1 is that above a certain level of per capita income – say about US$5,000 – the association between increases in life expectancy and income becomes weaker. More money cannot buy a country much better health. A tentative policy conclusion might therefore be that policies that increase the material affluence of the populations of these richer, mainly developed countries will have limited effects on people's health status. I will return to this part of the graph in section 3.

For now, I want to look more closely at the relationship between income and health in the developing world. What we notice from the graph in Figure 24.1 is that there are a number of countries whose position deviates from the trend line. There are some countries which do rather better than one would expect in terms of life expectancy for their level of income – these countries lie above the curve. Conversely, there are some countries whose position suggests they are doing somewhat worse in terms of health outcomes than their income would predict. These countries lie below the curve.

How can these outliers be explained? First, average per capita income is a broad measure which conceals many different types of social organization. Because it is an average it does not tell us about the inequalities in income between richer and poorer groups within a country. Even if two countries have the same per capita income, that income might be distributed very unequally in one, with the top 20 per cent of the population taking a far bigger slice of the national resource 'cake' than the poorest 60 per cent or even 80 per cent. The incidence of poverty will therefore be higher than in countries where income is distributed more evenly. Health outcomes are likely to be dragged downwards as a result.

Governments can influence patterns of income distribution. In very poor countries, unequal access to land is often a key determinant of poverty. Land reforms can therefore help alleviate destitution. Governments can also formulate economic policies that promote higher levels of employment (and hence better incomes) among the poor. Sen (1998, 1999) argues that these were key measures taken by many poor countries that have achieved good health at low levels of income. Conversely, failure to reduce inequalities has been a feature of the performance of those countries lying below the curve.

There may be a second reason for the differences seen in Figure 24.1. Average per capita income makes no distinction for how resources are used by populations and their governments. For any given level of wealth, governments might choose to spend their resources in very different ways. Some may focus spending on the provision of health and other health-sustaining services, such as water and education. Other governments might prioritize spending on defence or other activities which produce few or no benefits for health. Anand and Ravallion (1993) argue that lower levels of poverty and higher levels of public spending on health account for much of the better performance of some countries, although there is continuing dispute about this (for the debates see, for example, Filmer et al., 1997; Wang, 2003; Mackintosh and Koivusalo, 2004). Because of the labour-intensive nature of health care, it is possible for low-wage economies to undertake quite extensive programmes of health services (Sen, 1998).

Finally, a focus on average incomes may conceal deeper patterns of social organization that mediate the impact of a given level of wealth. One example which is particularly conducive for health is the level of female literacy (itself the result of complex interactions between government priorities, public pressure and cultural influences). Female literacy – through its influence on the ability of women to process health-related information and through its effects on women's incomes – tends to benefit the health of young children. The dramatic gains in life expectancy that have been achieved in places such as China, Kerala and Sri Lanka have partly been won through large reductions in deaths among the under-fives.

Another example which is certainly depressing health gains in some of the countries below the curve, such as South Africa and Namibia, is extremely high levels of HIV/AIDS. Indeed many countries, especially in Eastern and Southern Africa, but also elsewhere, are witnessing reversals of a number of health indicators as a result of the pandemic.

These debates about the potential of economic growth to improve health are echoed in discussions about Britain's own economic development in the nineteenth and early twentieth centuries. In the 1970s, the demographer Thomas McKeown produced evidence which showed that, contrary to popular perception, improvements in health in the UK over that period were not due to scientific advances such as more efficacious medicine and surgical techniques or immunization or to public health measures, but rather to a raised 'standard of living' which led to better nutrition.

However, McKeown's argument has been disputed by the social historian Simon Szreter. He points out that the social disruption caused by rapid industrialization (which led to massive rural to urban migration and overcrowding in urban areas) led to declines in life expectancy in the Victorian cities, *even in the context of rising wage levels* (Szreter, 1995). Szreter further argues that the mortality declines identified by McKeown often resulted from the application of public health measures by governments (under public pressure) in order to ameliorate the appalling conditions in the cities.

What all of these discussions show is that economic growth alone will be not be enough to improve population health. Purposive action is needed to direct the fruits of growth towards social improvements that sustain health (Sen, 1998). In fact, even a lack of economic growth does not necessarily mean health has to suffer. By prioritizing and devoting what little money is available to the task of improving health, or by influencing the patterns of income distribution, or by utilizing their comparative advantage of low wages in labour-intensive services such as health and education, even very poor countries can achieve remarkable health outcomes.

3 Income and health – the developed country story

The second set of debates produced by the curve in Figure 24.1 centres around the countries with average incomes greater than US$5,000 per year. As you can see, there appears to be little life expectancy gain from increased incomes. There are, however, very real health inequalities within these countries which researchers regularly relate back to 'socioeconomic status', as inquiries such as those undertaken by different governments in the UK show (Whitehead et al., 1992; Acheson, 1998). Yet absolute poverty and the very direct effects this has on health do not exist to anywhere near the same extent as they do in developing countries. So what is causing the health gradient within richer nations?

The answers to this question are complex. Research shows that low incomes can still have an effect on the presence of health deprivation even in richer countries. Poorer people are likely to have worse health, and may also have worse access to health and other health-sustaining services. They are more likely to be unemployed, to live in sub-standard housing, have jobs with greater health risks, and to undertake 'bad behaviours' such as smoking and drinking than wealthier parts of the population (Fox and Benzeval, 1995). There has been some debate as to whether 'income' is in fact a proxy for something else, such as education, and there is mixed evidence as to whether education or income are independently influential on health status (Deaton, 2002).

Yet there is more to the story of health disparities than low incomes. Epidemiological evidence from the Whitehall Studies shows a health gradient between top and bottom parts of the civil service, with health outcomes differing 'step-wise' at each grade of employment (Marmot, 1996). So, those at the top of the service have the best health, and those at the next grade down have worse health than those at the top, and so on. Clearly, this gradient is not related to the effects of low incomes (although low income may play a role in producing worse health in the lower ranks of the civil service). Researchers have therefore suggested that specific factors pertaining to the work environment, including control over the demands created by work, the ability to utilize skills and the availability of support from work colleagues are important for creating better health outcomes (Whitehead, 1995).

This evidence shifts the debate away from the material effects of low income on health in developing countries to consideration of psychosocial factors that may be influencing health outcomes. A further, though controversial, analysis appears to add weight to this shift in emphasis. Some researchers have argued that *levels of income inequality* are a primary determinant of health in rich nations. We have already seen that income inequality does matter in so far as societies with a greater proportion of poor people (as there will be in countries with high income inequality) will necessarily have a higher burden of ill-health. The controversial aspect of this thesis comes with the idea that what really matters is the way in which wide disparities in income affect the disposition – and therefore the health – of society as a whole (both richer and poorer people).

The social epidemiologist Richard Wilkinson, an important exponent of this view, argues that health is affected not only by material factors, but by the quality of social relations, a person's sense of status and childhood environment (Wilkinson, 1996, 2005). Societies with greater income inequalities tend to have higher rates of suicide and violence, fewer communitarian bonds, oppressive hierarchies of power, and high intra-family stress, which can lead to a worse environment for the developing child.

Wilkinson (2005) cites an impressive array of studies to bolster these linkages, but there are still sharp debates about the basic connection between income inequality and health status. The economist Angus Deaton argues bluntly that 'the best recent data support none of the original international correlations' (2002: 23), and sociologists have pointed out that stronger communities and other types of associative bond can be oppressive of individual freedoms in ways which harm health (Kunitz, 2001). Clearly, the debates in these areas will continue.

What this summary again shows is that while low income may be a determinant of health inequalities in the rich countries, it is coupled with other factors which may be equally important in determining unequal outcomes, including education, and position in a hierarchy (within a workplace, for example, or society as a whole). These 'confounders' make designing policy interventions to address health inequalities rather difficult. Would it be better, for instance, to provide universal high-quality education or re-distribute incomes in order to promote health? What interventions need to take place within the workplace to give people more sense of control? Does policy need to focus on the empowerment of the individual, or on working practices, or on the way in which economic policy affects the design of those working practices?

4 Assessing the health effects of economic change – the case of globalization

In the final part of this chapter I now want to put some of this evidence to use in assessing the claims made by public health experts about the effects of globalization. The two major and competing claims are these: first, globalization increases wealth in the world and therefore boosts health; and secondly, an argument that is commonly made by those opposed to, or wishing to reform, globalization, that it is leading to greater income inequalities within and between nations, and that this is a danger to health. To assess the evidence for these claims I will need to mix some economics with the health analysis.

A good example of the first type of claim was made by Richard Feachem, the former Head of the Health, Nutrition and Population Division at the World Bank (and, at the time of writing, Executive Director of the Global Fund for AIDS, Tuberculosis and Malaria). Writing in the *British Medical Journal*, Feachem argued that:

> globalization, economic growth and improvement in health go hand-in-hand. Economic growth is good for the incomes of the poor, and what is good for the incomes of the poor is good for the health of the poor. Globalization is a key component of economic growth. Openness to trade and the inflow of capital, technology and ideas are essential for sustained economic growth. (Feachem, 2001: 505)

I hope that you can see from this quote that the debates on income we have looked at earlier have real policy relevance.

However, the outcomes of globalization in terms of both economic growth and better health are not as clear-cut as Feachem suggests. Much of the economic debate relies on evidence about the effects of one (important) part of globalization, namely openness to trade. And the evidence here is mixed. East Asian countries appear to have done extremely well from increased trade on world markets. Using their comparative advantage of an abundance of unskilled labour – coupled with improvements in education and good economic management – they have managed to increase their exports of simple manufactured goods, such as textiles, clothing and toys, and have also proceeded up the 'value-chain' to produce more expensive goods, such as televisions, cars and computer components. There have been historically unprecedented declines in income poverty partly as a result.

However, openness to trade in African countries has had rather different effects. With poor producers dependent on the export of low-value primary commodities (such as coffee, cocoa, maize, and so on), whose price is volatile and tends to fall over time, African countries have seen extremely poor growth rates and absolute poverty has risen. In Latin America, a more 'economically-advanced' region, exporters have faced strong competition from East Asian countries in manufactured goods and failed to generate wealth from the creation of new industries and services. As a result, poverty rates have been stagnant across the region. It should also be noted that both African and Latin American agricultural producers have faced strong competition from heavily subsidized US and EU farmers.

What these different stories tell us is that globalization and openness to trade do not necessarily bring increased income. Mirroring the reversals in poverty reduction efforts in Latin America and Africa there has been a slow-down in the rate of improvement in a number of health indicators, such as infant and child mortality and life expectancy (Cornia and Menchini, 2005), and sometimes there have been outright reversals of past improvements. However, we must take care in attributing this to globalization. Other factors, such as HIV/AIDS and poor governance, account for some of it. We also know from our previous discussions that lack of economic growth is not necessarily a barrier to health improvement. However, there are cases (as we can see from Box 24.1) where openness to trade does appear to be associated with worsening in poverty and health; and more generally, the vulnerability of those economies (particularly in Africa) to the divergent fortunes of world trade makes it clear that those who call for more globalization must be prepared to acknowledge the risks it entails for countries without established welfare states that can protect populations during the process.

Box 24.1   Trade can lead to poverty and worse health: a case study from Mexico

In the run-up to the North American Free Trade Agreement (NAFTA), the Mexican government ended its subsidies to 'small-scale producers of basic crops', including corn, the main ingredient of tortillas, Mexico's staple food. When NAFTA opened the Mexico–USA border, corn from the USA flooded the Mexican market. Large-scale agribusiness is massively subsidized in the USA: in 2001, corn cost US$3.41 a barrel to produce in the USA, but sold on the world market for $2.28. Currency crises and IMF conditional loans also played a role in the rapid decline of Mexico's corn prices. Following the collapse of the peso in 1995, the bail-out organized by the Clinton administration included a US$1 billion export credit that obliged Mexico to purchase US corn. Predictably, Mexican imports of US corn to Mexico rose by 120 per cent in a year.

Mexican corn production stagnated while prices declined. Small farmers were hardest hit, becoming much poorer than they were in the early 1990s, despite efforts by the Mexican government to reintroduce some of the subsidies. Some 700,000 agricultural jobs disappeared over the same period. The lack of demand for farm labour depressed wages by 2001 to less than half of what they were 20 years earlier. Rural poverty rates rose to over 70 per cent; the minimum wage lost over 75 per cent of its purchasing power; infant mortality rates of the poor increased; and wage inequalities became the worst in Latin America.

Source: Global Health Watch, 2005, http://www.ghwatch.org/2005report/A.pdf.

What is perhaps more surprising is that this slow-down in health improvements has also occurred in some of the highest-performing developing countries in terms of economic growth – including the two with the largest populations, India and China (together containing around one-third of the world's people). Both of these countries have embarked on courses of internal market reforms, coupled with opening-up to the global economy. Both have enjoyed periods of economic growth, in China's case at historically unprecedented levels for much of the past three decades. China has massively reduced income poverty, although inequality has increased, particularly inequality between rural and urban areas. In India, poverty reduction has also occurred, but at a slower rate and has been equally uneven in its effects. Yet both of these countries have experienced slow-downs in improvements in the infant mortality rate in the last 10–20 years, as Table 24.1 makes clear. It is not the case that the improvements are 'bottoming out' at a low level of infant mortality, as the comparative data for Sri Lanka and South Korea in Table 24.1 show.

What this data suggests is that, first, gains in economic growth in India and China, which are partly associated with globalization, have not been used to support more rapid health improvements. Secondly, it may also be suggestive of a change in emphasis on the part of policy-makers in these countries – away from policies that support populations towards focusing on policies that respond to (global) market incentives (Drèze and Sen, 2002).

Some have gone further than this and suggested that globalization actively re-orients government expenditures in all countries away from investment in the social fabric and towards investment in attracting foreign investment and trade. This strong argument is

Table 24.1   Improvements in the infant mortality rate (selected countries)

| | *Infant mortality rate (per 1,000 live births)* | | | | | *Annual rate of decline (per cent)* | |
	1960	1981	1991*	1999	1960–81	1981–91	1991–99
China	150	37	31	30	6.7	2.0	0.0
India	165	110	80	71	1.9	3.3	1.5
South Korea	85	33	23	8	4.5	3.6	13.2
SriLanka	71	43	26	15	2.4	5.0	6.9

* data for China from 1990
Source: Drèze and Sen, 2002. By permission of Oxford University Press.

debated by some economists who argue that openness to world trade and the instability this brings forces countries to spend more on welfare states to protect their population (Rodrik, 1998). Arguments continue in this area, especially around the ability of the poorest countries to create appropriate safety nets in resource-constrained environments.

What about the other claims of those critical of globalization – those who say that globalization is producing greater inequalities between and within countries and that this will have deleterious impacts on health? For reasons of space we will concentrate simply on the issue of *within* country inequalities, as the evidence is strongly contested – for two reasons. First, the measurement of income inequalities is quite variable and different methods produce different results. And secondly, drawing out the health implications of these changes may be difficult.

Thompson (2004) concurs with Cornia and Menchini (2005) that there has been a widespread rise in *within-country* income inequalities in the era of globalization. What has caused this may be partly due to globalization (openness to trade, for example, increasing competitive pressures on low-skilled workers in richer countries), but is also due to a set of policy stances associated with globalization. To understand this, let us remind ourselves of the definition of globalization set out at the beginning of this chapter, *as a process whereby (national) economic decisions are increasingly influenced by global conditions*. Some analysts have noted how the threat of global competition has been associated with a reduction in the power of trade unions and reductions in the welfare state – key planks of protection for low-income workers – as governments call for 'more flexible' labour markets. As mentioned before, the association between globalization and the size of welfare states is the subject of some debate, but the battles over the power of trade unions and labour market regulations have certainly been experienced in many developed countries, and do help to explain why income inequality has increased in some of them.

The evidence on whether health inequalities are increasing in the wake of this increase in income inequalities is not conclusive, however. Yet we know from the analysis in sections 2 and 3 that an increase should worry public health advocates. First, it might imply a larger number of people struggling to survive on low incomes with the associated effects on their health. And secondly, if we accept the Wilkinson hypothesis, an increase in income inequalities could lead to adverse social outcomes which affect mental and physical health. The fact that there is little good analysis of the relationship between globalization, income inequalities and health inequalities is rather worrying.

5 Conclusion

In summary, then, the claims of the globalization pessimists have some grounding in the available evidence: there is no straightforward relationship between globalization, income and health, and nor, judging from the analysis in sections 2 and 3, should we expect there to be. What we do know is that any gains from globalization need to be captured by governments and reinvested purposively in 'health-producing' areas. Simply hoping that income rises among certain population groups will lead to better health is optimistic. Governance is critical.

At the same time, those critical of globalization should not automatically assume that it is global economic conditions which worsen the health of the poor. First, the linkages are not always clear, and there is a need to examine the direct impacts of economic change through better research on the way health is affected by the shifts in incomes, prices and government expenditures that are induced by globalization. And secondly, it is also clear that even when beset by the forces of global change, governments can do a lot to protect the health of the vulnerable: not all nations have suffered to the same extent. National policy management of global change in the interests of health *is* possible, although the capacity of the very poorest nations to do this is severely constrained.

Acknowledgement

With thanks to David Hewitt for data analysis. Any faults with its use and interpretation remain the author's.

References

Acheson, D. (1998). *Independent Inquiry into Inequalities in Health Report*. London: HMSO.

Anand, S. and Ravallion, M. (1993). Human development in poor countries: on the role of private incomes and public services. *Journal of Economic Perspectives,* 7 (1): 133–50.

Cornia, G.A. and Menchini, L. (2005). The pace and distribution of health improvements during the last 40 years: some preliminary results. Available at: http://www.wider.unu.edu/conference/conference-2005-3/conference-2005-3-papers/Cornia%20&%20Menchini.pdf (accessed 19 December 2005).

Deaton, A. (2002). Policy implications of the gradient of health and wealth. *Health Affairs*, March/April.

Drèze, J. and Sen, A. (2002). *India: Development and Participation*. Oxford: Oxford University Press.

Feachem, R. (2001). Globalization is good for your health, mostly. *British Medical Journal,* 323: 504–6.

Filmer, D., Hammer, J. and Pritchett, L. (1997). Health policy in poor countries: weak links in the chain. World Bank Policy Research Working Paper 1874. Washington, DC: World Bank. Available at: http://www.worldbank.org/html/dec/Publications/Workpapers/WPS1800series/wps1874/wps1874.pdf (accessed 19 December 2005).

Fox, J. and Benzeval, M. (1995). Perspectives on social variations in health. In Benzeval, M., Judge, K. and Whitehead, M. (eds), *Tackling Inequalities in Health: an Agenda for Action*. London: King's Fund.

Global Health Watch (2005). *Global Health Watch 2005–2006: an Alternative World Health Report*. London: Zed Books. Available at: http://www.ghwatch.org/2005report/A.pdf (accessed 19 December 2005).

Kunitz, S. (2001). Social capital: the mixed health effects of personal communities and voluntary groups. In Leon, D. and Walt, G. (eds), *Poverty, Inequality and Health: an International Perspective*. Oxford: Oxford University Press.

Mackintosh, M. and Koivusalo, M. (2004). *Health Systems and Commercialization: In Search of Good Sense*. Geneva: UNRISD. Available at: http://www.unrisd.org/unrisd/website/document.nsf/(httpPublications)/32A160C292F57BBEC1256ED10049F965?OpenDocument (accessed 19 December 2005).

Marmot, M. (1996). The social pattern of health and disease. In Blane, D., Brunner, E. and Wilkinson, R. (eds), *Health and Social Organization: Towards a Health Policy for the 21st Century*. London: Routledge.

Rodrik, D. (1998). Why do more open economies have bigger governments? *Journal of Political Economy,* 106: 997.

Sen, A. (1998) Mortality as an indicator of economic success and failure. *The Economic Journal,* 108 (January): 1–25.

Sen, A. (1999). *Development as Freedom*. Oxford: Oxford University Press.

Szreter, S. (1995). The importance of social intervention in Britain's mortality decline *c.* 1850–1914: a re-interpretation of the role of public health. In Davey, B., Gray, A. and Searle, C. (eds), *Health and Disease: a Reader* (2nd edition). Milton Keynes: Open University Press.

Thompson, G. (2004). Global inequality, economic globalization and technological change. In Brown, W., Bromley, S. and Athreye, S. (eds), *Ordering the International: History, Change and Transformation*. London: Pluto Press.

Wang, L. (2003). Determinants of child mortality in LDCs: empirical findings from demographic and health surveys. *Health Policy,* 65 (3): 277–99.

Whitehead, M. (1995). Tackling inequalities: a review of policy initiatives. In Benzeval, M., Judge, K. and Whitehead, M. (eds), *Tackling Inequalities in Health: an Agenda for Action*. London: King's Fund.

Whitehead, M., Townsend, P. and Davidson, N. (eds) (1992). *Inequalities in Health: the Black Report and the Health Divide*. London: Penguin.

Wilkinson, R. (1996). How can secular improvements in life expectancy be explained? In Blane, D., Brunner, E. and Wilkinson, R. (eds), *Health and Social Organization: Towards a Health Policy for the 21st Century*. London: Routledge.

Wilkinson, R. (2005). *The Impact of Inequality: How to Make Sick Societies Healthier*. London: Routledge.

Chapter 25

Othering of Refugees: Social Exclusion and Public Health

Natalie J. Grove, Anthony B. Zwi and Pascale Allotey

Introduction

Understanding and appreciating the experiences associated with forced migration is crucial to responding effectively to the health needs of refugees, asylum seekers and irregular migrants. In this chapter we explore how the relatively few forced migrants who resettle in developed countries are received, and in particular how forced migrants are constructed and portrayed as the 'other'.[1] We examine the role of public discourse and of political, legal and media contributions to creating and reinforcing the position of forced migrants as 'not belonging'. The effects of this process and the marginalisation that results have an impact on the health of migrants and that of host populations. We conclude by suggesting that public health must reframe thinking about forced migrants and respond to this 'othering' at health service delivery and policy level.

Forced migration: motivations for movement and responses of resistance

The Refugee Convention 1951 (http://www.unhcr.ch/1951convention/) defines refugees as 'persons outside their country of origin who are unable or unwilling to return because of a well founded fear of persecution for reasons of race, religion, nationality, membership of a particular social group, or political opinion'. While it has been argued that this definition is narrow and outdated, excluding many people who fear harm and are in need of protection, it remains dominant (see Table 25.1 for further definition of terms). African nations, who

This chapter is based on: Grove, N. and Zwi, A. (2006) Our health and theirs: forced migration, othering and public health, *Social Science and Medicine*, 62: 1931–42.

Table 25.1   Forced migrants: definition of terms

Refugee	A *refugee* is a person who, 'owing to a well-founded fear of being persecuted for reasons of race, religion, nationality, membership of a particular social group, or political opinion, is outside the country of his nationality, and is unable to or, owing to such fear, is unwilling to avail himself of the protection of that country'. (Article 1, The 1951 Convention Relating to the Status of Refugees.)
Asylum seeker	An *asylum seeker* is a person who has left his/her country of origin, has applied for recognition as a refugee in another country, and is awaiting a decision on his/her application.
Illegal immigrant	*Illegal immigrants* are people who enter a country without meeting legal requirements for entry, or residence. On the other hand, refugees often arrive with the 'barest necessities' and without personal documents.
Internally displaced person	An *internally displaced person (IDP)* may have been forced to flee his/her home for the same reasons as a refugee, but has not crossed an internationally recognised border.

Source: UNHCR (http://www.unhcr.org.au/basicdef.shtml)

together host up to 30 per cent of the global refugee population, have sought to address some of these shortcomings in their own 1969 Convention on the Specific Aspects of Refugee Problems in Africa, which expanded the definition of refugees to include persons who are forced to flee their home as a result of external aggression, occupation, foreign domination or other events that have seriously disturbed the public order.

Humanitarian protection in developed countries has not been particularly responsive to the changing circumstances of forced migration. Developed nations are adopting ever-narrower interpretations of the Convention and enforcing often punitive policies, including providing only temporary protection, repatriating people against their will, and employing mandatory and indefinite detention of unauthorised arrivals. These policies seek to limit the extent of protection afforded and discourage further migration. Understanding the differences in the labelling of different categories of forced migrants is critical because such discourses are strongly linked to the rights and protections, and therefore the well-being, of forced migrants within host countries.

A British survey in 2003 found that on average people thought that the UK housed 23 per cent of the world's refugees. The actual figure is closer to 2 per cent (MORI/ Migration Watch UK (2003) *British Views on Immigration.* London: MORI).

Box 25.1   Irregular migration

Among irregular arrivals who are fleeing refugee-like circumstances, some seek protection and asylum once inside the borders of another country while others attempt to remain undetected in a place where they lack authorisation. Fear of repatriation, distrust of asylum procedures, and anxiety about being detained contribute to the decision to

(Continued)

live an irregular or illegal existence (Gibney, 2000). While some effort has been made to understand the difficulties and challenges that irregular migrants encounter in their journey to host countries, comparatively little is known of their circumstances once they 'settle' and seek to establish themselves in a state where they have no legal status. Forced migrants who reside without documentation or authorisation may be among the most vulnerable of all groups (Prem Kumer and Grundy-Warr, 2004). Lacking legal standing, they are subject to exploitation and deception by employers, traffickers, irregular migration networks and members of their own communities (Gibney, 2000).

Othering

'Othering' is a process that 'serves to mark and name those thought to be different from oneself' (Weis, 1995). It defines and secures one's own identity by distancing and stigmatising an(other). Its purpose is to reinforce notions of our own 'normality', and to set up the difference of others as a point of deviance. We come to know *who we are* by establishing *who we are not*, and who is not us. The person or group being 'othered' experiences this as a process of marginalisation, disempowerment and social exclusion.

Over the last three decades, increasing movements of people as a result of globalisation and greater ease of travel, particularly between developed countries, have increased awareness of the 'other.' In Europe, the notion of a 'European identity' has served to heighten the awareness of those seen as not belonging (Licata and Klein, 2002). Clear distinctions are made between migrants (including nationals of other European countries), refugees, asylum seekers and illegal immigrants, with each category associated with increasing levels of intolerance (van der Veer, 2003). It is therefore apposite to adopt a framework of 'othering' to explore how refugees as a group are 'constructed' in their place of destination, and how they are set apart from mainstream communities.

In the following section we illustrate some of the ways in which refugees and asylum seekers are currently being othered – from posing a threat of importing and transmitting disease through to representations of being 'queue jumpers'. These negative stereotypes are produced and reproduced, contributing to an increasingly hostile reception for refugees, particularly in developed countries.

The language of threat

Where people are outside of their 'proper' place of belonging and within our boundaries they are increasingly represented as a threat to notions of community and sovereignty, forcing questions of 'who is in' and 'who is out'.

(Grove and Zwi, 2006: 1934)

The adoption of metaphors of threat, of natural disaster, of invasion, of war, and of contagion, have helped construct people who are forced to move in an impersonal, destructive and destabilising light. Refugees are reported to *pour* across borders, arrive in *swarms*, *tides*, *waves* and *floods*, threatening to *swamp* and *overrun* host communities (Turton, 2003). At other times the language of war and battle is employed; emphasis is placed on the (necessarily) irregular and unpredictable arrival of asylum seekers, they are painted as invaders who warrant extreme measures to be taken to deter or detain (Pugh, 2004).

The 'illegal' nature of entry is used effectively to emphasise the difference between *us* and *them*: *we* are law-abiding, *they* are law-breaking. It is argued that positioning the asylum seeker as 'illegal' contributes to public acceptance of 'detention' and shifts the focus from protection *of* the refugee, to protection *from* the refugee (Sathanapally, 2004). Detention itself powerfully criminalises forced migrants in the eyes of the community in its similarity to imprisonment.

Importantly for public health, refugees are also portrayed as a threat to a robust and healthy society, presenting a threat of disease itself. Koutroulis (2003) discusses how the language of epidemics conjures threats of contagion and reinforces the need for quarantine and separateness, strengthening the role of mandatory detention. This leads to a remarkable inversion in how health concerns are perceived, such that the receiving population is seen to be under threat rather than attending to the health needs of those displaced. Refugees shift from being *at* risk (from a myriad of health problems encountered in their place of origin or during their journey to safety) to being *of* risk (to the communities and neighbours where they settle).

In these ways othering encourages us to interact with refugees and asylum seekers from a standpoint of defence: erecting barriers, screening out and deterring, defending borders, and effectively guarding against uncontrolled contact. By focusing not on individual lives and circumstances, but rather on mass movement, we are left unable to personalise the refugee or asylum seeker. As the perception of multiple threats mounts, a heightened level of border protection is invoked, and increasingly complex measures are used to exclude refugees.

Box 25.2   Resilience

Refugees and asylum seekers are rarely portrayed as individuals with agency, skill or resilience, with a capacity to contribute and be an asset to their new communities. Rather, as the language of 'burden-sharing' suggests, they are perceived as needy, helpless and a drain on resources.

Queue jumping and the uninvited guest

One of the most powerful ways in which asylum seekers and forced migrants are portrayed is as 'uninvited'. Typically, the focus is on supposed deception, trickery and fraud that may be required to enter or remain in a country without a valid visa. The responsibility of the state to uphold moral principles, and fulfil a range of legal duties and obligations under international law, is rarely acknowledged or explicitly stated.[2]

Notions of the 'uninvited guest' have been employed by politicians to justify sensational attempts at deterring 'boat people'. The Australian government has intercepted refugees at sea and refused entry into Australian waters of vessels thought to be carrying refugees. These actions were accompanied by Prime Minister John Howard's defiant declaration: 'we will choose who comes to these shores and the circumstances under which they come' (see www.australianpolitics.com/).

Alongside this is a narrative that refugees should adhere to the process set up by the UNHCR and host government, and should enter in an orderly 'queue' to be resettled. Such queue-jumping debates, however, deliberately distort the experiences of those fleeing persecution, and fail to acknowledge that for many there is simply no queue to join; that refugee camps which are intended to provide safety are often themselves the site of violent conflict and abuse;[3] and that waiting out time in camps may never produce the desired outcome of resettlement in a country of safety (Dauvergne, 2003).

The 'war on terror' unleashed after 11 September 2001 has reinforced suspicion, distrust and anxiety about migrants, refugees and asylum seekers, and somehow blended the victims and perpetrators of terror and violence. From Australia to Russia, the United Kingdom to South Africa, these trends have been harshly reinforced in recent years (Schuster, 2003; Salaita, 2005).

Charity, choice and response

Even following resettlement, the ongoing process of othering ensures that developing a sense of belonging is difficult and that the position of refugees *within* is tenuous. Definitions of community may expand and contract; acceptance may remain conditional on favourable local and global circumstances (Jenkins, 2004). Following the London bombings and the race riots on Sydney beaches, we see the boundaries of community redrawn – resettled refugees, asylum seekers and other minority ethnic groups, including many who were born and raised in the UK or Australia respectively, are effectively placed on the outside, away from the integral 'core of the community'.

Where communities have come to see the granting of asylum and safe haven as an act of charity rather than an obligation under international law (Pickering, 2001), forced migrants may be especially marginalised. Heightened pressure on refugees to convey gratitude for the generosity of receiving countries is problematic. Refugees are, by definition, victims of adversity. However, 'the fact that they are not inevitably poor, nor as pure or grateful as their hosts might wish, can be a source of difficulty' (Beiser, 1999: 170). This becomes apparent where refugees dare to assert their rights, to question or contest their treatment, to articulate different rules of engagement. Public criticism, acts of dissent or protest are all seen as indications of a less than genuine claim. Here, the othering that occurs through a dialogue of charity and hospitality traps the refugees and effectively silences them.

In a health context this is a central barrier in calling for adequate, appropriate and accessible services. Difficulties arise where refugees or their supporters call for specialised services. The training of health professionals and bilingual health workers and translators are seen as luxuries and privileges, in addition to the 'charity' already extended by the host community. The 'right to health' is sidelined in an argument about the ungrateful nature of the refugee and suspicions are then raised about the motivations for claiming asylum (see

Box 25.3). The logic then follows that denying access to services such as health may act as a deterrent to 'would-be asylum seekers'.

Box 25.3   Choice

A poll taken in 2003 asked respondents to select reasons they thought asylum seekers came to Britain. Only 50 per cent chose among their answers, 'because they have been persecuted in their home countries', while 44 per cent believed they came 'because they will have free access to health services', and 45 per cent because 'they want to live off social security payments' (http://www.mori.com/polls/2003/migration.shtml).

Forced migrants are, in fact, rarely in a position to weigh up the potential health facilities and services available in destination states, yet many wealthy countries have reduced access to health care in an effort to present themselves as an unattractive option to those seeking asylum. Despite increased health needs, the UK has introduced a 'fee for service' policy for 'failed asylum seekers', that is those who have applied for but failed to obtain refugee status. This policy raises concerns about basic health care becoming inaccessible, and the arbitrary determination of the right to access ultimately impinging on the ability of asylum seekers, refugees and other settled minority groups to access health care even when entitled to do so (Hargreaves et al., 2005). In Australia, restricting access to health services and introducing complicated procedures for processing protection visas has resulted in refugees spending months and sometimes years in the community without undergoing any basic health screening (Smith, 2001), thus reducing opportunities to treat communicable diseases and other health problems.

Overload

One of the difficulties facing refugees in developed countries is a public perception of 'overload' in relation to immigration numbers in general and refugees in particular (Tazreiter, 2003). These perceptions are perpetuated by sensationalist media which stimulate anxieties of being burdened by unmanageable floods of refugees. The reality, however, is that developing countries have absorbed by far the greatest responsibility for processing and accommodating refugees, and often apply broader and more generous definitions in the assessment of their needs (Lubbers, 2002).[4]

Granting temporary or conditional protection reinforces perceptions that *we* can only offer the bare minimum in terms of assistance, that developed countries have capacity to assist only over the short term, and that the full resettlement of refugees (and their families) is too great a burden to bear. This defies the spirit of the Refugee Convention, conflicts with the stated aim of the UNHCR to find durable solutions for those who have fled persecution, and paradoxically may result in a greater dependency and demand on social services and welfare systems (see Lynn, 2002, for discussion of this in the US context).

Box 25.4   Overload

The reality is that demand for refugee status is often overstated. Refugee numbers world-wide appear to have stabilised and the pressure to search for third countries willing to resettle large numbers of refugees has been moderated: in 2004, the numbers of refugees seeking asylum in industrialised countries declined for the third consecutive year and reached its lowest level in 16 years (UNHCR, 2005b).

In constructing refugees as the other, the crisis of competition for local resources is more easily developed – *they want* what *we have*. In the public mind, what is at stake is access to the National Health Service, beds in hospitals, pressure on waiting lists and so forth.

Public health and othering

Why does othering matter so much? Why should we be concerned with the way forced migrants are described and represented? What are the consequences of this discourse, and how might the public health movement respond?

Public health has an ethos of working with communities to promote health gain. Public health has been described as 'ultimately and essentially an ethical enterprise committed to the notion that all people are entitled to protection against the hazards of this world and to the minimization of death and disability in society' (Beauchamp, 1976: 13). It embodies a commitment to social justice (Levy and Sidel, 2006). Beaglehole et al. (2004: 2084) have defined public health as 'collective action for sustained population-wide health improvement'. This recognises the importance of addressing structural impediments to health, of identifying the determinants of ill health, ensuring access to services, addressing inequalities, and developing population-wide interventions. Working with marginalised groups to ensure inclusion, access and influence are core, as is advocating with and articulating the rights of disempowered communities.

There are compelling ethical and public health reasons to challenge the othering of forced migrants. Governments may seek to avoid their international responsibilities to protect those who are persecuted and displaced. This is made possible by a public that sees refugees and asylum seekers as a dehumanised threat, outside the boundaries of belonging and without legitimate claims to entitlements. Othering affects the way we think and respond to refugee issues. It distances and separates, prompts communities to act from a position of defence and reduces the complexity of forced migration and forced migrants to simple dichotomies: legal–illegal, genuine–fraudulent, deserving–abusive, needy–autonomous, helpless–independent (Hardy and Phillips, 1999). It encourages 'us' to see their needs as separate, and in conflict with 'ours'. That the language and rationale of public health have been co-opted to such othering discourse requires a direct response and must be countered. Where fears of infection and disease are raised in support of restrictive refugee policies or detention of asylum seekers, public health practitioners must send a clear and consistent message, that refugees and asylum seekers *do not* in themselves present a health risk to communities. They must debunk myths about overloading and overwhelming health services, and provide a human context to the refugee situations, to the reality of conflict, displacement, camp life and the journeys and motivations of those who seek protection in developed countries.

Box 25.5   Public health consequences of othering

Othering affects interactions with health services in multiple ways:

- Access to health services: reduced by a lack of availability, cost, language and cultural barriers.
- Utilisation of services: limited because they are deemed inappropriate, untrust-worthy, or in some other respect unsafe.
- Disclosure to health workers: even when services are used, disclosure is under-mined by distrust and suspicion, especially where health workers are seen as part of the state's mechanisms of exclusion, through their relationship with other authorities or in screening and refugee-status determination processes.
- Presentation to services: delayed, late or absent as a result of fear, anxiety and lack of knowledge of how to access services.
- Health promotion and uptake of preventive health services: marginalised com-munities and individuals within communities are poorly reached by mainstream health messages and may find it difficult to engage in health promotion activities.

The public health community must also recognise that othering carries a 'real risk of the creation of vulnerable, marginalised under classes' (Allotey and Zwi, 2006, in press), with very real consequences for population health. History has demonstrated that othering, whether based on disability, gender, health status or ethnicity, has negative consequences for access to, and delivery of, health services (see, for example, Kitchin, 1998; Phillips and Drevdahl, 2003; Johnson et al., 2004; Kang et al., 2003). Public health need look no further than the lessons learned from dealing with the emergence of HIV/AIDS to recall how socially excluded groups, from gay and bisexual men, to sex workers and injecting drug users, were placed at heightened health risk by their social marginalisation.

In response to policies which seek to limit services available to forced migrants, public health must reiterate that there is no health benefit in denying care to refugees and asylum seekers. Restricting access to health services, or establishing conditions which result in reduced uptake of services, does not protect the broader community. Rather, if refugees do not receive appropriate and timely health care, then this may indeed place the wider community at risk over time – the 'burden' on the health system that such policies seek to prevent. Othering also promotes dis-ease, anxiety and stress, feeding into adverse psychosocial outcomes and a greater need for services in the long term.

Public health must apply the lessons learned from other marginalised and excluded minority groups – what is good for the individual (access to and utilisation of health services) is good for the public's health. This is most obvious in relation to infectious disease, but is equally true for early detection and intervention of chronic conditions and mental health concerns.

In the context of refugees and asylum seekers, public health can ensure that services are sensitive and responsive to needs, and play a role in conveying a sense of understanding, sensitivity and respect for the experiences, fears and desires of forced migrants.

Key points of action (see Box 25.6) include advocating for a comprehensive range of health services to be made available to all forced migrants during and following the determination of their status as refugees, and improving responsiveness of services and resourcing transcultural health research to inform better practice (Ekblad, 2004). Better integration of health and community services and improved continuity of care and referral will enhance outcomes. Health services require key infrastructure which includes the support of interpreting and translating services, outreach workers, and targeted prevention and health promotion programmes. Providing client-held records, developing gender and culturally sensitive programmes and interventions, and encouraging general practitioners to play a greater role in providing long-term health care to refugees and asylum seekers will also be of value (Coker, 2004). Educating medical and public health professionals to grapple with complex, global issues, such as population displacement, will help students to see their responsibilities as extending beyond their own local communities into advocacy and activist roles (Davidson et al., 2004).

Box 25.6   Public health responses to othering

- Upstream interventions to reduce poverty and social injustice.
- Advocacy to oppose othering and narratives which exclude and marginalise.
- Enhanced policy, programme and service responsiveness to needs of particular migrant communities.
- Integration of health promotion with caring services; health services with social welfare and education.
- Cultural and language sensitivity within service provision and communication strategies.
- Better training of health workers to appreciate the context from which migrants come and into which they have settled.
- Support for strengthening migrant community organisations and advocacy activities.

Conclusion

This chapter calls on public health practitioners to respond to the othering of forced migrants by putting forward a counter-narrative and discourse of inclusion and caring, of recognition of the complexities of the contexts out of which forced migrants come, and of the challenges they face in securing protection. It argues for public health to return to its social activism origins in an effort to promote social justice, critique the inadequacies of current policies and systems, and seek more inclusive means of promoting rights, responsibilities and community. Finally, it reminds health practitioners of one of the core lessons learned in working with vulnerable groups – that respect for human rights at an individual level is key to effective public health at a population level. It is not us against them; we are not separate, distant, different; *they* are not *the* other. Rather, we are intimately connected and interdependent. This is highlighted by the fact that what is good practice in refugee health is good community health for all.

Notes

1   It should be noted that the vast majority of involuntary migration involves the displacement of people within, rather than across, borders. The UNHCR recorded 7.6 million 'persons of concern', internally displaced (IDPs) and stateless persons, at the end of 2004, but recognised this as likely to significantly underestimate the problem (UNHCR, 2005a). Furthermore, of those that do manage to flee their country, around 90 per cent will remain within the same region and it is a very small minority who eventually settle in developed countries. How this small minority of forced migrants are received in rich, western nations is the focus of this chapter.

2   Under Article 14 of the Universal Declaration of Human Rights, everyone has the right to seek and enjoy asylum, while Article 31.1 of the 1951 Convention Relating to the Status of Refugees states that countries should not impose penalties on individuals coming directly from a territory where their life or freedom is threatened on account of their illegal entry.

3   The precarious existence of refugees, even after they have escaped the initial violent conflict, is increasingly recognised. The establishment of categories such as Women at Risk acknowledge the high rates of abuse, rape and exploitation that women, and particularly unaccompanied women refugees, suffer.

4   However, this hospitality is not unmarred by resistance from nationals of host countries (Adepoju, 2002). See Crisp (2003) for a discussion of developing countries' declining commitment to asylum, the 'increasingly hostile reception accorded to refugees in developing regions', and possible explanations for this.

References

Adepoju, A. (2002) Fostering free movement of persons in West Africa: achievements, constraints, and prospects for intraregional migration. *International Migration*, 40: 3–28.

Allotey, P. and Zwi, A. (2006, in press) Population movements. In Kawachi, I. and Wamala, S. (eds), *Globalization and Health: Challenges and Prospects*. New York: Oxford University Press.

Beaglehole, R., Bonita, R., Horton, R., Adams, O. and McKee, M. (2004) Public health in the new era: improving health through collective action. *Lancet*, 363: 2084–6.

Beauchamp, D.E. (1976) Public health as social justice. *Journal of Inquiry*, XII: 3–13. Quoted in Levy, B.S. and Sidel, V.W. (2006) The nature of social injustice and its impact on public health. In Levy, B.S. and Sidel, V.W. (eds), *Social Injustice and Public Health*. New York: Oxford University Press, pp. 5–21.

Beiser, M. (1999) *Strangers at the Gate: the 'Boat People's' First Ten Years in Canada*. Toronto: University of Toronto Press.

Coker, M. (2004) Asylum seekers and refugees in the United Kingdom. In Healy, J. and McKee, M. (eds), *Accessing Health Care: Responding to Diversity*. Oxford: Oxford University Press, pp. 183–206.

Crisp, J. (2003) Refugees and the global politics of asylum. *The Political Quarterly*, 74 (1): 75–87.

Dauvergne, C. (2003) Challenges to sovereignty; migration laws for the 21st century. *New Issues in Refugee Research, Working Paper No. 92*. Geneva: UNHCR Evaluation and Policy Analysis Unit.

Davidson, N., Skull, S., Burgner, D., Kelly, P., Raman, S., Steel, Z., Vora, R. and Smith, M. (2004) An issue of access: delivering equitable health care for newly arrived refugee children in Australia. *Journal of Paediatrics and Child Health*, 40: 569–75.

Ekblad, S. (2004) Migrants: universal health services in Sweden. In Healy, J. and McKee, M. (eds), *Accessing Health Care: Responding to Diversity*. Oxford: Oxford University Press.

Gibney, M. (2000) Outside the protection of the law: the situation of irregular migrants in Europe. *Refugee Studies Working Paper No. 6*. Oxford: Oxford University Press.

Grove, N. and Zwi, A. (2006, in press) *Our* health and *theirs*: forced migration, othering and public health. *Social Science and Medicine*, available online on 19 October, 2005, http://www.science direct.com/science/journal/02779536.

Hardy, C. and Phillips, N. (1999) No joking matter: discursive struggle in the Canadian refugee system. *Organization Studies*, 20: 1–24.

Hargreaves, S., Holmes, A. and Friedland, J. (2005) Charging failed asylum seekers for health care in the UK. Lancet, 365: 732–3.

Jenkins, F. (2004) Bare life: asylum-seekers, Australian politics and Agamben's critique of violence. *Australian Journal of Human Rights*, 10 (1): 79–95.

Johnson, J., Bottorff, J., Browne, A., Grewal, S., Hilton, B. and Clarke, H. (2004) Othering and being othered in the context of health care services. *Health Communication*, 16 (2): 255–71.

Kang, E., Rapkin, B., Springer, C. and Haejin Kim, J. (2003) The 'Demon Plague' and access to care among Asian undocumented immigrants living with HIV disease in New York City. *Journal of Immigrant Health*, 5 (2): 49–58.

Kitchin, R. (1998) 'Out of place', 'knowing one's place': space, power and the exclusion of disabled people. *Disability and Society*, 13 (3): 343–56.

Koutroulis, G. (2003) Detained asylum seekers, health care and questions of human(e)ness. *Australian and New Zealand Journal of Public Health*. 27 (4): 381–4.

Levy, B.S. and Sidel, V.W. (eds) (2006) *Social Injustice and Public Health*. New York: Oxford University Press.

Licata, L. and Klein, O. (2002) Does European citizenship breed xenophobia? European identification as a predictor of intolerance towards immigrants. *Journal of Community and Applied Social Psychology*, 12: 323–37.

Lubbers, R. (2002) Asylum for all: refugee protection in the 21st century. *Harvard International Review*, 24 (1): 60–5.

Lynn, D. (2002) Forging creative partnerships: the alliance of public health and public safety among immigrant populations. *Policy Studies Journal*, 30: 132–46.

Phillips, D. and Drevdahl, D. (2003) 'Race' and the difficulties of language. *Advances in Nursing Science*, 26 (1): 17–29.

Pickering, S. (2001) Common sense and original deviancy: new discourses and asylum seekers in Australia. *Journal of Refugee Studies*, 14 (2): 169–86.

Prem Kumer, R. and Grundy-Warr, C. (2004) The irregular migrant as Homo Sacer: migration and detention in Australia, Malaysia and Thailand. *International Migration*, 42 (1): 33–64.

Pugh, M. (2004) Drowning not waving: boat people and humanitarianism at sea. *Journal of Refugee Studies*, 17 (1): 50–69.

Salaita, S. (2005) Ethnic identity and imperative patriotism: Arab Americans before and after 9/11. *College Literature*, 32: 146–68.

Sathanapally, A. (2004). *Asylum Seekers, Ordinary Australians and Human Rights*. Working Paper 2004/3. Sydney: Australian Human Rights Centre, University of New South Wales.

Schuster, L. (2003) Common sense or racism? The treatment of asylum-seekers in Europe. *Patterns of Prejudice*, 37: 233–55.

Smith, M. (2001) Asylum seekers in Australia. *Medical Journal of Australia*, 175: 587–9.

Tazreiter, C. (2003) *Asylum-seekers as Pariahs in the Australian State: Security against the Few.* WIDER Discussion Paper No. 2003/19. Helsinki: United Nations University.

Turton, D. (2003) Refugees, forced resettlers and 'other forced migrants': towards a unitary study of forced migration. *New Issues in Refugee Research, Working Paper No. 94.* Geneva: UNHCR Evaluation and Policy Analysis Unit.

UNHCR (2005a) *2004 Global Refugee Trends.* Geneva: UNHCR Division of Operational Support.

UNHCR (2005b) *UNCHR Press Release: Asylum Claims Fall to Lowest Level since 1998*, 1 March 2005, http://www.unchr.ch/cgibin/texis/vtx/home/opendoc.htm?tbl=NEWS&id=4224411d4& page=news (accessed 30 March 2005).

Van der Veer, K. (2003) The future of western societies: multicultural identity or extreme nationalism? *Futures*, 35: 169–87.

Weis, L. (1995) Identity formation and the process of 'othering': unravelling sexual threads. *Educational Foundations*, 9: 17–33.

Part V
Promoting Public Health at a Local Level

Introduction

Stephen Handsley

With its commitment to tackling and reducing health inequalities, the thrust of the English Government's White Paper, *Choosing Health: Making Healthier Choices Easier*, is on improving the determinants of poor health such as housing and the local environment, and improvements in health care and prevention services. To achieve this, it sees local communities as the catalyst for action and change, with local authorities working alongside local communities, business and voluntary groups to promote public health. This echoes the view of the World Health Organisation (WHO) which, similarly, has called for an investment in people and communities as the most effective way of tackling health inequalities and promoting healthier lifestyles.

Part V of the Reader contains chapters focusing both on the practice and process of multidisciplinary public health at a local level. Its primary focus is on the potential of participatory and community action approaches to promoting public health. However, Part V is also concerned with the implementation and effectiveness of these approaches and the ways in which community-based health interventions are assessed and evaluated.

In Chapter 26, Gunjit Bandesha and A. Litva use a locally based Asian Health Development Project (AHDP) to unpick and unpack the concept of community participation in health. Highlighting the challenges faced by a range of stakeholders involved in community-based health projects, they explore both the benefits of and barriers to participation and discuss some of the problems associated with converting the rhetoric of community participation in health into reality.

By their very nature, efforts to practise and promote public health at a local level call for an appreciation and understanding of the settings approach. Indeed, settings have become an important cornerstone for successful multidisciplinary public health as healthy interventions and initiatives seek to be responsive to local needs and living circumstances of potential beneficiaries as outlined in the 1986 *Ottawa Charter*. Using prisons as an example of a healthy setting, in Chapter 27 Michelle Baybutt, Paul Hayton and Mark Dooris explore the public health possibilities and opportunities offered by health-promoting prisons in England and Wales. Discussing the reform and modernisation of prison health services in England and Wales, they outline some of the contextual issues and highlight key health concerns; introduce the concept, principles and practice of health-promoting prisons at international, national and regional levels; and explore key challenges and opportunities.

Developing healthy communties involves first recognising the social and cultural dynamics which embody context-specific networks that people and institutions use to achieve their goals. In short, working out what makes communities tick? For some, social capital is an important ingredient in this endeavour. In Chapter 28, Andy Gibson first unpacks the concept of social capital before moving on to discuss its links with health inequalities. He then goes on to explore the way in which a deeper understanding of social capital is essential for those working in multidisciplinary public health, both at policy and at the practical level.

In the same way that an understanding of social capital is integral to community-based multidisciplinary public health in the 21st century, an appreciation of evaluation and assessment are of equal importance in the practice and process of promoting public health at a local level. In Chapter 29, Paul Bridgen discusses some of the problems involved in evaluating community empowerment. Using policy development in the UK since 1997 as a case study, he seeks to delineate the concept of community empowerment from other community-based approaches to health improvement and suggests that the urban political science literature provides some useful insights with regard to the operationalisation of community empowerment in process-focused evaluative research.

On a similar theme, in Chapter 30 Maurice Mittelmark suggests that, for healthy policy-making at a local level to be a success, it must be accompanied by a rigorous and robust process of health impact assessment. For Mittelmark, this process involves harnessing the participatory capacity of communities and integrating them with public health practitioners and policy-makers in a mutual attempt to identify negative health impacts while addressing health inequalities.

While promoting public health at a local level is all about addressing many of the social, environmental and physical factors which lead to health inequalities, concern for mental health is undoubtedly of equal importance. In the final chapter of this section, Lynne Friedli explores some of the issues involved, not only in promoting mental health but also in changing people's perceptions of mental health. The chapter argues for a radical transformation in the way we think about mental health and suggests that what is required is a major shift in focus from prevalence of psychiatric morbidity to one which measures the mental health and well-being of populations. Such a shift will, Friedli concludes, create new opportunities to consider the mental health impact of social and economic policy and to add a new dimension to political debate about the future direction of society in the UK, Europe and beyond.

Chapter 26

Perceptions of Community Participation and Health Gain in a Community Project for the South Asian Population: a Qualitative Study

Gunjit Bandesha and A. Litva

Introduction

The concept of community participation in health first appeared over three decades ago in the developing world as part of a movement for social justice.[1] It was envisaged that basic health needs could be met more appropriately and efficiently by the greater involvement of people themselves.[2] Community empowerment is considered central to the process of participation, enabling people to have a greater say and more control over their own lives and local health-care decisions. In working with marginalized communities, community participation could reduce health inequalities and improve equity.[3] In 1991, the World Health Organization[4] summarized the benefits of participation:

1   coverage – involves more people than non-participatory projects;
2   efficiency – promotes better co-ordination of resources;
3   effectiveness – goals and strategies are more relevant as a result of participation;
4   equity – promotes a notion of providing for those in greatest need;
5   self reliance – increases people's control over their own lives.

Edited from: Bandesha, Gunjit and Litva, A. (2005) Perceptions of community participation and health gain in a community project for the South Asia population: a qualitative study, *Journal of Public Health* 27 (3): 241–5. By permission of Oxford University Press, on behalf of Faculty of Public Health.

Primary Care Trusts (PCTs) in England are challenged with converting the rhetoric of community participation in health into reality, [5] yet the precise nature of participation remains elusive and little is known of the actual benefits of participation.[1, 6] As PCTs move from policy to implementation, local understanding of the concepts of participation and its associated health gain need to be explored *in situ* in order to ensure that rhetoric can translate into reality.

The Asian Health Development Project (AHDP) was set up in a small town in Greater Manchester to access and respond to the health needs of the local South Asian community. A 'community participation' approach was used to achieve 'potential health gain'. A number of initiatives were used to engage the community, including training programmes on health and health services, a diabetes awareness project with cookery classes, first aid courses and exercise classes. Many professionals from the PCT, Hospital Trust and the local authority were involved in these initiatives. This chapter presents the findings of a study that explored the perceptions of participation and its associated health gain among lay and professional stakeholders of the AHDP.

Methods

Semi-structured interviews were conducted with 13 professional stakeholders who had been involved in the project (project workers, managers, nurses, dieticians), exploring their perceptions of participation and health gain in the project. A non-probabilistic maximum variation sampling strategy was used to provide multiple perspectives. Interviews were conducted by G.B. and lasted between 60 and 90 minutes. Questions were adapted to each interview but concentrated on the nature and extent of participation by the local community and the health benefits the community had gained as a result of the project.

Three focus groups were conducted with each of the subgroups of the local South Asian community (Indian, $n = 5$; Pakistani, $n = 5$; and Bangladeshi, $n = 4$), exploring perceptions of participation and health gain in the project. All the participants were female (reflecting the gender of the majority of the participants of the project) and ranged in age from 25 to 46 years. The average length of focus groups was 90 minutes. To validate emerging themes from the focus groups, four in-depth interviews were conducted with lay informants using an opportunistic sampling strategy.

All interviews and focus groups were audio-taped and transcribed verbatim. Analysis was carried out using a content analysis for emerging themes based on Denzin's Interpretive Interactionism framework.[7] Emerging themes were grouped into categories and are reported below.

Results

Perceptions of participation: partner or problem?

Lay participants felt they had no control over the project or its resources and considered themselves as recipients of the project's work rather than active shapers or partners in the process. This is illustrated by one Pakistani lay informant:

It's not up to us to decide what the project does ... we aren't involved like that ... we just wait to see what they put on.

In contrast, professionals frequently described the project as a partnership, but made little reference to the distribution of power in the project.

Barriers to participation: engaging the community

Lay participants recognized that many people did not want to, nor had the time to, participate in the project. Once again, this is neatly illustrated in this quote from a Pakistani lay informant:

They have the children to look after, the cooking, the cleaning ... they don't want to go and some of them say they're too old to go.

The project was not considered a priority compared with the other problems families had to deal with. Professionals too spoke of the difficulty they had in getting people to attend events associated with the project. Professional F:

It's hard to get people to come to these sort of things ... but it was like a Saturday morning and the project was good, but it just didn't attract the numbers.

The project failed to engage the most deprived Bangladeshi section of the community and was seen by some as widening inequity in the local South Asian population.

Barriers to participation: engaging health professionals

Engaging health professionals was seen as equally problematic. Professionals admitted the project had been unsuccessful in involving local GPs over its 5-year duration, mainly due to pressure of work. Professional C:

We have GPs who are over-stressed and under some pressure ... so they haven't got involved because they have their noses to the grindstone a lot of the time.

There were similar fears and uncertainty among professionals about methods that challenged traditional ways of working. Professional E:

It's always a power thing with GPs ... they don't want to be told what to do ... we had discussions with them at the project ... but it was always a question of this is peripheral, it's not something that's going to touch their day-to-day lives, so they could afford to ignore it.

Barriers to participation: language and cultural awareness

Some professionals expressed reservations that community participation was not possible without good interpreting services. Others viewed participation as an empowering process (not simply about getting health messages through) that could overcome language and cultural barriers. Lay informants agreed that non-English speakers were less likely to participate in community projects. However, according to Professional D:

> Language is not a barrier to people participating ... with mother-tongue support, people are glad their language is spoken and therefore think information is accessible and are therefore able to participate.

Lay informants, however, were frustrated by the lack of cultural awareness and sensitivity in the project. Others felt that some health professionals held stereotypical views of Asian women and made assumptions about beliefs and behaviour, as illustrated by one Pakistani lay informant:

> They see you in your own clothes with your head covered and think she can't speak English ... by just looking at you, you can see their attitude changes ... and when you open your mouth and can speak English ... they say, 'Oh, you can speak English' and they're really surprised.

Barriers to participation: time and resources

Professionals working to short deadlines and used to more immediate results felt frustrated at the slow pace of change in participation projects. Others recognized that slow, steady progress was the only way to ensure reliable and sustainable results and to avoid 'quick fixes' that were not relevant. There was consensus among health professionals that community participation was not a cheap option and considerable resources were required by projects to achieve their potential and demonstrate cost-effectiveness. According to Professional I:

> You have got to have recurrent funding ... you are competing with a lot of other priorities, so you have got to have a clearer idea about what your outcomes are and be able to show them.

Benefits of participation: a more informed population

There was agreement between lay and professional informants that the project had raised awareness on health issues and services and created a more informed population. Community members felt they had learned a lot and some had moved on to further training and employment opportunities:

> I think we have all learned a lot you know ... about first aid and diabetes and that ... and that might help you to get a good job in the future ... you never know. (Pakistani lay informant)

> I feel I know my rights now ... I know what the services are supposed to do and I won't be afraid in asking for it. (Indian lay informant)

Health impact of project: psychological benefits

Lay informants felt more confident through participating in the project while professional informants felt that the project had raised the self-esteem of those who participated. Confidence was perceived to have improved through gaining knowledge and skills and making new friends:

> I did this course, just six weeks, but it gave me [an] idea [of] how to handle six children in crèche ... so that has given me more confidence ... plus all courses have given me strength and build my confidence inside ... I learn something new. (Indian lay informant)

Health impact of the project: social cohesion

Professional informants believed participation in the project had enhanced the sense of social cohesion in the community. Professional L:

> We have got evidence of very much more increased participation in the regeneration agenda from minority ethnic communities ... we are getting at least a quarter of people from ethnic communities, which in the beginning we might have only got one or two people coming.

This was seen to have been achieved by greater engagement of the South Asian community in regeneration initiatives and neighbourhood forums. Lay informants had made new friends on the project, but did not feel the project had made any difference to the community at large or improved community cohesion in any way:

> Most of the women in our community don't come to the project ... I don't think the community really notices any difference because of the project. People just carry on with their lives, like before. (Indian lay informant)

Health impact of the project: lifestyle changes

There was disagreement between lay and professional informants as to whether the project had resulted in any lifestyle changes among participants. Some professional informants were optimistic about the project's impact, while others recognized the project's limitations in affecting the broader social determinants of health. Lay informants did not make the link between health knowledge gained and changes in lifestyle:

> Our people do eat unhealthy you know ... too much oil and sweet things and that ... but the project can't do anything about that ... people can't change their habits. (Pakistani lay informant)

Healthy living ideas from the project were difficult to put into practice and often met with resistance from other family members:

> We all know oil and salt is bad for us, but we still do it, don't we. My husband likes the oil to be seen on the plate and if he can't see it, he'll say what have you done? (Bangladeshi lay informant)

Health impact of the project: better use of health services

Some professional informants felt the local population were more appropriate users of services as a result of the project. However, the project was perceived to have had little influence over local service providers and the allocation of resources:

> I wouldn't say the project has got to the stage where you could show changes in the direction of resources or services, as a result of involvement of South Asian people. (Professional K)

The project was considered to have failed in its remit to influence local service providers.

Discussion

This study used qualitative methods to explore the views of lay and professional informants. It suggests that there are important differences in perceptions of participation and its associated health gain. There are fundamental differences in the understanding of the term 'partnership with the community'. Lay informants did not consider the AHDP as a partnership. The equal nature of partnerships with the community is contested in the literature,[8] with unrealistic expectations leading to disillusionment and frustration. The issue of power is considered central to the process of participation,[9] but professionals tend not to have to account for the weight they attach to local views.[10] The 'I plan, you participate'[11] philosophy may lead to failure in local participation projects.

Engaging communities can be problematic and deprived communities may not be willing participants, particularly if the benefits of projects are not apparent and tangible. The Bangladeshi community, which is the most deprived in the area, participated the least in the project. Cultural insensitivity may hamper projects with the South Asian Community, but the heterogeneous needs of the South Asian community need to be acknowledged to ensure participation projects do not exacerbate inequalities. Campbell and McLean.[12] warned that expressed ethnic allegiance does not mean people will have common needs and interests that will unite them in local health initiatives. Madan[13] suggests that participating communities are 'made, not born' and the project needs to rethink its strategy for engaging all sections of the community.

Previous studies have shown professional uncertainty and an inability to relinquish power can also hinder participation projects.[14,9] Health-care professionals who are taught little on empowering and emancipatory approaches may find it difficult to participate themselves and enable participation from the public. Training in participatory education for professionals may address lay concerns about communication issues and enhance participation by professionals.

Lay informants perceived health gain on an individual level in terms of knowledge gained and confidence achieved. Self-confidence and self-esteem are developed through the participation process[15] and the project appears to have been successful in this area. However, there is no necessary link between knowledge gained and behaviour change. The project did not result in any socio-environmental changes, having relied more on an educational approach, rather than a community-development approach. Consequently, lay informants did not admit to any lifestyle changes.

There was disagreement as to whether empowerment at an individual level had transmitted to health gain at a community level. Strong social networks[16] are thought to create healthier conditions, particularly among poorer communities, but there was disagreement amongst lay and professional informants as to whether the project had improved social cohesion in the local community. The notion of community is contested in the literature and studies show that implicit assumptions regarding sharing are often not held out in practice.[17] The local South Asian community is culturally diverse and geographically scattered and professional notions of increased social cohesion require further exploration.

Appropriate and accessible health services impact on health gain, but the project was perceived to have had little influence on local services. There was little change within statutory organizations as a result of the project. Partnership models in some community initiatives may represent mediation of continued disadvantage, because they tend to be based on relationships of unequal power and allow statutory organizations to assume that projects will manage minority ethnic issues without any need for internal change themselves.[18]

The weaknesses of this study included the limited access to the local population, which determined the opportunistic sampling strategy used for the focus groups. Although our results suggest that the views of the subsections of the community were consistent with one another, our small sample size may have limited access to a variety of opinions, reflecting the heterogeneous nature of the South Asian community. Key themes were identified and supported by the literature, which improves the generalizability of the results to other settings.

The allure of community participation has captured the attention of policy-makers in the UK with its promise of improvements in public health. However, the strategy, which was initially thought to be common sense and straightforward, is increasingly recognized as being quite complex.[10] This study uncovers issues of misunderstanding and conflict in one participation project. However, further systematic approaches are required to evaluate the policy *in situ* and demonstrate accountability for scarce health service resources.

References

1   Macauley, A.C., Commanda, L.E., Gibson, N., McCabe, L., Robbins, M. Twohig, L. Participatory research maximises community and lay involvement. *British Medical Journal*, 319: 774–778.

2   Zakus, J.D., Lysack C.L. (1998) Revisiting community participation. *Health Policy Plan*, 13: 1–12.

3   Billings (2000) Community development: a critical review of approaches to evaluation. *Journal of Advanced Nursing*, 31: 472–480.

4   World Health Organization (1991) *Community Involvement in health development: Challenging Health Services*. Geneva: WHO.

5   Department of Health (2002) *National Health Service and Health Care Professions Act*. London: HMSO.

6   Rifkin, S.B., Lewando-Hundt, G. and, Draper, A.K. (2000) *Participatory Approaches in Health Promotion and Health Planning. A literature review*. London: Health Development Agency.

7   Denzin, N.K. (1989) *Interpretive interactionism*. Newbury Park, CA: Sage.

8   Heenan, D. (2004) A partnership approach to health promotion: a case study from Northern Ireland. *Health Promotion International*, 19: 105–113.

9 Dockery, G. (1996) Rhetoric or reality: participatory research in the National Health Service in the UK. In Koning, K., Martin, M. (eds), *Participatory Research in Health*. London: Zed Books.

10 Milewa, T. (1997) Community participation and health care priorities: reflections on policy, theatre and reality in Britain. *Health Promotion International*, 12: 161–168.

11 Lahiri-Dutt, K. (2004) 'I plan, you participate': a southern view of community participation in urban Australia. *Community Development Journal*, 39: 13–27.

12 Campbell, C., McLean, C. (2003) Social capital, local community participation and the construction of Pakistani identities in England: implications for health inequalities policies. *Journal of Health Psychology*, 8: 247–262.

13 Madan, T.N. (1987) Community involvement in health policy, sociostructural and dynamic aspects of health beliefs. *Social Science and Medicine*, 25: 615–620.

14 Nicher, M. (1986) The primary health centre as a social system, PHC, social status and the issue of teamwork in South Asia. *Social Science and Medicine*, 23: 347–355.

15 Freeman, R., Gillam, S., Shearin, C., Pratt, J. (1997) *Community development and involvement in primary care*. London: King's Fund.

16 Wallace, S. (1993) Evaluation of the BBC/HEA Health Show. *Health Education Journal*, 52: (4).

17 Jewkes, R., Murcott, A. (1996) Meanings of community. *Social Science and Medicine*, 43: 555–563.

18 Atkin, K., Rollings, J. (1993) *Community care in a multi-racial Britain: a critical review of the literature*. London: HMSO.

Chapter 27

Prisons in England and Wales: an Important Public Health Opportunity?

Michelle Baybutt, Paul Hayton and Mark Dooris

Introduction

During the last decade, the public health importance of prisons has increasingly been recognised both nationally and across Europe (Department of Health, 2002; Gatherer et al., 2005). This chapter explores the public health opportunities offered by prisons. It discusses the reform and modernisation of prison health services in England and Wales; outlines contextual issues and highlights key health concerns; introduces the concept, principles and practice of health-promoting prisons at international, national and regional levels; and explores key challenges and opportunities.

Background: reforming prison health in England and Wales

In 1996, a highly critical review of prison health care was published by HM Chief Inspector of Prisons for England and Wales (1996). This found services – then operated by Her Majesty's (HM) Prison Service, largely independently of the National Health Service (NHS) – to be isolated, reactive, inefficient and dominated by a medical model of health, with inadequately qualified staff experiencing low morale, poor communications and lacking appropriate professional training and development. As a result, there were huge variations in standards of care across the prison estate, with prisoners' health needs not being properly assessed or met, and public health opportunities not being exploited. The report proposed a radical overhaul, with responsibility for prison health care moving from the Prison Service to the NHS.

The subsequent publication of *The Future Organisation of Prison Health Care* (Joint Prison Service and National Health Service Executive Working Group, 1999) paved the way for rapid reform and modernisation. In 2000, responsibility for health policy development and standards transferred from HM Prison Service (an Agency located within the Home Office division of government) to the Department of Health, and in 2003, funding for prison health services followed. Whereas previously, only secondary and specialist prison health care was the responsibility of the NHS, since 2006, all health services within HM prisons are commissioned by the NHS.

The prison health reforms have been characterised by a commitment to *partnership* and *equivalence*. While funding and responsibility for commissioning and ensuring delivery of services has shifted to the NHS, local-level partnerships have been established between prisons and Primary Care Trusts (PCTs) to oversee needs assessment and joint planning of services. Nationally, the Head of Prison Health has relocated from the Prison Service to the Department of Health, but has remained a member of the Prison Service Management Board reporting to government ministers in both the Department of Health and the Home Office. This approach has encouraged PCTs to recognise prisoners as part of their local community, with the underlying objective of providing services based on assessed need and at least broadly equivalent to those for other citizens.

In implementing the reforms, a number of challenges have been evident. Organisationally, financially and culturally, the Prison Service and the NHS have faced different pressures and experienced conflicting priorities (e.g. between the goals of imprisonment and the aims of health care in an intrinsically non-therapeutic environment). Furthermore, negative public perceptions of prisons and prisoners have provided the additional challenge of justifying the provision of equivalent health care services to a group of the population widely deemed 'unworthy'. Prisons (as closed institutions) have little experience of working with external health providers, while the NHS has little experience of commissioning primary care in the prison setting and limited understanding of the wider issues associated with working in the offender management system – and the uncertainty and insecurity experienced by many NHS staff during reorganisation (Department of Health, 2001) has only added to the complexity of mainstreaming prison health. In addition, the lack of reliable local data on prison health needs has provided a challenge to local prison/PCT partnerships to develop improved quality and outcome measures, and to better align prison health with national standards and targets.

Prison health in England and Wales: current context and issues

The prison population

In general, prisons in England and Wales are overcrowded and experience a high turnover. Important points to note are that:

- There are 139 prisons in England and Wales, varying in size from 145 to 1,500 prisoners and in security level from Category A (highest security risk) through to Category D (lowest security risk).

- HM Prison Service has a rapidly increasing prison population, currently standing at around 77,000. However, as many prisoners serve short sentences, there are probably twice that number actually passing through our prisons each year.
- The UK has the highest imprisonment rate in western Europe – 141 per 100,000, up from 90 per 100,000 in 1992.
- Approximately 12 per cent of prisoners are foreign.
- Around 17 per cent of prisoners are on remand (or unsentenced).
- There are 16,000 young people in prison under the age of 21 years of age, about 2,500 of whom are aged 15–17 and are therefore classed as children.
- 4,000 prisoners are women.
- Prisoners are far more likely than the general population to have grown up in care, poverty or an otherwise disadvantaged family; to have few educational qualifications and low basic skills; and to have poor mental and physical health.
- Linked to this – and in common with prisons across Europe – our prisons contain an over-representation of the most socially excluded members of society, including black and minority ethnic groups, injecting drug users, homeless people, commercial sex workers, people experiencing mental illness, and more generally people with untreated chronic conditions. (Social Exclusion Unit, 2002, 2004; HM Prison Service, 2006; International Centre for Prisons Studies, 2006)

It would be a mistake, however, to generalise too much across the prison population, as each prison presents its own particular health needs. The population in our prisons is in fact a real mix: over half of the adult male population is serving four years and over, and, of these, some 6,000 are serving life or indeterminate sentences. However, those serving shorter sentences – often six months or less – move through the system very quickly. The public health opportunities offered by prisons are clearly constrained by length of stay, and it is therefore of crucial importance that health needs analysis takes place at the local/PCT level. The reform of prison health care has encouraged PCTs to treat prisons as populations within their local community, so that plans can be tailored to meet local circumstances.

Key health concerns

In England and Wales, Prison Health's current objective is to improve the health of prisoners and tackle health inequalities by:

- improving the standard of prison health services through greater integration with the wider NHS;
- reducing or mitigating the effects of unhealthy or high-risk behaviours; and
- promoting effective links with health and related services in the community to improve throughcare. (Department of Health, HM Prison Service and Welsh Assembly Government, 2003: 3)

Reports from the Department of Health (2002) and Social Exclusion Unit (2002, 2004) identify a number of key health concerns for prisons, highlighting the enormous potential for promoting public health and tackling health inequalities:

- *Mental health*: 72 per cent of male and 70 per cent of female sentenced prisoners have two or more mental health disorders – 14 and 35 times the level in the general population respectively. Self-harm and suicide are serious problems: 20 per cent of male and 37 per cent of female sentenced prisoners have attempted suicide, and between 2002 and 2003 there were 105 suicides in prison.
- *Smoking*: 77 per cent of male and 82 per cent of female sentenced prisoners smoke.
- *HIV*: 0.3 per cent of male prisoners and 1.2 per cent of female prisoners are HIV positive.
- *Alcohol and drug use*: a large number of prisoners have a history of hazardous alcohol and drug use: 24 per cent have injected drugs and, of these, 20 per cent are infected with hepatitis B and 30 per cent with Hepatitis C.

Concept, principles and practice of health promoting prisons

Background

The provision of equivalent health services means that, as well as providing health care, prisons should also provide health education, patient education, prevention and other health promotion interventions to meet the assessed needs of the prison population. Furthermore, it is recognised that good health and well-being are central to successful rehabilitation and resettlement, and that this requires a prison environment that is supportive of health and a 'whole prison approach' that moves beyond a focus on health services (Department of Health, 2002).

The healthy settings approach

The concept and practice of 'healthy settings' have developed over the past 20 years to become a key element of public health strategy (Dooris, 2004). The settings approach has its roots within the World Health Organisation (WHO) Health for All strategy and, more specifically, within the *Ottawa Charter for Health Promotion* (WHO, 1986), which encouraged a move towards a more holistic model of health. With its five-fold focus on building healthy policy, creating supportive environments, strengthening community action, developing personal skills and reorienting services, the Charter stated that 'health is created and lived by people within the settings of their everyday life; where they learn, work, play and love'.

The WHO has defined 'settings for health' as 'the place or social context in which people engage in daily activities in which environmental, organisational and personal factors interact to affect health and well-being'. Adopting an ecological model of health, a systems perspective and a 'whole system' focus on organisation development and change, the settings approach aims to address this interplay of factors and to integrate a commitment to health within the culture, structures and routine life of settings (Dooris, 2006).

Health-promoting prisons: European, national and regional perspectives

At a European level, the Health in Prisons Project (HIPP) was initiated by WHO in 1995, launching an international movement concerned to promote health and tackle health inequalities in the prison setting (Gatherer et al., 2005). Following the settings approach as previously developed in relation to cities, schools and hospitals, the healthy prison concept reinforces the fact that the health and well-being of prisoners is not the sole responsibility of those providing health care. Moreover, for health promotion in this setting to be more fully realised, action in a number of strategic areas needs to be advanced at a European level (WHO, 2004), encouraging all countries:

- to establish integrated working between public health and prison health systems in order to promote overall wider public health and reduce health inequalities;
- to encourage prisons to operate within the widely recognised national and international codes of human rights and medical ethics in their provision of services for prisoners;
- to assist the reduction of re-offending by encouraging prison health services to contribute fully to each prisoner's rehabilitation and resettlement, especially in relation to drug addiction and mental health problems;
- to reduce the exposure of prisoners to communicable diseases, thereby preventing prisons becoming focal points of disease;
- to promote all prison health services, including health promotion services, to reach standards equivalent to those in the wider community.

With a Collaborating Centre based at the Department of Health in London, the HIPP aims to encourage innovation and evidence-based practice in prison health, to promote stronger links with public health and to improve the health of prisoners, staff, visitors, prisoners' families and local communities. It functions by networking key stakeholders, creating and disseminating knowledge and expertise, and working to influence prison health policies and programmes in member countries. Membership of the HIPP requires a national-level ministerial commitment with appropriate resourcing, and there are currently over 30 member countries.

Several major international conferences have been organised, including the first international conference on healthy prisons, held in Liverpool in March 1996 (Squires and Strobl, 1996) and the tenth anniversary conference in 2005 (WHO, 2006). In addition, a number of landmark documents have been produced, including the Consensus Statement on Mental Health Promotion in Prisons (WHO, 1999) and the Moscow Declaration on Prisons and Public Health of 2003 (WHO, 2003), and WHO has also created an awards scheme to recognise best practice in prisons and health.

Within England and Wales, the health-promoting prison agenda has been progressed through the publication of a strategy and action plan, *Health Promoting Prisons: A Shared Approach* (Department of Health, 2002). Grounded in the concept of decency and recognising that prisons should be safe, secure, reforming and health promoting, this explicitly adopts the healthy settings model and whole prison approach, with the aims of:

- building the physical, mental and social health of prisoners (and, where appropriate, staff);
- helping prevent the deterioration of prisoners' health during or because of custody;
- helping prisoners adopt healthy behaviours that can be taken back into the community.

The Whole Prison Approach is understood to comprise three key elements:

- policies in prisons which promote health (e.g. a no smoking policy);
- an environment in each prison which is actively supportive of health;
- prevention, health education and other health promotion initiatives which address assessed health needs within each prison.

Human rights and decency are important foundations for promoting health because they underpin all aspects of prison life. If the following measures are attained, then a basis exists from which to promote health:

- treatment for prisoners that is within the law;
- maintaining facilities that are clean and properly equipped;
- providing prompt attention to prisoners' proper concerns;
- protecting prisoners from harm;
- providing prisoners with a regime that makes imprisonment bearable;
- fair and consistent treatment by staff.

Health Promoting Prisons: A Shared Approach paved the way for *Prison Service Order (PSO) 3200 on Health Promotion* (HM Prison Service, 2003), which prioritised mental health, smoking, healthy eating, healthy lifestyles (including sex and relationships and active living) and drug and other substance misuse. The translation of a Department of Health strategy into an audited standard issued from within HM Prison Service was a crucial step forward for health-promoting prisons, embedding as it did a commitment to health within the offender management system.

At a regional level, progress in implementing PSO 3200 has varied, with the North West being the only region to have appointed a Regional Healthy Prisons Co-ordinator (with joint funding from the Department of Health and HM Prison Service). Since 2004, all 16 prisons in the North West have worked closely with the Co-ordinator, based within the Healthy Settings Development Unit at the University of Central Lancashire, to develop robust, locally agreed action plans that include activity in each of the key priority areas of PSO 3200 and ensure alignment with key national targets. The facilitation of networking and the consequent sharing of good practice and public health expertise have been key drivers in delivering a joined-up approach to public health across the 16 North West prisons and their local partnerships.

Health-promoting prisons: challenges and opportunities

The unique prison environment has special difficulties when it comes to promoting health. Most notably that prison is a home to one group of people and a workplace to another. For prisoners, at an individual level, prison takes away autonomy and may inhibit or damage self-esteem. Common problems include bullying and boredom, and social exclusion may be worsened as family ties are put under more stress by separation.

However, prison also provides a unique public health opportunity in terms of health promotion, health education and disease prevention (Department of Health, 2002):

- Prison offers access to disadvantaged groups who would normally be hard to reach. It is therefore a prime opportunity to address inequalities in health by means of specific health interventions as well as measures that impact upon the wider determinants of health.
- Each prison has the potential to be a healthy setting, whereby a holistic approach to spiritual, physical, social and mental health and well-being is developed within a single institution.

- To the many prisoners who have led chaotic lifestyles prior to prison, it is sometimes their only opportunity for an ordered approach to assessing and addressing health needs – in ways that connect to resettlement back into the community.
- Prison offers the opportunity to develop initiatives that add value to health and safety and human resource management, and more broadly promote staff health and well-being.

Within England and Wales, the transfer of commissioning responsibility for prison health care and the broader health-promoting prison agenda present complex challenges at a time of extensive reconfiguration within the NHS and the offender management system. Both the Prison Service and the NHS are large and complex organisations, each with their own cultures, norms and values. While this difference in many ways adds to the burden of effectively developing partnership approaches and managing change, it also offers the opportunity to harness the diversity of knowledge and experience to address the wider determinants of health, thereby reducing inequalities, tackling social exclusion and bringing about real health improvement and effective resettlement of ex-prisoners back into their communities.

Conclusion

In concluding, a number of observations can be made regarding the prison health reforms and the development of the health-promoting prisons agenda in England and Wales. First, the isolation of prison health care and the health-care staff and the *ad hoc* nature of provision are becoming a thing of the past. Nationally, the Department of Health leads policy and planning to tackle the major health needs of prisoners through ensuring provision of primary care, mental health, dental and other services, and a workforce strategy is in place to ensure the appropriate recruitment, development and retention of staff. All doctors employed to work regularly in prison are now qualified as General Practitioners (the vast majority working part-time within prison, part-time within the community) and many nurses have been attracted to work within the prison setting.

Secondly, there has been increased funding for capital building projects and for tackling key health issues such as mental health. Prison Health has worked with colleagues across government to put in place a clear gateway to specialist mental health services, fully accessible to the offender management system (e.g. 300 additional NHS mental health nurses have been recruited to form mental health in-reach teams).

Thirdly, although a number of problems remain, such as ignorance and prejudice in the public's perceptions of prisoners, the continuing struggle for adequate resources and underlying problems of overcrowding, the prison health reforms have provided useful levers for sustainable change.

Fourthly, the medical model of health provision has been reformed and prison health is beginning to be viewed as part of the mainstream agenda. It is now the norm for relevant major public health initiatives to include prisoners as part of their target audience: for example, *Choosing Health: Making Healthy Choices Easier* (Department of Health, 2004) further strengthened the health-promoting prison agenda, the first time such a publication has included a section on prison health and made explicit reference to prisoners in the context of specific topic-based proposals (e.g. smoking). This acknowledgement of the role of prisons in improving public health can be illustrated in relation to the problems posed by illegal drug use. It is now normal to consider the positive contribution that the offender management system can make, with prisons being the largest single provider of detoxifications regimens for alcohol and drug users in England and Wales (over 55,000 each year), and prisoners with a drug problem being supervised and put in touch with support services when released back into the community (Marteau and Farrell, 2005). Prisons are also now the number one provider of Hepatitis B immunisations. Similarly, prison is also seen as an opportunity to encourage smoking cessation, where quit rates are sometimes better than in the community (Macaskill and Hayton, 2006, in press).

Lastly, this acknowledgement of the public health opportunities offered by prisons implies a broader realisation that health improvement forms a legitimate and important part of the effort to integrate prisoners back into society and reduce re-offending, which in turn contributes to both the crime and violence and well-being agendas through helping build healthy, safe and sustainable communities. In this context, the reforms support the broader vision of health-promoting prisons by addressing the human rights issue that imprisonment should not be harmful to health, and should instead adequately address need and actively promote health. By integrating the health improvement and decency agendas, there is an opportunity to ensure that prison health becomes part of public health, and to tackle inequalities, reduce social exclusion and contribute to the well-being of society as a whole – outcomes that should have huge appeal across the broad spectrum of political opinion.

References

Department of Health (2001) *Shifting the Balance of Power within the NHS: Securing Delivery.* London: Department of Health.

Department of Health (2002) *Health Promoting Prisons: a Shared Approach.* London: Department of Health), http://www.dh.gov.uk/PolicyAndGuidance/HealthAndSocialCareTopics/PrisonHealth/fs/en (accessed 9 June 2006).

Department of Health (2004) *Choosing Health: Making Healthy Choices Easier.* London: Department of Health.

Department of Health, HM Prison Service and Welsh Assembly Government (2003) *Prison Health Handbook.* London: Department of Health, http://www.dh.gov.uk/PolicyAndGuidance/Health AndSocialCareTopics/PrisonHealth/fs/en (accessed 9 June 2006).

Dooris, M. (2004) Joining up settings for health: a valuable investment for strategic partnerships? *Critical Public Health,* 14 (1): 49–61.

Dooris, M. (2006) Healthy settings: challenges to generating evidence of effectiveness. *Health Promotion International,* 21 (1): 55–65.

Gatherer, A., Moller, L. and Hayton, P. (2005) WHO European Health in Prisons Project after ten years: persistent barriers and achievements. *American Journal of Public Health,* 95 (10): 1696–700.

HM Inspectorate of Prisons (England and Wales) (1996) *Patient or Prisoner? A New Strategy for Health Care in Prison.* London: Home Office.

HM Prison Service (2003) *Prison Service Order (PSO) 3200 on Health Promotion.* London: HM Prison Service, http://www.dh.gov.uk/PolicyAndGuidance/HealthAndSocialCareTopics/Prison Health/fs/en (accessed 9 June 2006).

HM Prison Service (2006) *Population Figures – February Monthly Bulletin.* London: HM Prison Service, http://www.hmprisonservice.gov.uk/ (accessed 9 June 2006).

International Centre for Prisons Studies (2006) *World Prison Brief: Prison Brief for United Kingdom – England & Wales.* London: International Centre for Prisons Studies, King's College, University of London, http://www.prisonstudies.org/ (accessed 9 June 2006).

Joint Prison Service and National Health Service Executive Working Group (1999) *The Future Organisation of Prison Health Care.* London: Department of Health, http://www.dh.gov.uk/Policy AndGuidance/HealthAndSocialCareTopics/PrisonHealth/fs/en (accessed 9 June 2006).

Macaskill, S. and Hayton, P. (2006, in press) *Stop Smoking Support in HM prisons: the Impact of Nicotine Replacement Therapy.* Stirling: Institute for Social Marketing, Stirling University/Open University).

Marteau, D. and Farrell, M. (2005) Clinical management of substance misuse in prisons. In Gerada, C. (ed.), *The Management of Substance Misuse in Primary Care.* London: Royal College of General Practitioners.

Social Exclusion Unit (2002) *Reducing Re-Offending by Ex-Prisoners.* London: Social Exclusion Unit.

Social Exclusion Unit (2004) *Mental Health and Social Exclusion.* London: Office of the Deputy Prime Minister.

Squires, N. and Strobl, J. (1996) *Healthy Prisons: a Vision for the Future.* Report of the First International Conference on Healthy Prisons. Liverpool: Department of Public Health, University of Liverpool.

WHO (1986) *Ottawa Charter for Health Promotion.* Geneva: World Health Organisation.

WHO (1999) *Mental Health Promotion in Prisons. Report on a WHO Meeting, The Hague, Netherlands, 18–21 November 1998.* Copenhagen: WHO Regional Office for Europe, http://www.euro.who.int/prisons (accessed 9 June 2006).

WHO (2003) *Declaration on Prison Health as Part of Public Health. Moscow – 24 October 2003.* Copenhagen: WHO Regional Office for Europe, http://www.euro.who.int/prisons (accessed 9 June 2006),

WHO (2004) *Strategic Objectives for the WHO Health in Prisons Project: 2004–2010.* Copenhagen: WHO Regional Office for Europe, http://www.euro.who.int/prisons (accessed 9 June 2006).

WHO (2006) *International Conference on Prison and Health: Proceedings – London, 17 October 2005.* Copenhagen: WHO Regional Office for Europe, http://www.euro.who.int/prisons (accessed 9 June 2006).

Chapter 28

Does Social Capital have a Role to Play in the Health of Communities?

Andrew Gibson

Introduction

Much of the research on social capital has explicitly attempted to link greater amounts of social capital with improved health status (Hawe and Shiell, 2000). This makes the concept of particular interest to public health practitioners. However, it is also important to recognise that the value of the social capital concept for public health, and its link to health and health inequalities, has been contested. Thus, while for some the new emphasis on social capital is welcomed as bringing the social back into economic development policy (Kawachi, 2002), for others it is criticised as representing a neo-liberalist approach to understanding social relations (Navarro, 2002). Hawe and Shiell (2000) suggest that social capital may merely represent a repackaging of what many public health practitioners have been doing for a long time.

Part of the dispute arises from ambiguity about what the concept of 'social capital' actually refers to. Despite a number of international meetings and conferences that have attempted to clarify the components of social capital, there is still a lack of theoretical clarity about the concept. Indeed, as Portes (1998) observes social capital is being applied to so many events and different contexts that it is in danger of losing any distinct meaning.

Despite this lack of clarity, Wakefield and Poland (2005) point out that policy-makers are increasingly paying attention to the potential role that public health practitioners can or should play in building social capital to promote health and diminish health inequalities. Thus, whatever one's view of the concept, social capital has become an increasingly important concept for public health practitioners to become familiar with. In fact, Wakefield and Poland (2005) suggest that an ability to frame one's work in these terms may become critical to developing a competitive edge in securing funding for public health interventions.

This chapter will begin by examining the work of Robert Putnam (1993, 1998, 2000), since he has perhaps been most influential in bringing the concept of social capital to prominence. The chapter will then take a closer look at research on the relationship between health and social capital before exploring its implications for social policy. Finally, the chapter will draw out the practical relevance of the concept for public health practitioners working within a community context.

What is social capital?

The earliest references to the phrase 'social capital' appear to be in L.J. Hanifan's *The Community Center,* published in 1920, although it could be argued that the term represents a reframing of concerns about the nature of civil society which date back much further (Portes, 1998). Important contributions have also been made by the French social theorist Pierre Bourdieu (1985) and the American sociologist James Coleman (1988). However, it is generally acknowledged by both advocates and critics alike that Robert Putnam, an American political scientist, has done most to bring the concept into prominence both within the social sciences and more broadly within social policy circles. In the UK setting, Richard Wilkinson (1996) directly acknowledges Putnam's work as the inspiration for his own use of the concept in his influential research on the cause of health inequalities. Although many researchers seem now to accept Putnam's definition of social capital, the subject area remains hotly debated (DeFilippis, 2001; Fine, 2001).

Putnam defines social capital as 'features of social life such as networks, norms, and social trust that facilitate co-ordination and co-operation for mutual benefit' (1993: 85). Putnam (2000) describes a number of beneficial effects that social capital has for society. He argues that high levels of social capital can improve economic performance and reduce corruption (Putnam, 1993). He also argues that it has positive effects on health, educational attainment, crime levels, and political participation (Putnam, 2000). Putnam makes use of data on levels of voter turnout, involvement in political parties, trade unions, and professional organisations, volunteering, church attendance, levels of trust in politicians and levels of 'neighbourliness' in order to support his argument empirically.

However, Putnam's work has been criticised on several grounds. For example, Skocpol (1996) has criticised the way that Putnam measures social capital. Putnam does this using a form of methodological individualism, that is in his research on the USA Putnam uses the General Social Survey to measure the level of social involvement of individuals and simply aggregates up from this. The difficulty with this approach is that it ignores the way in which power relationships, both internal and external to a community, influence its development. As DeFilippis (2001) points out, communities or regions are not solely a product of the internal attributes of the individual people living and working within them. All communities have internal social structures and power relations that also interact with the rest of the world. It is not simply social networks that make people rich or poor. For DeFilippis, what needs to be changed is not necessarily the level or number of connections, but the power relationships.

Putnam also tends to treat social capital and civil society as virtually synonymous. He argues: 'social capital refers to the norms and networks of civil society that lubricate co-operative action among both citizens and their institutions' (Putnam, 1998: v). He assumes that social capital and civil society are positive things necessary for democratic government and economic health. However, as DeFilippis notes, the nature of civil society is something that has been hotly debated. For Hegel, civil society was inherently conflictual (Hegel, 1965). This idea was developed by Marx, but reworked from a materialist perspective. For both Marx and Engels, property and class interests make a universalist civic society impossible, at least under capitalism (Callinicos, 1999). The Italian revolutionary Gramsci viewed the associations of civil society as one of the principal means via which the ruling classes generate and sustain their 'hegemony' over labour and the peasantry (Gramsci, 1971/1929–35). More recently, some feminist authors have made similar arguments about how conceiving civil society in terms of beneficial relationships and shared interests is inherently oppressive to those people who do not share in these interests or benefits (Benhabib and Cornell, 1987; Young, 1990). As DeFilippis points out, Putnam in his own work in Italy (Putnam, 1993), stresses the importance of things like soccer club membership. Unfortunately Italian soccer has been bedevilled by racism.

Putnam's assumption that social capital is normatively good is also open to question. In order to illustrate the benefits of social capital Putnam quotes Coleman's (1988) example of the diamond industry in New York, and how market transactions involving large quantities of jewels are facilitated by the social networks of trust within the Jewish community that controls the industry. However, as DeFilippis (2001) points out, the description he offers ignores the reality of exploitation within ethnic enclave economies, for example see Waldinger (1986). It also ignores the fact that anyone who is not a member of the ethnic enclave creating the market is excluded from that market, irrespective of their ability. One could argue in response that those who are excluded should develop their own connections to the relevant social networks in order to overcome this. However, as DeFilippis (2001) points out, if everyone is connected to the same networks and realises the same benefits, the advantages of network membership disappear. For DeFilippis, social capital must be premised on the ability of certain groups to realise it at the expense of others in order for it to operate as a form of capital.

Bridging and bonding social capital

Putnam has attempted to deal with some of these criticisms by introducing the concepts of bridging and bonding social capital, which he borrows from Gittell and Vidal (1998). 'Bonding social capital' refers to social networks designed to increase the bonds within a certain group. Putnam gives church-based women's reading groups, ethnic fraternal organisations and fashionable country clubs as examples. 'Bridging social capital' refers to social networks which attempt to build ties between groups. Putnam (2000) gives the civil rights movement, many youth service groups and ecumenical religious organisations as examples of 'bridging social capital'.

According to Putnam, most groups have elements of both of these, but often they may be characterised by a predominance of one form of social capital or another. In particular he sees a lack of 'bridging social capital' as problematic since 'bonding social capital', along with holding a particular group together, can be used to exclude outsiders. Bonding capital can therefore be used to perpetuate inequality and exclusion.

However, Putnam's argument still leaves the issue at the level of the community and whether or not it possesses enough 'bridging social capital'. It fails to recognise the importance of the social and cultural systems in which relationships between groups are embedded. In particular, critics have stressed a lack of attention to class dynamics (Forbes and Wainwright, 2001; see also Muntaner et al., 2000; Navarro, 2002), although parallel arguments could be made about attention to issues of gender and race.

Social capital and health inequalities

The links between social capital and health have come into increasing prominence in the literature on income inequality and health (Hawe and Shiell, 2000). The relationship between health and socio-economic status (SES), using a wide range of measures, is well established (Whitehead, 1987; Townsend and Davidson, 1988; Independent Inquiry into Inequalities in Health, 1998). The evidence points to a continuous gradient rather than a threshold effect, thus suggesting that the adverse health effects of health inequalities are widespread, rather than confined to the poorest sections of society.

However, in most developed countries health inequalities have not decreased despite rising national wealth (as measured by increasing GNP per capita) and improvements in longevity. This has provoked discussion about the possible ways that social factors other than material deprivation may affect health outcomes. Some researchers (Wilkinson, 1996; Kawachi and Kennedy, 1997; Kawachi et al., 1997) argue that inequality is bad for health, independent of the impact on individuals of material factors such as income levels. This emphasises the negative impact on health of the *experience* of inequality. For example, Wilkinson has attempted to demonstrate a strong correlation between violent crime rates, income inequality and levels of ill health (Wilkinson et al., 1998). He has sought to explain these findings by arguing that living in a highly unequal society leads to feelings of humiliation, disrespect and shame among those who are lower down the social hierarchy. He argues, drawing on the work of Putnam (1993), that increased inequality erodes levels of social cohesion/social capital within society and increases the significance of differences in social status. These factors in turn lead to increases in psychosocial stress of various kinds, which translate into patterns of ill health and into violent crime. From this perspective, psychosocial stress impacts on health both directly, via the effects of stress on disease development, and indirectly via its contribution to the incidence of health-damaging behaviours such as excessive alcohol consumption.

In support of Wilkinson's argument, Ichiro Kawachi et al. (1997) report a strong correlation between group membership and social trust, and both income inequality and total mortality. Kawachi and Kennedy (1997: 1037) argue that 'income inequality leads to increased mortality via disinvestment in social capital'. They argue that a large gap between rich and poor people leads to higher mortality through the breakdown of social cohesion. This may have a direct effect on health via various psychosocial mechanisms or an indirect effect through the experience of violence.

However, Muntaner and Lynch (1999) develop a critique of Wilkinson's work from a neo-Marxist perspective by placing emphasis on the effects of class relations and other sources of inequality in power, for example gender, in generating inequalities in health. Vicente Navarro (1999) similarly argues that poor social cohesion is the result and not the cause of health and social inequalities.

Social capital and its implications for social policy

Given the degree of controversy that surrounds the concept of social capital, it is worth asking why the concept has become so influential in social policy circles. Hawe and Shiell (2000) suggest that the answer lies in the rhetorical power of the concept and the uses to which politicians can put it. They suggest that social capital, like its sister concept of community, has attracted the interest of both the 'left' and 'right' because those on the 'left' see in social capital a concept which can be mobilised to criticise the worst excesses of neo-liberal individualism, while the 'right' see it as a concept capable of putting a human face on the economic rationalism of the market, without resorting to welfare expenditure.

Similarly, Levitas (2000) argues that Tony Blair has attempted to distance himself from both Margaret Thatcher's claim that there is no such thing as society and from Old Labour's association with state intervention by emphasising the importance of community. Community has become a key concept in New Labour's ideology:

> At the heart of my belief is the idea of community. I don't just mean the local villages, towns and cities in which we live. I mean our fulfilment as individuals lies in a decent society of others. My argument … is that the renewal of community is the answer to the challenges of a changing world. (Blair, 2000)

Levitas (2000) argues that the emphasis on 'the renewal of the community' has important implications for social policy and helps explain the current fashionability of concepts such as social capital. However, she is concerned that building social capital may become an alternative policy objective to economic regeneration, one which largely relies on the unpaid labour of community members themselves, while at the same time potentially stigmatising those communities judged to be deficient in social capital.

Public health, community development and social capital

A corollary of the argument that social capital is positively linked with health is the assumption that communities experiencing high levels of ill health may do so, at least in part, because of a lack of social capital. This assumption seems to lie behind policy-makers' increasing focus on the potential health benefits of building social capital within disadvantaged communities. However, a growing body of work challenges this assumption. For example, Patricia Fernandez-Kelly's research in West Baltimore (1994, 1995) and Stack's research in poor communities in both urban and rural settings (e.g., 1974, 1997) and Vicky Cattel's studies of working-class communities in East London (2001) all highlight the essential role that local social networks play in helping individuals survive in disadvantaged communities. In some ways social capital is perhaps more central to the life experiences of people coping with disadvantage than to other social groups, since, as Wakefield and Poland (2005) point out, access to social capital may facilitate access to goods and services which would otherwise be unaffordable, for example child care.

Research also suggests that the benefits of local forms of social capital extend beyond the provision of material support. Halpern (1993) and Gibson (2006) suggest that the development of strong, internally cohesive groups with an identity that separates them from others can have an important beneficial impact on health. These types of relationship are central to people's experiences of themselves and fundamental to the development of self-esteem. The development of group identity may, therefore, be essential to the ability of disadvantaged and excluded groups to develop consciousness of, and resistance to, dominant groups and their exclusionary practices.

Gibson (2006) therefore argues that it is not lack of social capital *per se* that is the problem in deprived communities, but the fact that unlike middle- and upper-class forms of social capital, working-class social networks are unlikely to give their members access to the types and level of resources needed to significantly improve their social situation. An approach which fails to recognise this runs the risk of pathologising the behaviour of marginalised or disadvantaged social groups.

However, it is also important to recognise the potentially negative effects of the development of strong local forms of social capital. For example, certain forms of social capital can operate to reinforce relative social positions within a local community, acting to exclude those with different norms and values. Social capital networks may act to exclude some individuals on the basis of their ethnicity. Furthermore, the self-policing aspect of local social capital networks can result in significant pressure being exerted on individuals to conform to group norms. This might be a particular problem for some of the most marginalised members of already disadvantaged communities, leading to a double form of social exclusion.

Equally significant for public health practitioners are the potential social distances that separate them from the people they strive to help. The bias towards measuring levels of social capital via monitoring participation in certain, essentially middle-class activities, is apparent in the social capital literature. For example membership levels in organisations such as Parent Teacher Associations, service clubs, established religious institutions, and sports leagues are often quoted as indicators of levels of social capital. As Foley and Edwards (1999) point out, participation in these kinds of organisation is class-specific, with members of the middle and upper classes more likely to participate. Similarly, Bourdieu (1984) argues that groups in lower social positions are most likely to experience the labelling of their social activities as undesirable or even as pathological and deviant, while those in higher social positions experience their activities as socially valued. Wakefield and Poland (2005) therefore suggest that the forms of participation that are sometimes uncritically encouraged by public health practitioners may reflect their own taken-for-granted class-based assumptions rather than those of the populations with which they seek to engage. As a result, even when opportunities to participate in community-based activities are widely offered, only individuals with specific habits, dispositions and self-perceived competency are likely to feel at home.

Furthermore, the proposal to build 'bridging social capital' in order to deal with the problem is unlikely to be helpful. Wakefield and Poland (2005) suggest that, in practice, what actually happens under the guise of developing bridging social capital is that only particular individuals, who originate from within dominated groups, but who have acquired at least some familiarity with the dominant culture and values (e.g., through education), are enabled to participate. In addition, the forms of participation advocated often have a direct or indirect financial cost (e.g., membership fees or child care costs during meetings), resulting in the exclusion of those people who lack the economic capital required to participate. Attempts at building 'bridging social capital' can therefore have the unintended consequence of concentrating the power of marginalised groups into the hands of a few spokespersons or established community leaders, while at the same time introducing social distance between those speaking and those being spoken for (Bourdieu, 1984).

Moreover, in a society divided along lines of class, race and gender, the development of shared norms and networks is likely to be extremely difficult. For example, locally based forms of social capital may be a product of resistance to domination and exploitation (Gibson, 2006). It is therefore not surprising that, as a result of these experiences, social trust, one measure of social capital, appears to be lowest among disadvantaged social groups and higher among those in dominant social positions.

Wakefield and Poland (2005) argue that rather than focusing on social capital *per se*, an approach that builds social capital in and through explicit campaigns to reduce economic and other disparities between groups may be more likely to reduce social exclusion than a more communitarian approach.

Conclusion

A number of complex issues remain for public health practitioners interested in community development (Wakefield and Poland, 2005):

1. An approach which assumes that disadvantaged communities lack social capital runs the risk of pathologising the behaviour of marginalised groups.
2. Consensus approaches to problem-solving within communities are unlikely to be inherently representative of the needs and wishes of marginalised groups.
3. The emphasis frequently placed on developing horizontal connections between groups is problematic, since disadvantaged groups are unlikely to have enough resources to pool to solve their own problems.
4. The position of public health practitioners working within a community context is possibly paradoxical since there is potential to inadvertently encourage community members to adopt dominant norms of participation and social engagement.

Despite these reservations, an understanding of the role played by local forms of social capital in defending disadvantaged groups from the psychosocial and material impact of stigmatisation, while at the same time recognising the potentially negative consequences of these processes may be of help. Such an approach, as long as it recognises the relationship between local forms of social capital and wider social structures of inequality, could help public health practitioners intervene in communities in ways that more effectively promote health.

References

Benhabib, S. and Cornell, D. (eds) (1987) *Feminism as Critique*. Minneapolis: University of Minnesota Press.

Blair, T. (2000) *Speech to the Annual Conference of the Women's Institute*, 7 June, London.

Bourdieu, P. (1984) *Distinction: a Social Critique of the Judgement of Taste*. Translated by Richard Nice. Cambridge, MA: Harvard University Press.

Bourdieu, P. (1985) The forms of capital, in J.G. Richardson (ed.), *Handbook of Theory and Research for the Sociology of Education*. New York: Greenwood Press.

Callinicos, A. (1999) *Social Theory: a Historical Introduction*. Cambridge: Polity Press.

Cattell, V. (2001) Poor people, poor places, and poor health: the mediating role of social networks and social capital. *Social Science and Medicine*, 52: 1501–1516.

Coleman, J. (1988) Social capital in the creation of human capital. *American Journal of Sociology*, 94, supplement, S95–S120.

DeFilippis, J. (2001) The myth of social capital in community development. *Housing Policy Debate*, 12 (4).

Fernandez-Kelly, P. (1994) Towanda's triumph: social and cultural capital in the transition to adulthood in the urban ghetto. *International Journal of Urban and Regional Research*, 18: 88–111.

Fernandez-Kelly, P. (1995) Social and cultural capital in the urban ghetto, in A. Portes (ed.), *The Economic Sociology of Immigration: Essays on Networks, Ethnicity and Entrepreneurship*. New York: Russell Sage Foundation Press.

Fine, B. (2001) *Social Capital versus Social Theory: Political Economy and Social Science at the Turn of the Millennium*. London: Routledge.

Foley, M.W. and Edwards, B. (1999) Is it time to disinvest in social capital? *Journal of Public Policy*, 19: 141–173.

Forbes, A. and Wainwright, S.P. (2001) On the methodological, theoretical, and philosophical context of health inequalities research: a critique. *Social Science and Medicine*, 53: 801–816.

Gibson, A. (2006) Health and community: is the concept of social capital helpful? PhD thesis, Faculty of Health and Social Care, Milton Keynes, Open University.

Gittell, R. and Vidal, A. (1998) *Community Organising: Building Social Capital as a Development Strategy*. Thousand Oaks, CA: Sage.

Gramsci, A. (1971/1929–35) State and civil society. In Q. Hoare and G.N. Smith (eds and trans.) *Selections from the Prison Notebooks*. New York: International Publishers.

Halpern, D.S. (1993) Minorities and mental health. *Social Science and Medicine*, 36: 597–607.

Hegel, G.W.F. (1965) *Philosophy of Right*. Oxford: Clarendon Press.

Hanifan, L.J. (1920) *The Community Center*. Boston: Silver, Burdett & Co.

Hawe, P. and Shiell, A. (2000) Social capital and health promotion: a review. *Social Science and Medicine*, 51: 871–885.

Independent Inquiry into Inequalities in Health (1998) *Independent Inquiry into Inequalities in Health* (the Acheson Report). London: HMSO.

Kawachi, I. (2002) Social capital and health: why social resources matter. Keynote address, first international conference on inner city health, Toronto, Ontario, 3 October 2002.

Kawachi, I. and Kennedy, B.P. (1997) Health and social cohesion: why care about income inequality? *British Medical Journal*, 314: 1037–1040.

Kawachi, I., Kennedy, B.P., Lochner, K. and Prothrow-Stith, D. (1997) Social capital, income inequality, and mortality. *American Journal of Public Health*, 87: 1491–1498.

Levitas, R. (2000) Community, utopia and New Labour. *Local Economy*, 5 (3): 188–197.

Muntaner, C. and Lynch, J. (1999) Income inequality, social cohesion, and class relations: a critique of Wilkinson's neo-Durkheimian research program. *International Journal of Health Services*, 29: 59–81.

Muntaner, C., Lynch, J., and Smith, G.D. (2000) Social capital and the third way in public health. *Critical Public Health*, 10: 107–124.

Navarro, V. (1999) Health and equality in the world in the era of 'globalisation'. *International Journal of Health Services*, 29 (2): 215–226.

Navarro, V. (2002) A critique of social capital. *International Journal of Health Services*, 32: 423–432.

Portes, A. (1998) Social capital: its origins and applications in modern sociology. *Annual Review of Sociology*, 24: 1–24.

Putnam, R. (1993) *Making Democracy Work: Civic Traditions in Modern Italy.* Princeton, NJ: Princeton University Press.

Putnam, R. (1998) Forward. *Housing Policy Debate*, 9 (1): v–viii.

Putnam, R. (2000) *Bowling Alone: the Collapse and Revival of American Community.* New York: Simon & Schuster.

Skocpol, T. (1996) Unravelling from above. *The American Prospect*, March–April, 20–25.

Stack, C. (1974) *All Our Kin.* New York: Harper & Row.

Stack, C. (1997) *Call to Home: African Americans Reclaim the Rural South.* New York: Basic Books.

Townsend, P. and Davidson, N. (1988) *Inequalities in Health: the Black Report.* Harmondsworth: Penguin.

Wakefield, E.L. and Poland, B. (2005) Family, friend or foe? Critical reflections on the relevance and role of social capital in health promotion and community development. *Social Science and Medicine,* 60: 2819–2832.

Waldinger, R. (1986) *Through the Eye of the Needle: Immigrants and Enterprise in New York's Garment Trades.* New York: New York University Press.

Whitehead, M. (1987) *The Health Divide: Inequalities in Health in the 1980s.* London: Health Education Council.

Wilkinson, R. (1996) *Unhealthy Societies: the Afflictions of Inequality.* London: Routledge.

Wilkinson, R., Kawachi, I. and Kennedy, B. (1998) Mortality, the social environment, crime and violence. *Sociology of Health and Illness*, 20 (5): 578–597.

Young, I.M. (1990) *Justice and the Politics of Difference.* Princeton, NJ: Princeton University Press.

Chapter 29

Evaluating the Empowering Potential of Community-based Health Schemes: the Case of Community Health Policies in the UK since 1997

Paul Bridgen

The 'New' Labour government and community empowerment

A central feature of New Labour's approach to social policy in the United Kingdom (UK) since 1997 has been its emphasis on community involvement in local policy formation and implementation. Across a broad range of policy areas the Blair government has stressed the importance of participatory approaches to policy-making. Health policy, particularly health promotion, and neighbourhood renewal are two policy areas where this emphasis on community involvement has been particularly pronounced. With regard to health promotion, New Labour has explained that 'supporting community-based action will serve to empower individuals and improve levels of self-determination' (DoH, 1999). Elsewhere, favourable references have been made to 'community empowerment' (Social Exclusion Unit, Policy Action Team, 2000) and 'community development approaches' (NHS Executive, 1999; Social Exclusion Unit, 2000).

Rhetoric of this type is not new and scepticism has greeted the claims New Labour has made for its policy approach. One way of testing these claims is by evaluating the policy initiatives that follow from them. However, as a number of authors have noted (e.g.

Edited from: Bridgen, P. (2004) Evaluating the empowering potential of community-based health schemes: the case of community health policies in the UK since 1997, *Community Development Journal*, 39 (3): 289–302. By permission of Oxford University Press.

Laverack and Wallerstein, 2001), evaluating the empowering potential of community-based health promotion schemes is not a straightforward task, not least because of the conceptual ambiguity surrounding community empowerment. This chapter discusses the problems involved in evaluating community empowerment, using policy development in the UK since 1997 as a case study. It seeks more clearly to delineate the concept of community empowerment from other community-based approaches to health improvement and suggests that the urban political science literature provides some useful insights with regard to the operationalization of community empowerment in process-focused evaluative research.

The UK policy framework

New Labour's rhetoric about community involvement and empowerment has influenced a number of policy initiatives in the UK health field. In this regard, Health Action Zones (HAZs) and the New Deal for Communities (NDC) are obvious examples, although as will be seen, Primary Care Trusts (PCTs) share some similar features.

HAZs were first established in 1997 in areas of particular deprivation and poor health (a second wave was approved in 1998) (DoH, 1997). They are meant to constitute 'holistic' partnerships in a given geographic area involving the various agencies (statutory, voluntary, public and private) interested in health improvement. Their aims are to 'tackle health inequalities and modernise services through local innovation' (DoH, 1998a; Haznet, 1998). NDCs are smaller, neighbourhood-based initiatives that again emphasize partnerships between local agencies and the public in areas of particular deprivation, but that also aim to raise educational achievement and tackle worklessness and crime, as well as improve health (DETR, 1999). PCTs are part of the core NHS (DoH, 1997). They are freestanding, statutory NHS bodies that have responsibility for: the management, development and integration of all primary care services; health improvement in their local area; and the purchase of secondary care. They are the most important body in UK's local politics of health arena.

In both HAZs and NDCs the commitment to 'bottom-up' approaches means public involvement has been a central feature. Thus, 'communities' are meant to be 'at the heart of the partnership' (DETR, 2001) and a Community Empowerment Fund has been established to support community development (Sullivan, 2001; Bauld and Judge, 2002). The means for involving the community have varied, but most NDCs include sizeable community representation on the executive bodies of the project. In the Southampton (Thornhill) NDC, for example, each working party overseeing the various projects is chaired by a resident and most cannot take a binding decision unless there is at least a 60/40 split of residents and officers (Thornhill NDC, 2001). 'Community empowerment' is regarded by leading officials as the aim and the model of the programme. PCTs, on the other hand, while more 'top-down' in their approach, have been constituted as 'stakeholder organizations', with governing boards that include a mix of professional groups and representation from other local agencies and the public (Rowe, 2002).

Empowerment or manipulation?

Despite this policy framework and the rhetoric that accompanies it, considerable doubts remain about what all of this amounts to in practice. After all, community empowerment has become a malleable concept that has been used rhetorically to justify a variety of health policy approaches in different parts of the world. While it gained popularity with the emergence of the 'new public health' movement in the 1970s, it was then successfully incorporated into the New Right's consumerist discourse in the 1980s (Farrant, 1991; Saltmann, 1994; Mayo with Anastacio, 1999).

There is little doubt that New Labour's policy initiatives in the UK have involved greater emphasis on participatory democratic approaches than those sponsored by its Conservative predecessor. However, what evidence is there that under the Blair government community empowerment, as a method of promoting health, has taken on or has the potential to take on meanings more in line with the original conception of the 'new public health' movement?

One way of answering this question is by evaluating the empowering potential of the community-based schemes introduced by New Labour. Are HAZs and NDCs empowering the communities in which they have been established? Do they have the potential to do so? The problem with this approach, however, is that measuring community empowerment is no easy task. Relatively little attention has been given in the health promotion literature to how such an evaluation might be conducted. Indeed, as Laverack and Wallerstein suggest, 'a lack of practical methodologies, field-tested in different settings and cultural contexts, has been the main obstacle to making (empowerment) operational in health promotion programmes' (2001). What is clear is that any attempt to undertake this task faces a number of important problems.

In this regard, the first problem concerns the term community empowerment itself. Considerable debate continues about its theoretical underpinnings, policy implications and potential as a tool for improving health (particularly that of the least advantaged in society). A variety of 'empowerment' schemes are recommended in the literature, but there is little consensus about whether all of these schemes actually empower their communities and, if they do, how and why they might improve health.

This conceptual ambiguity raises problems for evaluation because differences in the meaning given to community empowerment by evaluators will affect the operationalization of the concept, and thus judgements about the empowering potential of schemes. Developments that might be taken as signifying empowerment under one conceptualization might not be considered as so significant under another. Thus, any attempt to evaluate the empowering potential of the area-based schemes has first to make clear how this term is being understood and, on this basis, indicate the community developments on which judgements are based.

Moreover, it is also important with regard to conceptual clarification, to untangle 'community empowerment' from other terms, such as 'capacity building' and 'social capital'. These have sometimes been used interchangeably with 'community empowerment', but in fact there is no straightforward relationship between any of these concepts. The next two sections will consider this conceptual debate and argue that to have any real value or meaning, community empowerment must involve some attempt to increase the influence of the community over the external policy developments that affect it. This is not to say that community-based schemes that seek to achieve other goals are not worthwhile: it is merely to make clear that they cannot meaningfully be understood as schemes that seek to *empower* their *communities*. Some seek to empower but only on an individual basis; others are community-based but are not primarily concerned with shifting power relations.

Although conceptual clarification can give a clearer sense of what is being looked for in the evaluation process (despite problems still remaining in this regard) it still leaves a number of difficulties to be addressed. These difficulties are similar to those experienced in the evaluation of all complex community initiatives (Mackenzie, Lawson and Mackinnon, 2002). For example, it is widely recognized that any changes to the external environment as a result of a community-based scheme are only likely to occur in the longer term. Given this, and the complexity and openness of such schemes, it is almost impossible to determine the extent to which the scheme itself is responsible for any change. For these and other reasons, the health promotion literature generally recommends that evaluation of community empowerment schemes should focus on measures of process rather than outcome.

However, the problem with these types of approach is that the process measures currently recommended are insufficiently developed or precise to allow the separation of empowering from non-empowering community-based health promotion schemes. What require much more systematic investigation are the types of processes that community-based schemes need to develop to increase their ongoing influence over the external policy environment. This issue will be the subject of the final section.

Communities, power and health

There are a wide variety of community-based participatory approaches to health improvement recommended in the literature, many of which claim community empowerment as an objective. However, not all of these schemes are founded on any clear definition of power or explanation of its relationship to health. This section will consider those approaches that *are* based on such foundations. The next will consider other types of community-based approach. Only those approaches associated with the community psychology and community health movement, it will be suggested, can be understood as being concerned in any meaningful way with the empowerment of communities.

While there are two main literatures linking power (or powerlessness) and health – the first being mainly psychological, while the second makes a more indirect connection that focuses on the effect of power on the distribution of health-enhancing resources, there is only scope here to discuss the latter approach.

The community health movement

[...] While the psychological literature cites powerlessness, or 'a lack of control over destiny' as a key driver to ill-health for individuals in marginalized situations (Wallerstein, 1992), it the relationship between individual empowerment and social and political change which forms the other strand of the community empowerment literature, associated with the community health movement. Here, the need for – and purpose of – community success in bringing about social and political change is far more clear-cut. This is because the community health movement's primary interest in power has less to do with the question of individual-level powerlessness, and more to do with the consequences of powerlessness for the distribution of health-enhancing resources (e.g. knowledge, skills, health services, material resources). The lack of power held by particular individuals or groups in society is regarded as a major explanation for their health experience and, in particular, the existence of health inequalities. Community empowerment is thus seen as part of a strategy to alter the distribution of health-enhancing resources. This might involve improving the access of disadvantaged communities to health services or encouraging the development of previously unrecognized individual or community skills. However, ultimately given that the main explanation for health inequalities is structural (Townsend, Davidson and Whitehead, 1988), its essential purpose is to help bring about directly or indirectly a redistribution of income.[1] Broader social or political change is vital. Indeed, the alleged failure of community-based schemes to succeed in this regard has been used by structuralist critics of the community health movement to question its value as a tool for addressing health inequalities (Wainwright, 1996). [...]

Capacity building and social capital

While some community-based health promotion interventions have been explicitly based on the ideas summarized above, this is not true for all of them, even some of those which claim community empowerment as an objective. Two other concepts – capacity building and social capital – have also been influential. These have often been used interchangeably with community empowerment, but as this section will suggest, they are different in important respects both in terms of their theoretical underpinnings and as a guide to policy development.

Considerable interest has been shown in community capacity building in the mainstream health promotion literature. This literature, which has its origins in health education, focuses on encouraging the broadest possible dispersal of health promoting knowledge and skills, particulary to disadvantaged social groups. Thus, one study (Hawe et al., 1998) found that health workers understood the purpose of capacity building as, amongst other things, to create 'a more favourable attitude towards health promotion'. To this end, capacity building involves a variety of activities in a number of domains and settings. A community-based aproach is just one such activity, under which 'individual community members are drawn into forming new organizations or joining existing ones to improve the health of community members' (Crisp et al., 2000, p. 100). This type of approach is sometimes described as an empowering process, in that it involves mobilizing the existing health-enhancing resources of the community (de graaf, 1986, quoted in Crisp et al., 2000, p. 100).

However, the claim that schemes of this type are empowering has been extensively criticized (Bunton, Nettleton and Burrows, 1995). The focus of this criticism is on the role of external organization and 'experts' in community health promotion and the tension between professional and lay knowledge. While the importance of the latter is often emphasized in this literature, the role of health and welfare professionals has led some commentators (Crisp et al., 2000) to regard community inolvement in such schemes as just another way of 'getting people to accept expert messages' (Blackburn, 1993). In short, they manipulate rather than empower. Indeed, health promotion workers themselves have expressed concerns about hidden agendas and 'paternalism' (Hawe et al., 1988, pp. 290–2)

For the most part the health focus of these schemes is individualistic and behavioural, with the main goal being the encouragement, albeit with community leadership, of more 'healthy lifestyles' (e.g. smoking cessation, reductions in alchohol consumption, etc.). While this might have beneficial effects on health, it could also be regarded as disempowering because it individualizes explanations of the causes of ill-health among disadvantaged communities. If there is a link with the powerlessness and health literature, it is mainly with the subjective psychological strand. As a result, there is less focus on structural explanations for health inequalities and consequently little emphasis on the promotion of social and political change.

This is also true of the Putnam-influenced literature on social capital and health (Putnam, 2000; Campbell, with Wood and Kelly, 1999). Community-based interventions inflenced by this concept have also on occasions been associated with a community empowerment agenda, mainly because of Putnam's emphasis on increasing civic engagement. However, Putnam's interest in civic engagement is mainly focused on the existence (or otherwise) and broader public effect of social networks. He is less concerned about the distribution of power within these relationships, particulary as this affects the ability of the least powerful to access social resources (Bridgen, 2006). In the health sphere, increasing social capital has been regarded as beneficial mainly because improved social networks act as support mechanisms that promote or protect health in particular groups (Campbell, with Wood and Kelly, 1999; Murray, 2000). In short, community activity is mainly regarded as an end in itself, not a necessary step on the way to the achievement of broader social or political change.

Structural change, policy development and governance

Determining empowering potential

As the previous section has shown, it is possible to distinguish between different approaches to community-based participatory health promotion on the basis of their theoretical underpinnings. Determining in practice which schemes have empowering potential and which do not, however, is more difficult.

As has been seen, the evaluation literature recommends in this regard a focus on measures of process. However, there is a major problem with this recommendation: community interventions based on different underpinning principles might look very similar in terms of process and their effect on individual perceptions of powerlessness. Moreover, some schemes might be based on a mix of ideas. Thus, while processes which aim to increase community competence, organization, cohesiveness etc. *might* be a step towards the enhancement of the community's ability to bring about broader social and political change, this is not necessarily the case. Movement along the community empowerment continuum is not inevitable.

What is required is some way of distinguishing between 'empowerment' programmes that see capacity-building developments as ends in themselves and those that regard these developments as means to a more ambitious end. This raises a further question: can programmes that do not display the characteristics of an empowering approach as outlined above nevertheless develop into empowering programmes? Policy development and 'unintended benefits' in implementation are certainly not unknown, even in programmes that are essentially conservative (Stoker, 2000). However, do certain characteristics *have* to be present to make such a metamorphosis possible?

Laverack and Wallerstein suggest that 'empowerment approaches' can be distinguished from other participatory schemes because they 'have an explicit agenda to bring about social and political changes and this is embodied in their sense of liberation, struggle and community activism' (2001, p. 182). They propose that this formulation be used in conjunction with a consideration of nine 'organizational domains' that influence community empowerment. These are: 'participation; leadership; problem assessment; organizational structures; resource mobilization; links to others; asking why; programme management; and the role of outside agents'. However, this proposed approach, while suggestive, requires further elaboration and development if it is really to offer, as its authors claim, a 'straightforward way to … measure community empowerment'. The content and relevance of these 'domains', for example, requires greater explication. Neither is it clear precisely what evaluators should be looking for in each domain, nor how 'progress' in each should be ranked.

What, in particular, requires greater specification is the nature of political change required if a community is to increase its power in external policy debates or over the distribution of health-enhancing resources in local and/or national negotiations? As Hawe suggests, '[s]tructural change', as it might affect these power relations, has been 'poorly defined in community interventions … (and) needs more clarification prior to evaluation' (1994, pp. 206–207). She argues (quoting Heller, 1989) that 'rather than simply "changing the cast of characters of those in power", it is changing how committees operate, how decisions are made and how *organizations negotiate with outside bodies* that makes the difference to the way services are provided or achievements gained'. Connections with outside bodies would seem particularly important if communities are really to influence significantly external policy developments that affect their area. This point has recently been emphasized by Mutaner et al. (2001) in a critique of Putnamesque approaches to community participation. They highlight the importance of 'the bridging connections (to broader social networks) and linking social connections (to social institutions) that help determine which individuals and groups have access to and control over the health-enhancing resources in society'.

Consideration of these processes should be at the centre of evaluations of the empowering potential of community-based programmes. An important part of any process-based evaluation of a community empowerment programme should be to judge the extent to which the establishment (or improvement) of 'bridging connections' between the community and external social and political institutions is part of the programme's agenda. For example, with regard to NDCs in the UK, the relationship established between them and PCTs, which hold local responsibility for the distribution of a wide range of health-enhancing resources, would seem of particular interest.

Policy networks and community empowerment

Recent debates about the concept of governance in urban political science provide a valuable analytical tool. This literature has focused mainly on local government and urban regeneration, but is nevertheless relevant to any policy field that involves a large number of actors and in which there exist power dependencies. Thus, governance has been defined as:

> governing, achieving collective action in the realm of public affairs where it is not possible to rest on recourse to the authority of the state ... It focuses attention on a set of actors that are drawn from but also beyond the formal institutions of government. A key concern is processes of networking and partnership. (Stoker, 2000, p. 3)

It is in these 'policy networks' that policy outcomes are shaped; they 'prescribe the issues which are discussed' and how they are dealt with; they have 'a distinct set of rules', shared values and ideology which 'privilege certain policy outcomes' (Marsh and Smith, 2000, p. 6). The local politics of health in the UK clearly shares some of the characteristics described by the governance literature, particularly since the establishment of PCTs, HAZs and NDCs, and given New Labour's emphasis on partnership working (DoH, 1998b).

If community-based schemes in the UK are to affect their external policy-making environment, it is these local policy networks of health that they will need to penetrate. The central question for community empowerment programmes thus becomes: how open are these networks to influence and/or change, and what types of circumstances and structures are needed to bring this about?

Policy networks have been theorized as an alternative to pluralist, Marxist and elitist theories of policy-making. Thus, while they are 'likely to reflect the broader pattern of structural inequality in society' and the degree to which they are open varies, they can nevertheless be subject to external influence and structural change, both of which can affect policy outcomes (Marsh and Smith, 2000, p. 7). A key development in the governance debate has been the move away from a hierarchical, concentrated and socially controlling conception of power. Rather, the emphasis is on the way power is socially produced, dispersed and composite, with influence 'not flowing from a single institutional or structural source in a single direction', but rather *enacted* in interactions' (McGuirk, 2000; see also Harding, 1997). External influence is possible because networked 'power configurations are less stable, less deterministic and more mutable, than bureaucratic conceptions of power would suggest'. Thus, it is possible for those outside a network to empower themselves by 'finding and exploiting instability in the relevant networks', 'building new associations and exploiting the need to share resources'.

Moreover, 'the interests or preferences of members of a network may not be defined merely, or perhaps even mainly, in terms of that membership' (Marsh and Smith, 2000, p. 6). Thus, an individual agent might have a 'foot in both camps' and be able to push forward in one policy network an agenda shaped in another. In a variety of fields, structural change in policy networks – with implications for policy outcomes – has been shown to have occurred on the basis of the actions of other networks operating in the same political field (Daugbjerg, 1998). A determined coalition of external actors or organizations can alter the way an erstwhile dominant policy network functions.

If altering the structure of policy networks and, on this basis, influencing policy development is theoretically possible (and this certainly remains a contested debate in the policy network literature), this has important implications for the evaluation of the empowering potential of locally based interventions. The types of question an evaluator might thus consider are as follows: to what extent is the intervention seeking to penetrate the broader health policy network in their area? If so, how is it seeking to do so? Is it relying on individual contacts or have new organizational structures been put in place? Are coalitions being constructed with other sympathetic local political actors?

Such an approach undoubtedly requires further elaboration and investigation. Policy network theory does not provide a checklist of variables that can be used to evaluate community empowerment programmes in terms of their external relationships. In this regard, as has already been suggested, it is now generally accepted that comprehensive community initiatives (CCIs), such as HAZs and the NDC for example, are not susceptible to such traditional forms of evaluation. However, the governance literature does provide a way of thinking more clearly about (i) the relationship between community empowerment programmes and their external political environment, and (ii) the types of processes that would be required if the former was significantly to alter the latter. As this chapter has suggested, it is this part of the community-empowerment model that requires elaboration if community-based schemes that are seeking, in any meaningful sense, to 'empower' are to be distinguished from those schemes which have more limited, if not necessarily undesirable, aims.

Note

1. The different theoretical underpinnings of the community and pyschology health literatures have implications for the participatory role of the community but limitations of space preclude an investigation of this issue.

References

Bauld, L. and Judge, K. (eds) (2002) *Learning from Health Action Zones*, Aeneas Press, Chichester, UK.

Blackburn, C. (1993) Making poverty a practice issue, *Health and Social Care in the Community*, 1: 297–304.

Bridgen, P. (2006) Social capital, community empowerment and public health: policy developments in the United Kingdom since 1997, *Policy and Politics*, 34 (1): 27–50.

Bunton, R., Nettleton, S. and Burrows, R. (eds) (1995) *The Sociology of Health Promotion*, Routledge, London.

Campbell, C. with Wood, R. and Kelly, M. (1999) *Social Capital and Health*, Health Education Authority, London.

Crisp, B.R., Swerissen, H. and Duckett, S.J. (2000) Four approches to capacity building in health: consequences for measurement and accountability, *Health Promotion International*, 15 (2): 99–107.

Daugbjerg, C. (1998) Similar problems, different policies: policy networks and environmental policy in Danish and Swedish agriculture, in D. Marsh, *Comparing Policy Networks*, Open University Press, Buckingham, UK.

DETR (1999) *New Deal for Communities: an Overview*, Department of the Environment Transport and Regions, London.

DETR (2001) *New Deal for Communities. Annual Review, 2000–2001*, Department of the Environment Transport and Regions DETR, London.

DoH (1997) *The New NHS: Modern, Dependable*, Department of Health, London.

DoH (1998a) Frank Dobson gives the go-ahead for first wave of Health Action Zones, Press release: reference 98/120, 31 March 1998, Department of Health, London, accessed at: http://tap.ccta. gov.uk/doh/intpress.nsf/page/98-120?OpenDocument.

DoH (1998b) *Partnership in Action (New Opportunities for Joint Working between Health and Social Services)*, Department of Health, London.

DoH (1999) *Saving Lives: Our Healthier Nation*, White Paper, Cmnd 4386, The Stationery Office, London.

Farrant, W. (1991) Addressing the contradictions: health promotion and community health action in the United Kingdom, *International Journal of Health Services*, 21 (3): 423–439.

Harding, A. (1997) Is there a 'new community power' and why should we need one?, *International Journal of Urban and Regional Research*, 21: 638–655.

Hawe, P. (1994) Capturing the meaning of 'community' in community intervention evaluation: some contributions from community psychology, *Health Promotion International*, 9 (3): 199–210.

Hawe, P., King, L., Noort, M., Grifford, A.M. and Lloyd, B. (1998) Working invisibly: health workers talk about capacity-building in health promotion, *Health Promotion International*, 13 (4): 285–95.

Haznet (1998) *Background*, Haznet, London, accessed at: http://www.haznet.org.uk/haz/background/background.asp.

Laverack, G. and Wallerstein, N. (2001) Measuring community empowerment: a fresh look at organizational domains, *Health Promotion International*, 16 (2): 179–185.

McGuirk, P.M. (2000) Power and policy networks in urban governance: local government and property-led regeneration in Dublin, *Urban Studies,* 37 (4): 651–672.

Mackenzie, M., Lawson, L. and Mackinnon, J. (2002) Generating learning, in L. Bauld and K. Judge (eds), *Learning from Health Action Zones*, Aeneas Press, Chichester, UK.

Marsh, D. and Smith, M. (2000) Understanding policy networks: towards a dialectical approach, *Political Studies*, 48 (1): 4–21.

Mayo, M., with Anastacio, J. (1999) Welfare models and approaches to empowerment: competing perspectives from Area Regeneration Programmes, *Policy Studies*, 20: 5–21.

Murray, M. (2000) Social Capital formation and healthy communities: insights from the Colorado healthy communities initiative, *Community Development Journal*, 35 (2): 99–108.

Mutaner, C., Lynch, J. and Davey Smith, G. (2001) Social capital, disorganized communities, and the Third Way: understanding the retreat from structural inequalities in epidemiology and public health, *International Journal of Health Services*, 31: 213–237.

NHS Executive (1999) *Patient and Public Involvement in the New NHS*, accessed at: http://www.doh.gov.uk/involve.htm.

Putnam, R.D. (2000) *Bowling Alone: the Collapse and Revival of American Community*, Simon & Schuster, New York.

Rowe, R. (2002) Governance and accountability in Primary Care Groups and Trusts – is 'third way' welfare reform working?, a paper delivered to the UK Social Policy Association conference, Middlesbrough, UK.

Saltmann, R.B. (1994) Patient choice and patient empowerment in Northern European health systems: a conceptual framework, *International Journal of Health Services*, 24 (2): 201–229.

Social Exclusion Unit (2000) *National Strategy for Neighbourhood Renewal: a framework for consultation*, SEU, London.

Social Exclusion Unit, Policy Action Team (2000) *Community Self Help: a Report of Policy Action Team 9*, Home Office, London.

Stoker, G. (2000) Introduction, in G. Stoker (ed.), *The New Politics of British Local Governance*, Macmillan, Basingstoke, UK.

Sullivan, H. (2001) Modernisation, democratisation and community governance, *Local Government Studies*, 27: 1–24.

Thornhill NDC (2001) *Stepping Out: a New Future for Thornhill, Southampton*, accessed at: http://www.southampton.gov.uk/newdeal/contents.htm.

Townsend, P., Davidson, N. and Whitehead, M. (1988) *Inequalities in Health: the Black Report and the Health Divide*, Penguin, London.

Wainwright, D. (1996) The political transformation of the health inequalities debate, *Critical Social Policy*, 16: 67–82.

Wallerstein, N. (1992) Powerlessness, empowerment and health: implications for health promotion programs, *American Journal of Health Promotion*, 6: 197–205.

Chapter 30

Promoting Social Responsibility for Health: Health Impact Assessment and Healthy Public Policy at the Community Level

Maurice B. Mittelmark

Introduction

The 1997 Jakarta Declaration on Health Promotion into the 21st Century called for new responses to address emerging threats to health. The declaration placed a high priority on promoting social responsibility for health and identified equity-focused health impact assessment as a priority. Continuing on this theme, it is argued here that comprehensive implementation of equity-focused health impact assessment is the essential building block in constructing socially responsible policy and practice. An especially important arena for healthy public and private policy development is the local community and its settings, such as schools and workplaces.

There are several compelling reasons why local level policy-making is an important ingredient in the mix of health promotion strategies. Policy-making at macro levels may not be sensitive to the diversity of local conditions that directly affect the health and well-being of residents of different communities. Beyond that, important health-related planning policy-making and action originate at the local level. Also, the motivation of local leaders to practise healthy policy-making should be high, since they are affected by their own decisions. There is evidence, too, that a participatory community health development process can shift peoples' thinking beyond the illness problems of individuals to consideration of how programmes and policies could support or weaken community health, and illuminate

Edited from: Mittelmark, M.B. (2001) Promoting social responsibility for health: health impact assessment and healthy public policy at the community level, *Health Promotion International*, 16 (3): 269–274. By permission of Oxford University Press.

a community's capacity and control to improve local conditions for a healthier society. Each of these points is taken up below.

Even the best-intentioned national or international healthy public policy initiatives may fail to have the intended impact at the local level, and may even result in serious harm because of ignorance of local conditions. National policy-makers cannot anticipate with a high degree of confidence how their health-related policy will affect life and well-being at the community level. Local level analysis of social and health impacts could prevent policy 'boomerangs' by suggesting reasonable modifications to policy so that implementation fits local conditions and needs.

A case study illustrating this problem has its starting point in the early 1970s. More than 6000 people living in Iraq were hospitalized and 400 died after eating bread made from wheat flour containing a high dose of mercury from a fungicide (Egeland and Middaugh, 1997). This extremely serious poisoning episode aroused substantial concern internationally. In the United States, national officials reacted quickly, setting a recommended maximum daily dose of mercury of only one-fifth that of the limit recommended by the World Health Organization (WHO) (although there is evidence that twice the WHO-recommended maximum dose is safe). Public health workers in Alaska strongly questioned the wisdom of this move because many public health officials base their fish consumption advisories on mercury consumption recommendations from the national government. However, from the community perspective, severely limiting the consumption of seafood may do more harm than good. Aside from the known beneficial health effects of eating fish, poeple in many areas of remote Alaska rely on subsistence fishing. Restrictive advisories could damage the social, economic and personal well-being of entire villages. The point here is not to enter the debate on what levels of mercury in the food chain are safe or not, but merely to illustrate the importance of the local perspective on health-related decision-making that happens outside the community.

Another part of the rationale for an emphasis on health promoting policy-making at the community level is that much of the critical decision-making affecting health and well-being occurs at the community level. For an example of this, consider public sector schools. National policies in many countries dictate the required health curriculum, the formal training and competency levels of teachers, the examination procedures and so forth. But only policy-making in the schools can determine what the learning culture and environment will be. Will the very serious mental health problem of bullying be tolerated as inevitable, or will the teachers, parents and students develop policies and practices that sanction bullies in a serious way? Will the routines of the educational process, the food served in school and the school facilities support, or be of detriment to, the health of staff and students?

For those who are far removed from school days, consideration of the work environment makes the point equally well. Many countries today have national policies to protect workers' health. Nevertheless, many people have been in (or know about) a workplace where the culture 'grinds' people down, destroying morale, lowering productivity and causing excessive turnover, sick leave and 'burn-out'. Alternatively, enlightened management in many workplaces realizes that the path to sustained productivity is (policy resulting in) worker participation in decision-making, provision of training for advancement, development of working conditions that actually improve health, and so on. No amount of policy-making at the national level can affect the culture of workplace environments to the degree that policy at the local level can.

Moving up from the level of schools and workplaces to the community level, the case is equally strong that local healthy policy-making is essential for success. Hancock pointed out long ago that at the local community level there are important social ties between public policy-makers and those affected by policy (Hancock, 1985). Community policy-makers live where they work. They are identifiable with their policies. They (and their families and friends) are affected by their own decisions. The bureaucracies of communities are less complex than at national and regional levels, and there is greater likelihood of inter-sector collaboration at the local level.

Health impact assessment

Health impact assessment is an essential tool for healthy policy-making and practice. Health impact assessment addresses the basic question 'how are existing or planned policies, programmes or projects actually affecting, or likely to affect, people's health, for good and for bad?'. Answers to this question could help policy-makers and programme managers make the decisions and changes needed in order to perform their work in the most socially responsible manner possible.

The arena of health impact assessment is young and developing very rapidly (Scott-Samuel, 1996). International cooperation and coordination are being stimulated by, among others, the WHO European Centre for Health Policy (Lehto and Ritsatakis, 1999). They describe a general approach to health impact assessment that has the following five elements.

1   Health impact assessment examines direct and indirect impacts on health of policies, strategies, programmes or projects.
2   The initial stage is screening using available information to determine if there is confidence that impact is negligible, or if more information is needed.
3   If more information is needed, scoping is done to determine what level of resources and expertise are required to develop the needed information (ranging from a rapid appraisal using additional expertise to an in-depth impact analysis or an extensive impact review).
4   Generation of an assessment report.
5   Modification of the policy/project if indicated.

Despite the jargon (screening, scoping), models such as this should (with appropriate user interfaces) be useable in almost any setting and be accessible to any group of interested citizens, regardless of level of formal training. Science, business and government should have access to the technology, but so should average citizens, including those living in difficult conditions. However, the trend of ever more technical and complicated methods of impact assessment threatens to exclude average citizens from participation. In the best of worlds, science develeops knowledge and some of that knowledge can be put to use by average people to solve practical problems. That is technology born from science. Too frequently, however, as the technology becomes more complex, elites take over and the technology transforms into quasi-science.

This has happened in the environmental impact assessment arena and threatens to happen to health impact assessment. The jargon is becoming inaccessible to the average person and the methodology is becoming very complex. However, technological development and user-friendliness can co-exist, as in the information technology field, which has demonstrated how very complex technology can be made universally accessible through appropriate interfaces. User interfaces of the simplest kind are needed if health impact assessment is to reach where it is most needed. Health promotion should strive to build an approach to health impact assessment that any person or group with average education and intelligence can master with some study and practice.

At certain levels, developments in the health impact assessment arena are gratifying. There exist today a number of stimulating examples of national and international level inter-sector collaborations for healthy public policy and health impact assessment. The European Regional Office of WHO, for example, is beginning work with European partners to build capacity for health impact measurement and monitoring and health policy development (Lehto and Ritsatakis, 1999). In Australia, a national framework for health impact assessment has existed for several years (National Health and Medical Research Council, 1994). An impressive example of action at the national level is the National Assembly of Wales' recent formal commitment to health impact assessment as a central strategy in tackling determinants of health that cut across policy areas (Health Promotion Division, 1999). The Scottish Council Foundation's Healthy Public Policy Network has developed a vision for health improvement that includes explicit recognition of the health effects of policy-making in non-health sectors such as housing and transport (Stewart, 1998).

In Canada, the Federal/Provincial/Territorial Committee on Environmental and Occupational Health has published a very comprehensive handbook on health impact assessment (Minister of Public Works and Government Services Canada, 1999). In the United Kingdom, a network to promote impact assessments of government policy has been established and has begun to conduct methods seminars to develop the tools required.

There are positive developments also at the community level. For example, the Newfoundland and Labrador Heart Health Program (http://www.infonet.st-johns.nf.ca/providers/nhhp/docs/policy.html) have produced a practical 'Making Public Policy Healthy' guide book that citizens and community groups can use to create, support or oppose local policies. Many Healthy Cities initiatives around the world include some form of impact analysis among their strategies (WHO, no date, a).

The people assessing their health (PATH) project

A particularly stimulating exemplar comes from Eastern Nova Scotia, Canada (Gillis, 1999). The 'People Assessing Their Health' (PATH) project was undertaken in a region of Canada that is geographically isolated and faces difficult socio-economic circumstances. Community health impact assessment was used to increase public understanding of the determinants of health and empower citizens to play an active part in decisions influencing their health.

The first stage in the work was the local development of community health impact assessment tools (CHIATs) tailored to the special needs of each of the communities. All three CHIATs were intended to provide answers to the same question: 'What does it take to make and keep our community healthy?'. Other objectives were to develop the CHIATs in such a way as to:

- examine a broad range of factors that determine health, rather than only specific interests;
- identify what community members consider important in building a healthy community;
- encourage all community members to become involved in decisions about local programmes and policies;
- reflect community concerns and priorities; and
- provide information useful to community health boards to guide decisions about the organization of primary health care.

The process used included four steps. At the first step, public meetings were held to determine who in the community was interested in becoming involved, a local committee then selected a local person to coordinate the project, teams were trained in communication and group facilitation techniques, and local steering committees were formed.

In the second step, facilitators conducted citizen meetings, starting from the premise that community people know what it takes to make their community healthy. The process included measures that encouraged community members to consider the broadest possible range of determinants of health, and they were not steered (or distracted) by a pre-determined list compiled by public health 'experts'.

In the third step, steering committees designed their CHIATs based on data collected during step two. Information typically included was a statement of the values and principles that guided the work, a vision statement for a healthy community, a summary of key determinants of health, a list of factors important in building and sustaining a healthy community, and priorities for action. Community workshops were used to obtain feedback on drafts and the final CHIATs incorporated this feedback.

In the final step, steering committee members worked with local community leaders to ensure that the CHIATs were used in decision-making undertaken by community health planning groups and municipal decision-makers.

The outcomes were quite similar in each community. The most important health determinant identified in all three communities was jobs/employment opportunities. Other determinants identified were healthy child development, lifelong learning, lifestyle practices, physical environment, safety and security, social support, stable incomes and good health services. The CHIATs also pointed to factors thought to be key in building healthy and sustainable communities. These included: good communication; community involvement; local control; opportunities for leadership development; confidence in one's community; coordination and cooperation in service delivery; ethics, values and spirituality; and respect for one's culture and history.

The key lessons learned through the PATH experience are very likely applicable to other communities. The highly participatory process helped many people shift thinking beyond the illness problems of individuals to consideration of how programmes and policies could support or weaken community health. In all three communities, the process brought to light local socio-economic inequalities and illuminated community capacity and control to improve conditions for a healthier community. Finally, PATH demonstrated the value of developing CHIATs as a strategy to support community action on health.

PATH illustrates some core principles for community health impact assessment, and these are very consistent with community development strategies that have proven value (Mittelmark, 1999; Restrepo, 2000). PATH is a particularly good example of how ordinary citizens can have a place at the very heart of local decision-making, with the CHIAT process as a central element for positive change. PATH is of course not the answer for all communities. Some communities need processes to evaluate specific proposals, for example road-building projects, public safety issues or educational policies. Community health impact assessment need not take place at the community level, as in PATH, but could be focused in settings such as schools and workplaces. Inevitably, some communities/settings need impact assessment as a tool to help fight unwelcome change that threatens community well-being (new industry located in the wrong place, for example).

Conclusion

This chapter makes the claim that a key activity required to promote healthy policy-making at the local level is health impact assessment. Highly participatory local health impact assessment can be used to identify negative health impacts that call for policy responses, and to identify and encourage practices and policies that promote health. Socially responsible decision-making for improved equity-in-health is stimulated by community-level health impact assessment because it is a practical tool to help communities come to grips with local conditions that need changing if better health for all is to be realized.

The WHO's Healthy Cities networks that have been established around the globe are a solid basis upon which to advance this agenda (WHO, no date, a). Healthy Cities is a strong and growing movement that has long recognized the importance of systematic assessment of the health impact of local policies. In Europe, for example, with ~1100 cities and towns involved in the programme, both the 1990 Milan Declaration on Healthy Cities (WHO, no date, b) and the 1998 Athens Declaration for Healthy Cities (WHO, no date, c) emphasize the importance of intersectorality and accountability. The Milan Declaration is quite specific on this point, stating participants' pledges to:

> ... make health and environmental impact assessment part of all urban planning decisions, policies and programmes.

Follow-up on the good intentions expressed in public declarations is, however, not easy. Frankish et al. (1996) describe some of the difficulties and barriers that have been encountered in Healthy Cities' attempts to develop health impact assessment. The main lessons appear to be that highly complex approaches to health impact assessment are self-defeating, and that in any case there is no uniform way to conduct assessment. Relatively simple approaches, tailored in each instance to local circumstances, are called for. Healthy Cities and similar movements focused on villages, islands, prisons and hospitals (among others!) will undoubtedly continue to be innovation laboratories for healthy public policy-making. It is urged here that both within Healthy Cities and outside, the development of practical approaches to community health impact assessment should have a place high on the health promotion agenda in the coming period.

Acknowledgements

This chapter is a revised and substantially shortened version of a technical report prepared in cooperation with the World Health Organization, in support of the 5th Global Conference on Health Promotion: Bridging the Gap, Mexico, 5–9 June, 2000.

References

Egeland, G.M. and Middaugh, J.P. (1997) Balancing fish consumption benefits with mercury exposure. *Science*, 278: 1904–1905.

Frankish, C.J., Green, L.W., Ratner, P.A., Chomik, T. and Larsen, C. (1996) *Health Impact Assessment as a Tool for Population Health Promotion and Public Policy.* A report submitted to the Health Promotion Division of Health Canada. Institute of Health Promotion Research, University of British Columbia.

Gillis, D.E. (1999) The 'People Assessing Their Health' (PATH) Project: tools for community health impact assessment. *Canadian Journal of Public Health*, 90 (Suppl.1), S53–S56.

Hancock, T. (1985) Beyond health care: from public health policy to healthy public policy. *Canadian Journal of Public Health*, 76 (Suppl. 1), 9–11.

Health Promotion Division (1999) *Developing Health Impact Assessment in Wales: Better Health Better Wales.* National Assembly for Wales.

Lehto, J. and Ritsatakis, A. (1999) *Health Impact Assessment as a Tool for Intersectoral Health Policy.* A discussion paper for a seminar on 'Health impact assessment: from theory to practice', 28–30 October, Gothenburg, Sweden.

Minister of Public Works and Government Services Canada (1999) *Canadian Handbook on Health Impact Assessment.* Health Canada, Ottawa, Canada.

Mittelmark, M.B. (1999) Health promotion and the community-wide level: lessons from diverse perspectives. In Bracht, N. (ed.), *Health Promotion at the Community Level.* 2nd edn. Sage, Newbury Park, CA, pp. 3–26.

National Health and Medical Research Council (1994) *National Framework for Environmental and Health Impact Assessment.* Available at: http://www.health.gov.au/nhmrc/publicat/synopses/eh10syn.htm.

Restrepo, H. (2000) *Increasing Community Capacity and Empowering Communities for Promoting Health.* Fifth Global Conference on Health Promotion, Mexico City, Mexico, 5–9 June 2000. Available at: http://www.who.int/hpr/conference/products/reports/community.html.

Scott-Samuel, A. (1996) Health impact assessment – an idea whose time has come [editorial]. *British Medical Journal*, 313: 183–184.

Stewart, S. (ed.) (1998) *The Possible Scot: Making Healthy Public Policy.* Scottish Council Foundation, Edinburgh.

World Health Organization (WHO) (no date, a) WHO Healthy Cities Network. Available at: http://www. who.dk/healthy-cities/hcn.htm//#PhaseIII.

WHO (no date, b) The Milan Declaration on Healthy Cities. Available at: http://www.who.dk/policy/milan01.htm.

WHO (no date, c) Athens declaration for Healthy Cities. Available at: http://www.who.dk/healthy-cities/athensE.htm.

Chapter 31

Mental Health Promotion

Lynne Friedli

Public mental health

Public mental health takes a population-wide approach to understanding and addressing risk and protective factors for mental health and well-being, and has been defined as the art, science and politics of creating a mentally healthy society.

> Public mental health (of which mental health promotion is one element) provides a strategic and analytical framework for addressing the wider determinants of mental health, reducing the enduring inequalities in the distribution of mental distress and improving the mental health of the whole population. (Friedli, 2004: 2)

The focus on mental health as a public health issue is evidence of growing recognition that mental health influences physical health, health outcomes for a wide range of diseases (including coronary heart disease, Type 2 diabetes and cancer) and the extent to which people feel able and motivated to exercise choice and control and to adopt healthy lifestyles.

> How people feel is not an elusive or abstract concept, but a significant public health indicator; as significant as rates of smoking, obesity and physical activity. (Department of Health, 2001)

Mental health is a priority issue in the public health White Paper *Choosing Health*, with specific reference to 'new services to improve mental and emotional well-being' in the Delivery Plan (Department of Health, 2004a).

Policy context

> Transforming the NHS from a sickness service to a health service is not just a matter of promoting physical health. Understanding how everyone in the NHS can promote mental well-being is equally important. (Department of Health, 2001: para 6.7)

Recognition of the importance of mental health, emotional well-being and quality of life is both explicit and implicit in a very wide range of policy on health, education, culture, crime, regeneration, social inclusion and employment. There is also considerable public and media interest in issues related to mental health, for example happiness, the economics of well-being, quality of life, work/life balance and 'liveability' (Marks and Shah, 2004).

Although the situation across the UK varies, all four countries have a policy commitment to mental health promotion (Friedli, 2004), with perhaps the most comprehensive approach in Scotland (http://www.wellscotland.info/mentalhealth/national-programme. html). In England, the publication of the *National Service Framework for Mental Health* (Department of Health, 1999) marked a significant turning point. For the first time, health and social services were required 'to promote mental health for all, working with individuals, organisations and communities', as well as to tackle the stigma, discrimination and social exclusion experienced by people with mental health problems. This commitment was reinforced in *Choosing Health*: 'we will have delivered if we improve the mental health and well-being of the general population' (Department of Health, 2004a).

Tackling discrimination and social exclusion has tended to receive a stronger focus than promoting mental health for all (NIMHE, 2004; Social Exclusion Unit, 2004). Louis Appleby, National Director for Mental Health remarked on the lack of progress on Standard One and noted: 'We need to broaden our focus from specialist mental health services to the mental health needs of the community as a whole' (Department of Health, 2004b). The launch of *Making It Possible: Improving Mental Health and Well-being in England* (NIMHE, 2005) can be seen as an effort to achieve this broader focus and to provide greater leadership and support for a population-wide approach to improving mental health. *Making it Possible* sets a framework for action to:

- raise public awareness of how to look after our own mental health and other people's
- involve all communities and organisations, across all sectors, in taking positive steps to promote and protect mental well-being.

It argues that improving the mental health of the population will contribute to achieving a wide range of cross-government priorities for children and adults and to meeting Public Service Agreement (PSA) targets in health, education, neighbourhood renewal, crime, community cohesion, sustainable development, employment, culture and sport. *Making It Possible* has been given additional impetus by the inclusion of its key recommendations in the White Paper *Our Health, Our Care, Our Say: a New Direction for Community Services* (Department of Health, 2006).

Policy in Europe

Recent developments in Europe also appear to augur well for mental health promotion. The World Health Organisation (Europe)'s Declaration and Action Plan, which sets out the commitments and responsibilities of both the WHO and national governments, stresses the need for 'mental health activities capable of improving the well-being of the whole population, preventing mental health problems and enhancing the inclusion and functioning of people experiencing mental health problems' (WHO (Europe), 2005a). The Declaration was signed by the English Minister Rosie Winterton, along with 52 other European health ministers, in Helsinki in January 2005.

The European Union Green Paper on mental heath is a first response to the WHO (Europe) declaration on mental health, agreeing that 'there is no health without mental health', and acknowledging that mental health influences the fundamental goal of the EU to develop long-term prosperity (European Commission, 2005). While the proposed strategy will be at EU level, not at national level, its focus on public mental health should stimulate policy and action within member states (Stansfield, 2006).

Trends and debates

Shift from illness to health

What might be called the mental health promotion movement has contributed to, and has been informed by, a number of significant developments in thinking about mental health:

- the shift from treatment to recovery: what people need in order to hold on to or regain a life that has meaning for them
- interest in the relationship between social capital and health
- critiques of the use of economic development (GDP) as a sufficient indicator of national prosperity

Recovery aims to enable people with mental health problems to:

- maintain existing activities and relationships
- reduce the barriers that prevent people from accessing new things they want to do
- gain access to the material resources and opportunities that are their right (Perkins, 2002).

Its significance for mental health promotion is that it shifts the emphasis from mental illness services to the wider community and asks what a person needs to regain or hold on to a life that has meaning for them (Bates, 2002; Sayce, 2002).

Although the reform of mental illness services and addressing the stigma, discrimination and denial of human rights and civil liberties experienced by people with mental health problems remain central, these goals are now also being considered in the context of public mental health. This is an important development because the focus on stigma and discrimination has tended to preclude a wider debate about factors that are toxic to mental health, whether or not one has a diagnosis. We have a wealth of data on public attitudes to mental illness (Braunholtz et al., 2004; Gale et al., 2004), but very little on public knowledge of what harms and hinders mental well-being – the mental health equivalents of smoking and car exhaust fumes.

Well-being and regeneration

The economics of well-being challenges the equation of economic growth with life satisfaction and highlights the cost of economic growth, notably the psychosocial impact of inequality and materialism (Marks and Shah, 2004; Layard, 2005; Huppert, 2006). It draws on robust evidence that the structure and quality of social relations are fundamental to well-being and provides a context for analysing how the drivers of economic growth may undermine individual and community efforts to remain or become connected. The focus is less on individual psychological and cognitive attributes and more on the relationship between the organisation of society and how we feel. In the UK, a cross-government Whitehall Well-being Working Group has been established to explore how policies might change, with an explicit well-being focus (DEFRA, 2005).

Health assets or salutogenesis is an approach to public health that focuses on assets and resilience, rather than solely on deficit and vulnerability. It aims to maximise assets within a community, not just to reduce need. In mental health terms, it is the equivalent of measuring positive mental well-being, as opposed to surveys of psychiatric morbidity. This is important because strategies that focus on need may (inadvertently) reduce health assets, for example through fostering high levels of dependence on professional input. Conversely, an intervention that enhances health assets, for example social networks, may have no impact on disease. In other words, interventions to improve health may be entirely independent of interventions to prevent disease:

> Salutogenesis asks, 'What are the causes and distribution of health and well-being in this group, community or country population'. Epidemiology asks 'what are the causes and distribution of disease and early death in this group, community or population'. (WHO (Europe), 2005b)

Mental health promotion in practice: a case study

Social prescribing or community referrals

Social prescribing is a way of linking people (usually, but not exclusively, via primary care) with non-medical sources of support within the community (Friedli and Watkins, 2004). These might include opportunities for arts and creativity, physical activity, learning and volunteering, mutual aid, befriending and self-help, as well as support with, for example, benefits, debt, legal advice or parenting problems. Although there are many different models for social prescribing and a wide range of different projects, the basic principles of social prescribing provide an interesting example of different elements of mental health promotion, their strengths, weaknesses and the challenges they present.

Social prescribing provides a framework for developing alternative responses to mental distress and is part of a wider recognition of the influence of social and cultural factors on mental health outcomes. It is based in part on the importance of social support as a protective factor for both mental and physical health, and by evidence of the health benefits of participation, involvement and reciprocity, drawn from research on social capital. General practitioners have been the target of concerted efforts to improve the recognition and treatment of depression. In the absence of alternatives, GPs prescribe anti-depressants, at considerable cost, and, for mild to moderate depression, with little robust evidence of effectiveness (Mental Health Foundation, 2005). Concerns about potentially high levels of diagnosis and the rapid increase in prescription of anti-depressants have generated debates about alternative responses to mental distress in primary care. In particular, concern has been expressed about attaching a diagnosis to what may be, in effect, a socio-economic problem (Double, 2002).

Social prescribing has been quite widely used for people with mild to moderate mental health problems, with a range of positive outcomes, including enhanced self-esteem, reduced low mood, opportunities for social contact, increased self-efficacy, transferable skills and greater confidence (Aldridge and Lavender, 2000; James, 2001a, 2001b; Friedli et al., 2002). But there is also a growing interest in social prescribing as a route to reducing social exclusion, both for disadvantaged, isolated and vulnerable populations in general and mental health service users.

The most common examples of social prescribing are primary care-based projects which refer at-risk or vulnerable patients to a specific programme, for example *exercise on prescription, prescription for learning* and *arts on prescription*. However, it also includes a very wide range of initiatives in which primary care staff provide a signposting or gateway service, linking patients with sources of information and support within the community and voluntary sector (see Box 31.1 for an example).

Box 31.1   NHS Borders Galashiels Well-being Project: minor mental health problems in primary care

A volunteer-based service offering a range of existing community resources and developing the skills of local people. The Well-being Project is a service for people in primary care with mild to moderate stress, anxiety or depression, with psychosocial problems, who are not appropriate for referral on to secondary care. It benefits those who struggle with everyday life, by providing a tailored response to their needs and linking people to volunteers, voluntary organisations and local support services as well as providing self-help materials. The Project gives primary care staff the opportunity to offer a wider range of services and to relieve some of the pressure on their time. Referral is through GPs, health visitors, community nurses, practice nurses or other members of the primary care team.

Anecdotal feedback from primary care suggests a decrease in GP appointments, and a reduction in the severity of stress, anxiety and depression by people using the Project. However, lack of referrals from GPs remains a problem: 'we need to regularly remind them that the service is there', raising issues about true ownership of the service. (www.nhsborders.org.uk/view_item)

Since the Project started in June 2003, a total of 83 patients have been referred by health visitors and GPs. Sixty-seven review forms were sent to patients using the Project and 36 have been returned. Of these, 34 felt that the project had helped them in some way.

The Project is well documented and includes assessment, referral, evaluation and review forms.

Contact: wendy.lynn@borders.scot.nhs.uk

What would success look like?

The development of an evidence base for social prescribing has been limited by wide variations in how the term is used and understood as well as inconsistency in indicators used to measure success. The specific objectives of increasing the availability of, and access to, social prescribing might be:

*   An increase in public knowledge of positive steps for mental health (e.g. exercise, sensible drinking, stress management, building and maintaining social networks, talking things over).
*   An increase in social prescribing as a first-line treatment for symptoms of mild to moderate anxiety and depression.
*   A reduction in inappropriate prescribing of anti-depressants for mild to moderate depression, in line with NICE guidelines.
*   A reduction in frequent attendance (defined as more than 12 visits to a GP per annum).

The monitoring of outcomes for social prescribing might be done at primary care practice or Primary Care Trust level, measured through, for example, improved GHQ (General Household questionnaire) or SFS (Social Functioning Scores) scores, or through the use of other validated scales (e.g. the Affectometer II).

Short- and medium-term outcomes which could provide a basis for assessing whether social prescribing has made a difference might include:

*   increased uptake of arts, leisure, education, volunteering, sporting and other activities by vulnerable and at-risk groups, including people using psychiatric services
*   increased levels of social contact and social support among marginalised and isolated groups
*   reduced levels of inappropriate prescribing of anti-depressants for mild to moderate depression
*   reduced waiting lists for counsellors.

Conclusions

Some of the problems involved in demonstrating the benefits of social prescribing typify wider challenges in tracking progress in improving public mental health, both locally and nationally. Current measures of mental health are in fact predominantly measures of mental illness, drawn from surveys of psychiatric morbidity. Work is currently underway in Scotland to establish a set of national mental health and well-being indicators that can be used to create a summary mental health profile, as a starting point for monitoring future trends (Parkinson, 2006, in press). This will involve capturing the range of emotional and cognitive attributes associated with a self-reported sense of well-being (Hird, 2003; McAllister, 2005), and might include self-esteem, internal locus of control or mastery, resilience, satisfaction with life, optimism, social integration, sense of coherence and satisfying relationships (Huppert, 2006). It will also mean looking at potential indicators at a community level (e.g. social support, safety), and at a structural level (e.g. equity).

A shift in focus from prevalence of psychiatric morbidity to attempts to measure the mental health and well-being of populations has the potential to radically transform the way we think about mental health. It also creates new opportunities to consider the mental health impact of social and economic policy and to add a new dimension to political debate about the future direction of society in the UK, Europe and beyond.

References

Aldridge, F. and Lavender, P. (2000) *The Impact of Learning on Health*. Nottingham: NIACE.

Bates, P. (ed.) (2002) *Working for Inclusion: Making Social Inclusion a Reality for People with Severe Mental Health Problems*. London: Sainsbury Centre for Mental Health.

Braunholtz, S., Davidson, S. and King, S. (2004) *Well? What Do You Think (2004)?: the Second National Scottish Survey of Public Attitudes to Mental Health, Mental Well-being and Mental Health Problems*. Edinburgh: Scottish Executive Social Research, http://www.scotland.gov.uk/Publications/2005/01/20506/49641.

DEFRA (2005) *Securing the Future: UK Government Sustainable Development Strategy*. London: Department for the Environment, Farming and Rural Affairs, http://www.sustainable-development.gov.uk/publications/uk-strategy/uk-strategy-2005.htm.

Department of Health (1999) *National Service Framework for Mental Health*. London: The Stationery office.

Department of Health (2001) *Making It Happen: a Guide to Delivering Mental Health Promotion*. London: Department of Health, www.doh.gov.uk/index.htm.

Department of Health (2004a) *Choosing Health: Making Healthy Choices Easier*. London: The Stationery Office, http://www.dh.gov.uk/PublicationsAndStatistics/Publications/Publications PolicyAndGuidance/PublicationsPolicyAndGuidanceArticle/fs/en?CONTENT_ID=4094550& chk=aN5Cor.

Department of Health (2004b) *The National Service Framework for Mental Health: Five Years On*. London: The Stationery Office.

Department of Health (2006) *Our Health, Our Care, Our Say: a New Direction for Community Services*. London: The Stationery Office, http://www.dh.gov.uk/assetRoot/04/12/74/59/04127459.pdf.

Double, D. (2002) Education and debate: the limits of psychiatry, *British Medical Journal*, 324: 900–4.

European Commission (2005) *Green Paper: Improving the Mental Health of the Population. Towards a Strategy on Mental Health for the EU*. Brussels: Health and Consumer Protection Directorate General, http://europa.eu.int/comm/health/ph_determinants/life_style/mental/green _paper/mental_gp_en.pdf.

Friedli, L. (2004) Editorial. *Journal of Mental Health Promotion*, 3 (1): 2–6.

Friedli, L., Griffiths, S. and Tidyman, M. (2002) The mental health benefits of arts and creativity for African and Caribbean young men, *Journal of Mental Health Promotion*, 1 (3): 32–45.

Friedli, L. and Watkins, S. (2004) *Social Prescribing for Mental Health*. Durham: Northern Centre for Mental Health.

Gale, E., Seymour, L., Crepaz-Keay, D., Gibbons, M., Farmer, P. and Pinfold, V. (2004) *Scoping Review on Mental Health Anti-Stigma and Discrimination: Current Avtivities and What Works*. Leeds: National Institute for Mental Health in England.

Hird, Susan (2003) What is well-being? A brief review of current literature and concepts, *NHS Scotland*, April 2003, http://www.phis.org.uk/doc.pl?file=pdf/What%20is%20wellbeing% 202.doc.

Huppert, F.A. (2006) Positive mental health in individuals and populations, in F.A. Huppert, N. Baylis and B. Kaverne (eds), *The Science of Well-being*. Oxford: Oxford University Press, pp. 307–42.

James, K. (2001a) *Prescriptions for Learning Project Nottingham: First Evaluation Report*. Nottingham: National Insitute of Adult Continuing Education.

James, K. (2001b) *Prescribing Learning: a Guide to Good Practice in Learning and Health*. Nottingham: National Institute of Adult Continuing Education.

Layard, R. (2005) *Happiness: Lessons from a New Science*. London: Allen Lane.

Marks, N. and Shah, H. (2004) A well-being manifesto for a flourishing society, *Journal of Mental Health Promotion*, 3 (4): 9–15.

McAllister, F. (2005) *Wellbeing Concepts and Challenges*. Discussion paper for the Sustainable Development Research Network, http://www.sd-research.org.uk/documents/SDRNwellbeing paperfinal-20December2005_v3_000.pdf.

Mental Health Foundation (2005) *Up and Running? Exercise Therapy and the Treatment of Mild or Moderate Depression in Primary Care*. London: Mental Health Foundation.

NIMHE (2004) *From Here to Equality: a Strategic Plan to Tackle Stigma and Discrimination on Mental Health Grounds*. Leeds: National Institute for Mental Health in England, http:// www.shift.org.uk/mt/archives/blog_12/FIVE%20YEAR%20STIGMA%20AND%20DISC%20 PLAN.pdf.

NIMHE (2005) *Making It Possible: Improving Mental Health and Well-being in England*. Leeds: National Institute for Mental Health in England/Care Services Improvement Partnership.

Parkinson, J. (2006, in press) Establishing a core set of sustainable national mental health and well-being indicators for Scotland. *Journal of Public Mental Health*, 5 (1).

Perkins, R. (2002) Are you (really) being served?, *Mental Health Today*, September: 18–21.

Sayce, L. (2002) Inclusion as a new paradigm: civil rights, in P. Bates (ed.), *Working for Inclusion: Making Social Inclusion a Reality for People with Severe Mental Health Problems*. London: Sainsbury Centre for Mental Health, pp. 71–8.

Social Exclusion Unit (2004) *Mental Health and Social Exclusion*. London: Office of the Deputy Prime Minister.

Stansfield, J. (2006) Improving the mental health of the population: a strategy for Europe, *Journal of Public Mental Health*, 5 (1): 11–13.

WHO (Europe) (2005a) *Mental Health Action Plan for Europe*. Copenhagen: World Health Organisation. Regional Office for Europe, http://www.euro.who.int/document/mnh/edoc06.pdf and http://www.euro.who.int/document/mnh/edoc07.pdf.

WHO (Europe) (2005b) *Assets for Health and Development: Developing a Conceptual Framework*. Venice: European Office for Investment for Health and Development.

Index